New and Emerging Rheumatic Diseases

Editor

ERIN JANSSEN

RHEUMATIC DISEASE CLINICS OF NORTH AMERICA

www.rheumatic.theclinics.com

Consulting Editor
MICHAEL H. WEISMAN

November 2023 • Volume 49 • Number 4

ELSEVIER

1600 John F. Kennedy Boulevard • Suite 1800 • Philadelphia, Pennsylvania, 19103-2899
http://www.theclinics.com

RHEUMATIC DISEASE CLINICS OF NORTH AMERICA Volume 49, Number 4
November 2023 ISSN 0889-857X, ISBN 13: 978-0-443-13115-8

Editor: Joanna Gascoine
Developmental Editor: Karen Justine S. Dino

Rheumatic Disease Clinics of North America (ISSN 0889-857X) is published quarterly by Elsevier Inc., 360 Park Avenue South, New York, NY 10010-1710. Months of issue are February, May, August, and November. Business and editorial offices: 1600 John F. Kennedy Boulevard, Suite 1800, Philadelphia, PA 19103-2899. Periodicals postage paid at New York, NY and additional mailing offices. Subscription prices are USD 377.00 per year for US individuals, USD 865.00 per year for US institutions, USD 100.00 per year for US students and residents, USD 444.00 per year for Canadian individuals, USD 1081.00 per year for Canadian institutions, USD 100.00 per year for Canadian students/residents, USD 484.00 per year for international individuals, USD 1081.00 per year for international institutions, and USD 230.00 per year for foreign students/residents. To receive student/resident rate, orders must be accompanied by name of affiliated institution, date of term, and the *signature* of program/residency coordinator on institution letterhead. Orders will be billed at individual rate until proof of status received. Foreign air speed delivery is included in all *Clinics* subscription prices. All prices are subject to change without notice. **POSTMASTER:** Send address changes to *Rheumatic Disease Clinics of North America*, Elsevier Health Sciences Division, Subscription Customer Service, 3251 Riverport Lane, Maryland Heights, MO 63043. **Customer Service: 1-800-654-2452 (US and Canada). From outside of the US and Canada: 314-447-8871. Fax: 314-447-8029. For print support, e-mail: JournalsCustomerService-usa@elsevier.com. For online support, e-mail: JournalsOnlineSupport-usa@elsevier.com.**

Reprints. For copies of 100 or more of articles in this publication, please contact the Commercial Reprints Department, Elsevier Inc., 360 Park Avenue South, New York, New York, 10010-1710; Tel.: +1-212-633-3874, Fax: +1-212-633-3820, and E-mail: reprints@elsevier.com.

Rheumatic Disease Clinics of North America is covered in *MEDLINE/PubMed (Index Medicus), Current Contents/Clinical Medicine, Science Citation Index, ISI/BIOMED,* and *EMBASE/Excerpta Medica.*

Contributors

CONSULTING EDITOR

MICHAEL H. WEISMAN, MD
Adjunct Professor of Medicine, Stanford University, Distinguished Professor of Medicine Emeritus, David Geffen School of Medicine at UCLA, Professor of Medicine Emeritus, Cedars-Sinai Medical Center, Los Angeles, California, USA

EDITOR

ERIN JANSSEN, MD, PhD
Clinical Associate Professor, University of Michigan Medical School, Department of Pediatrics, Division Director, Division of Pediatric Rheumatology, Michigan Medicine, C.S. Mott Children's Hospital, Ann Arbor, Michigan, USA

AUTHORS

MILENA M. ANDZELM, MD, PhD
Instructor in Neuroimmunology, Department of Neurology, Boston Children's Hospital, Harvard Medical School, Boston, Massachusetts, USA

KELLY COLLEEN CUSHING, MD
Clinical Instructor, Division of Gastroenterology, U-M Inflammatory Bowel Disease Program, University of Michigan, Ann Arbor, Michigan, USA

ATIYE OLCAY BILGIC DAGCI, MD
Clinical Assistant Professor, Division of Pediatric Rheumatology, University of Michigan, C.S Mott Children's Hospital, Ann Arbor, Michigan, USA

JENNIFER R. BLASE, MD, PhD
Research Fellow, Pediatrics, University of Michigan, Ann Arbor, Michigan, USA

YAN DU, MD, PhD
Post Doctoral Researcher, Division of Immunology, Boston Children's Hospital, Harvard Medical School, Boston, Massachusetts, USA; Department of Rheumatology, The Second Affiliated Hospital of Zhejiang University School of Medicine, Hangzhou, Zhejiang, China

CHRISTOPHER FAILING, MD
Pediatric Rheumatologist, Sanford Health, Fargo, North Dakota, USA; University of North Dakota School of Medicine and Health Sciences, Grand Folks, North Dakota, USA

GEORGE E. FREIGEH, MD, MA
Allergist-Immunologist, Division of Allergy and Clinical Immunology, Department of Internal Medicine, University of Michigan, Ann Arbor, Michigan, USA

ANDREW GRIM, MD
Pediatric Rheumatology Fellow, Division of Pediatric Rheumatology, Department of Pediatrics, Michigan Medicine, Ann Arbor, Michigan, USA

EVAN HSU
Division of Immunology, Boston Children's Hospital, Harvard Medical School, Boston, Massachusetts, USA

ERIN JANSSEN, MD, PhD
Clinical Associate Professor, University of Michigan Medical School, Department of Pediatrics, Division Director, Division of Pediatric Rheumatology, Michigan Medicine, C.S. Mott Children's Hospital, Ann Arbor, Michigan, USA

SAARA KAVIANY, DO
Assistant Professor of Pediatrics, Department of Pediatrics, University of Chicago, Chicago, Illinois, USA

CHRISTOPH KESSEL, PhD
Assistant Professor of Immunology, Department of Pediatric Rheumatology and Immunology, Translational Inflammation Research, University Children's Hospital, Muenster, Germany

PUI Y. LEE, MD, PhD
Attending Physician, Rheumatology Program, Boston Children Hospital, Assistant Professor of Pediatrics, Harvard Medical School, Boston, Massachusetts, USA

MENG LIU, MD
Division of Immunology, Boston Children's Hospital, Harvard Medical School, Boston, Massachusetts, USA; Department of Rheumatology and Immunology, Guangdong Second Provincial General Hospital, Guangzhou, Guangdong, China

THOMAS F. MICHNIACKI, MD
Clinical Assistant Professor, Division of Hematology and Oncology, Department of Pediatrics, University of Michigan, Ann Arbor, Michigan, USA

SMRITI MOHAN, MD
Clinical Assistant Professor, Division of Rheumatology, Department of Pediatrics, University of Michigan CS Mott Children's Hospital, Ann Arbor, Michigan, USA

XIAO PENG, MD, PhD
McKusick-Nathans, Department of Genetic Medicine, Johns Hopkins School of Medicine, Baltimore, Maryland, USA

NADINE SAAD, MD
Assistant Professor, Division of Pediatric Rheumatology, Department of Pediatrics, Michigan Medicine, Ann Arbor, Michigan, USA

GRANT S. SCHULERT, MD, PhD
Associate Professor, Division of Rheumatology, Department of Pediatrics, Cincinnati Children's Hospital Medical Center, University of Cincinnati College of Medicine, Cincinnati, Ohio, USA

ANTHONY K. SHUM, MD
Professor, Medicine, Pulmonary Division, Department of Medicine, Cardiovascular Research Institute, University of California, San Francisco, San Francisco, California, USA

NOA SIMCHONI, MD, PhD
Clinical Instructor, Medicine, Pulmonary Division, Department of Medicine, University of California, San Francisco, San Francisco, California, USA

CORAL M. STREDNY, MD
Assistant, Program in Neuroimmunology, Division of Epilepsy and Neurophysiology, Department of Neurology, Boston Children's Hospital, Instructor of Neurology, Harvard Medical School, Boston, Massachusetts, USA

KEILA R. VEIGA, MD
Pediatric Rheumatologist, Division of Pediatric Rheumatology, Department of Pediatrics, New York Medical College/Maria Fareri Children's Hospital, Valhalla, New York, USA

TIPHANIE P. VOGEL, MD, PhD
Assistant Professor, Division of Rheumatology, Department of Pediatrics, Baylor College of Medicine, Center for Human Immunobiology, Texas Children's Hospital, Houston, Texas, USA

KELLY WALKOVICH, MD
Associate Professor, Department of Pediatrics, Pediatric Hematology/Oncology, University of Michigan Medical School, Ann Arbor, Michigan, USA

CHRISTINE S. WANG, MD, MSCS
Assistant Professor, Department of Pediatric Rheumatology, C.S. Mott Children's Hospital, University of Michigan, Ann Arbor, Michigan, USA

HOLLY WOBMA, MD
Clinical Fellow, Harvard Medical School, Division of Immunology, Boston Children's Hospital, Boston, Massachusetts, USA

Contents

Foreword: Emerging Concepts in Immune Dysregulation **xiii**

Michael H. Weisman

Preface: Emerging Concepts in Immune Dysregulation **xv**

Erin Janssen

Approach to Diagnosing Inborn Errors of Immunity **731**

Xiao Peng and Saara Kaviany

Inborn errors of immunity are now understood to encompass manifold features including but not limited to immunodeficiency, autoimmunity, autoinflammation, atopy, bone marrow defects, and/or increased malignancy risk. As such, it is essential to maintain a high index of suspicion, as these disorders are not limited to specific demographics such as children or those with recurrent infections. Clinical presentations and standard immunophenotyping are informative for suggesting potential underlying etiologies, but integration of data from multimodal approaches including genomics is often required to achieve diagnosis.

Type I Interferonopathies: A Clinical Review **741**

Christine S. Wang

This review will discuss when clinicians should consider evaluating for Type I interferonopathies, review clinical phenotypes and molecular defects of Type I interferonopathies, and discuss current treatments.

Suppressor of Cytokine Signaling 1 Haploinsufficiency: A New Driver of Autoimmunity and Immunodysregulation **757**

Meng Liu, Evan Hsu, Yan Du, and Pui Y. Lee

Suppressor of cytokine signaling 1 (SOCS1) is a negative regulator of cytokine signaling that inhibits the activation of Janus kinases. A human disease caused by SOCS1 haploinsufficiency was first identified in 2020. To date, 18 cases of SOCS1 haploinsufficiency have been described. These patients experience enhanced activation of leukocytes and multiorgan system immunodysregulation, with immune-mediated cytopenia as the most common feature. In this review, the authors provide an overview on the biology of SOCS1 and summarize their knowledge of SOCS1 haploinsufficiency including genetics and clinical manifestations. They discuss the available treatment experience and outline an approach for the evaluation of suspected cases.

Deficiency of Adenosine Deaminase 2: Clinical Manifestations, Diagnosis, and Treatment **773**

Andrew Grim, Keila R. Veiga, and Nadine Saad

Deficiency of adenosine deaminase 2 (DADA2) is a monogenic vasculitis syndrome caused by biallelic mutations in the adenosine deaminase 2 gene. The diagnosis of DADA2 is confirmed by decreased enzymatic activity of ADA2 and genetic testing. Symptoms range from cutaneous vasculitis and polyarteritis nodosa-like lesions to stroke. The vasculopathy of DADA2 can affect many organ systems, including the gastrointestinal and renal systems. Hematologic manifestations occur early with hypogammaglobulinemia, lymphopenia, pure red cell aplasia, or pancytopenia. Treatment can be challenging. Tumor necrosis factor inhibitors are helpful to control inflammatory symptoms. Hematopoietic stem cell transplant may be needed to treat refractory cytopenias, vasculopathy, or immunodeficiency.

COPA Syndrome from Diagnosis to Treatment: A Clinician's Guide **789**

Noa Simchoni, Tiphanie P. Vogel, and Anthony K. Shum

COPA syndrome is a recently described autosomal dominant inborn error of immunity characterized by high titer autoantibodies and interstitial lung disease, with many individuals also having arthritis and nephritis. Onset is usually in early childhood, with unique disease features including alveolar hemorrhage, which can be insidious, pulmonary cyst formation, and progressive pulmonary fibrosis in nonspecific interstitial pneumonia or lymphocytic interstitial pneumonia patterns. This review explores the clinical presentation, genetics, molecular mechanisms, organ manifestations, and treatment approaches for COPA syndrome, and presents a diagnostic framework of suggested indications for patient testing.

NF-κB and Related Autoimmune and Autoinflammatory Diseases **805**

George E. Freigeh and Thomas F. Michniacki

The NF-B pathway is a cardinal signaling pathway that has been implicated in the development of a diverse range of clinical diseases. Numerous cellular processes converge on this pathway, which results in cell proliferation and survival. Defects in this pathway and in its upstream regulators have been described as causing immunodeficiency. However, there is a growing body of literature connecting autoimmune and autoinflammatory conditions to NF-B pathway dysfunction. This review serves as a current appraisal of the literature of these disorders.

Expanding IPEX: Inborn Errors of Regulatory T Cells **825**

Holly Wobma and Erin Janssen

Regulatory T cells (Tregs) are critical for enforcing peripheral tolerance. Monogenic "Tregopathies" affecting Treg development, stability, and/or function commonly present with polyautoimmunity, atopic disease, and infection. While autoimmune manifestations may present in early childhood, as more disorders are characterized, conditions with later onset have been identified. Treg numbers in the blood may be decreased in Tregopathies, but this is not always the case, and genetic testing should be pursued when there is high clinical suspicion. Currently, hematopoietic cell transplantation is the only curative treatment, but gene therapies are in development, and small molecule inhibitors/biologics may also be used.

Understanding the Spectrum of Immune Dysregulation Manifestations in Autoimmune Lymphoproliferative Syndrome and Autoimmune Lymphoproliferative Syndrome-like Disorders **841**

Christopher Failing, Jennifer R. Blase, and Kelly Walkovich

As a disorder of immune dysregulation, autoimmune lymphoproliferative syndrome (ALPS) stems from pathogenic variants in the first apoptosis signal-mediated apoptosis (Fas) and Fas-ligand pathway that result in elevations of CD3+ TCRαβ+ CD4- CD8- T cells along with chronic lymphoproliferation, a heightened risk for malignancy, and importantly for the rheumatologist, increased risk of autoimmunity. While immune cytopenias are the most encountered autoimmune phenomena, there is increasing appreciation for ocular, musculoskeletal, pulmonary and renal inflammatory manifestations similar to more common rheumatology diseases. Additionally, ALPS-like conditions that share similar clinical features and opportunities for targeted therapy are increasingly recognized via genetic testing, highlighting the need for rheumatologists to be facile in the recognition and diagnosis of this spectrum of disorders. This review will focus on clinical and laboratory features of both ALPS and ALPS-like disorders with the intent to provide a framework for rheumatologists to understand the pathophysiologic drivers and discriminate between diagnoses.

Genetic Defects in Early-Onset Inflammatory Bowel Disease **861**

Atiye Olcay Bilgic Dagci and Kelly Colleen Cushing

Inflammatory bowel disease (IBD) represents a spectrum of disease, which is characterized by chronic gastrointestinal inflammation. Monogenic mutations driving IBD pathogenesis are more highly represented in early-onset compared to adult-onset disease. The pathogenic genes which dysregulate host immune responses in monogenic IBD affect both the innate (ie, intestinal barrier, phagocytes) and adaptive immune systems (ie, T cells, B cells). Advanced genomic and targeted functional testing can improve clinical decision making and present increased opportunities for precision medicine approaches in this important patient population.

Mechanisms and Emerging Therapies for Treatment of Seizures in Pediatric Autoimmune Encephalitis and Autoinflammatory/Autoimmune-Associated Epilepsy **875**

Milena M. Andzelm and Coral M. Stredny

There has been increasing understanding of the role of inflammation in seizures and epilepsy, as well as targeted immunomodulatory treatments. In children, immune-mediated seizures often present acutely in the setting of autoimmune encephalitis and are very responsive to immunotherapy with low rates of subsequent epilepsy. Conversely, seizures in autoimmune-associated epilepsies, such as Rasmussen syndrome, can remain refractory to multimodal therapy, including immunomodulation. In this review, the authors discuss the presentations of immune-mediated seizures in children, underlying mechanisms, and emerging therapies.

Molecular Pathways in the Pathogenesis of Systemic Juvenile Idiopathic Arthritis **895**

Grant S. Schulert and Christoph Kessel

Systemic juvenile idiopathic arthritis (sJIA) is a rare childhood chronic inflammatory disorder with risk for life-threatening complications including macrophage activation syndrome and lung disease. At onset, sJIA pathogenesis resembles that of the autoinflammatory periodic fever syndromes with marked innate immune activation, expansion of neutrophils and monocytes, and high levels of interleukin-18. Here, we review the current conceptual understanding of sJIA pathogenesis with a focus on both innate and adaptive immune pathways. Finally, we consider how recent progress toward understanding the immunologic basis of sJIA may support new therapies for refractory disease courses.

Targeted Treatment of Diseases of Immune Dysregulation **913**

Smriti Mohan

Increasing molecular knowledge of autoinflammatory and autoimmune disorders has enabled more targeted treatment of these conditions. Treatment of inflammasomopathies is often aimed at interleukin-1 (IL-1) blockade, with potential use of other inhibitors targeting cytokines such as IL-18 and IL-6. Interferonopathies and some disorders with overlap features of autoimmunity and autoinflammation may improve with Janus kinase inhibition. Autoimmune conditions may also respond to inhibition of different cytokines, as well as to inhibition of T and B lymphocytes. Effective treatment is increasingly possible through targeted/precision medicine approaches.

RHEUMATIC DISEASE CLINICS OF NORTH AMERICA

FORTHCOMING ISSUES

February 2024
The Giants of Rheumatology
Michael Weisman, *Editor*

May 2024
Rheumatic Immune-Related Adverse Events
Alexa Simon Meara and David Liew, *Editors*

RECENT ISSUES

August 2023
Vasculitis
Eli Miloslavsky and Anisha Dua, *Editors*

May 2023
Scleroderma: Best Approaches to Patient Care
Tracy Frech, *Editor*

SERIES OF RELATED INTEREST

Emergency Medicine Clinics
Available at: https://www.emed.theclinics.com/
Neurologic Clinics
Available at: https://www.neurologic.theclinics.com/

Foreword

Emerging Concepts in Immune Dysregulation

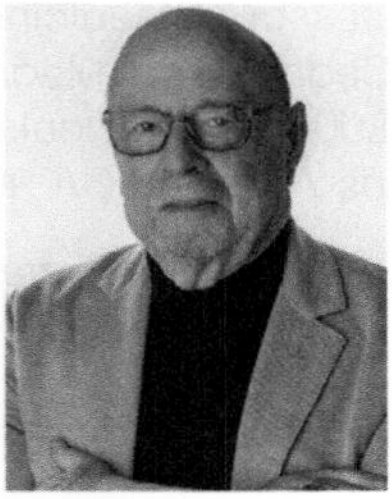

Michael H. Weisman, MD
Consulting Editor

From the standpoint of an Adult Rheumatologist, we have a lot to learn from our Pediatric Rheumatology colleagues. A start to this process is presented in an extraordinarily unique volume conceived and created by Erin Janssen. In the daily life of an Adult Rheumatologist, we are confronted by patients with what appears to be an adult-onset phenotype but with a large background of heterogeneity (lupus is the best example). The presentation of these childhood-onset cases and conditions related to inborn errors of immunity is there to teach us that our adult diseases probably begin long before the symptoms provoke their presentation to the health care system, and the heterogeneity we see is the result of a lengthy and poorly understood process. The study of these childhood-onset cases and current knowledge of recent developments in our understanding of these conditions will help not only raise the suspicion to make a specific diagnosis but also provide us with a landscape of the genetic underpinnings and molecular mechanisms that will lead to targeted treatment and potential prevention

Rheum Dis Clin N Am 49 (2023) xiii–xiv
https://doi.org/10.1016/j.rdc.2023.08.013
0889-857X/23/© 2023 Published by Elsevier Inc.

strategies. We are on the cusp of a much greater understanding of our specialty-related diseases and their management thanks to Erin and her colleagues.

Michael H. Weisman, MD
Adjunct Professor of Medicine
Stanford University
Distinguished Professor of Medicine Emeritus
David Geffen School of Medicine at UCLA
Professor of Medicine Emeritus
Cedars-Sinai Medical Center
10800 Wilshire Boulevard #404
Los Angeles, CA 90024, USA

E-mail address:
weisman@cshs.org

Preface

Emerging Concepts in Immune Dysregulation

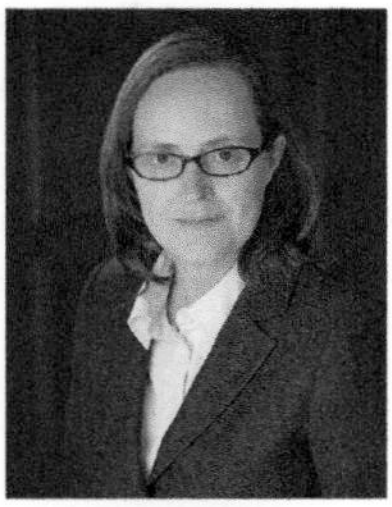

Erin Janssen, MD, PhD
Editor

As Rheumatologists, we have the privilege of following our patients over time and often observe changes in and/or the accumulation of their disease manifestations. As these changes occur, a single autoimmune manifestation may grow into polyautoimmunity or other conditions may arise, such as frequent infections, atopic disorders, or malignancies. Caring for these complex patients requires a deep understanding of the immune system and mechanisms of immune dysregulation. Knowledge of cutting-edge diagnostics and therapies is crucial for providing the best care to our patients. In addition, awareness of recently identified genetic associations and an understanding of the molecular pathogenesis underlying well-established conditions are vital.

In this issue of *Rheumatic Disease Clinics of North America*, we delve into several inborn errors of immunity (IEIs) that often present with autoimmunity and may be treated by a rheumatologist. In these articles, we provide information on when to have a high index of suspicion that an IEI may be present and how to investigate further. Type I interferonopathies, SOCS1 haploinsufficiency, deficiency of ADA2, COPA syndrome, NF-κB–related diseases of immune dysregulation, and Tregopathies were chosen due to their relevance to us as rheumatologists and recent developments in our understanding of these conditions. The issue also contains updated information regarding the genetic underpinnings and pathophysiology underlying autoimmune lymphoproliferative syndrome, systemic juvenile idiopathic arthritis, early-onset inflammatory bowel disease, and pediatric autoimmune encephalitis and autoinflammatory/autoimmune epilepsy. The issue is book-ended with articles on diagnosing IEIs and

Rheum Dis Clin N Am 49 (2023) xv–xvi
https://doi.org/10.1016/j.rdc.2023.08.012
0889-857X/23/© 2023 Published by Elsevier Inc.

the therapeutics that may be useful in their management. I hope you find this issue informative and use it to enhance your clinical practice.

Erin Janssen, MD, PhD
University of Michigan Medical School
Department of Pediatrics
Michigan Medicine
C.S. Mott Children's Hospital
1500 East Medical Center Drive, SPC 5718
Ann Arbor, MI 48109, USA

E-mail address:
ejanssen@med.umich.edu

Approach to Diagnosing Inborn Errors of Immunity

Xiao Peng, MD, PhD[a], Saara Kaviany, DO[b,*]

KEYWORDS

• Diagnostic evaluation • Inborn errors of immunity • Immune dysregulation
• Immune phenotyping • Genetic sequencing

KEY POINTS

- Evaluation for inborn errors of immunity (IEIs) requires a high clinical index of suspicion, as these disorders have diverse phenotypes.
- Immune phenotyping of patients with IEIs must be considered in the setting of potentially confounding variables such as environmental factors, ongoing treatments, and acute stressors such as infection.
- Next-generation sequencing (NGS) has had significant impact on the molecular diagnostic approach for patients with suspected IEIs.

INTRODUCTION TO INBORN ERRORS OF IMMUNITY

The increasing use of molecular diagnostics has led to rapid expansion of the genotypic and phenotypic landscape of inborn errors of immunity (IEIs). Like cancer, IEIs are proving to be individually rare, but collectively common. Although clinical diagnostic criteria remain lacking for most IEIs, a consensus now exists for nearly 500 IEIs, and the list of newly identified monogenic conditions encompassing diverse cellular processes continues to grow.[1] Even more humbling is the suggestion from human gene connectome analysis that at least another 2500 genes remain as likely causative candidates.[2] As reflected in the field's evolution away from the use of the term "primary immunodeficiency," IEIs are now understood to encompass manifold features including but not limited to immunodeficiency, autoimmunity, autoinflammation, atopy, bone marrow defects, and/or increased malignancy risk (**Fig. 1**). Moreover, more detailed natural history studies have noted immune abnormalities in patients with diverse genetic syndromes ranging from chromosomal aneuploidies to epigenetic disorders to inborn errors of metabolism. There are now over 100 described IEIs

[a] McKusick-Nathans, Department of Genetic Medicine, Johns Hopkins University School of Medicine, 600 North Wolfe Street, Blalock 1008, Baltimore, MD 21287, USA; [b] The University of Chicago & Biological Sciences, Department of Pediatrics, University of Chicago, 5841 South Maryland Avenue, Chicago, IL 60637, USA
* Corresponding author.
E-mail address: skaviany@bsd.uchicago.edu

Rheum Dis Clin N Am 49 (2023) 731–739
https://doi.org/10.1016/j.rdc.2023.06.001 rheumatic.theclinics.com
0889-857X/23/

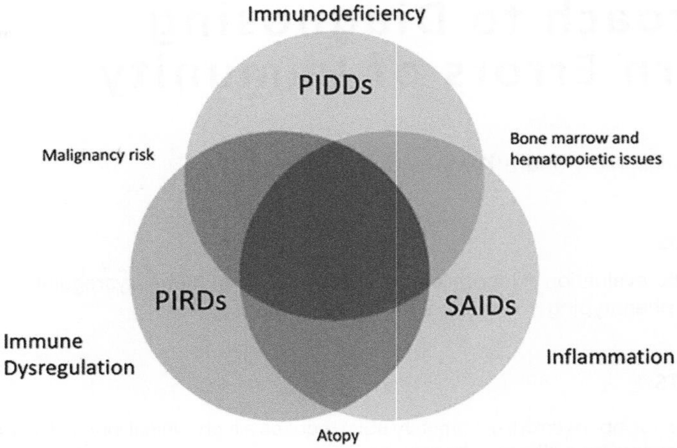

Fig. 1. Features shared by most IEIs. Not all IEIs may show all these features in equal measure, and the predominant features may evolve over time. PIDDs, primary immune deficiency disorders; PIRDs, primary immune regulatory disorders; SAIDs, systemic autoinflammatory disease.

predominantly featuring autoinflammation and/or immune dysregulation, many of which are not limited to pediatric patients.[3] Thus, even without the complications of expressivity and penetrance associated with disorders where host-environment interactions are so crucial to pathogenesis, it is already significantly challenging to identify these disorders. Multi-modal approaches are often required to achieve diagnosis although no assays are able to substitute for the essentiality of a detailed clinical timeline and history. Indeed, as we will discuss in the following sections, the success of novel-omics-based testing is predicated upon this.

The IEI realm is also unique in that clinicians have access to a growing repertoire of descriptive and functional assays that shed light on various facets of immune function. Thus, not only must we consider a patient's immune phenotypes on an organismal level but also on a cellular level.

It is also important to conceptually distinguish immunity as a process from the immune system—the former exists in virtually all living cells, while the latter, the "professionals" of immunity, has evolved in complexity through evolution. Thus, while we previously conceived immune disorders as affecting particular branches of "professional" immunity, that is, B cells, T cells, neutrophils, monocytes, or complement, we now realize that IEIs encompass a much more diverse group of disorders, affecting both innate and adaptive branches of the immune system but also the cell-intrinsic immunity of nonimmune cells.[1,4] Insight into the specific combinations of predispositions shown by patients with suspected IEIs, for example, the spectrum of infections (ie, bacterial, viral, fungal, etc) or the organ systems affected by inflammation (ie, skin, GI tract, CNS, etc), sheds light on the realm of IEI subtypes that should be considered and helps guide diagnostic strategy.

CLINICAL DIAGNOSIS OF IEI

Advances in various laboratory technologies—from flow cytometry- and imaging-based studies to DNA- and RNA-based sequencing to epigenomics, proteomics, or metabolomics—are already being used for hypothesis-generating research in IEIs and rapidly being adapted toward clinical diagnostic testing as well. Increasing use of first-line broad-spectrum next-generation sequencing (NGS) has already helped significantly expand the genotype-phenotype landscape of IEIs. We expanded the understanding of monogenic etiologies for heterogeneous clinical phenotypes, many of which had previously been thought to only be polygenic in etiology. Understanding the mechanisms associated with these monogenic IEIs has helped shed light on the pathophysiology of more polygenic forms of a similar disease. However, the limitations of NGS have likely also biased our understanding of the IEI genetic landscape toward certain types of "easier-to-detect" lesions residing within less-confounding genetic contexts.

Second, increased broad genetic testing has also shown that even "classic" IEI genes may be associated with a broader spectrum of phenotypic presentations than previously known. Moreover, family members with the same identified mutation can have significantly divergent presentations, raising the question of what additional genetic modifiers may exist. However, the wealth of new correlations has also led to significantly more ambiguity regarding relationships between specific genes and clinical phenotypes. This creates a challenging bottleneck regarding functional assessment of these findings, particularly if robust assays may not already exist for each gene. Finally, we are only beginning to understand the contributions of environment, commensals, and additional somatic drivers that arise in the course of each patient's unique natural history.

Given all the aforementioned challenges, IEI diagnoses can often be delayed. Moreover, even with achievement of molecular diagnosis, one may not always be able to extrapolate treatment strategies from one patient to another given their varied constellations of clinical concerns. IEIs are phenotypically complex, and even functional studies may reveal contradictory findings across cell types and individuals. Moreover, when patients' bodies must cope with having germline disease where the mutation exists in all cells, the precarious biological homeostasis they must achieve to stay alive is not easy to modulate. For many IEIs, immunomodulatory agents may help temporarily dampen the disease state, but curative options remain limited to hematopoietic stem cell transplant (HSCT) and/or gene therapy. The latter is not yet mature as a treatment option for the bulk of IEIs, while the former is also accompanied by its own significant risks. In addition, HSCT may not be curative for all facets of an IEI, particularly where the hematopoietic cells are not the only contributors to disease. Lastly, our pharmacologic space, although significantly more diversified over the past decade, currently still covers a very small area of the total biological space of an immune disease.

LABORATORY TESTING

Standard immunophenotyping approaches to assess adaptive immune function remain a linchpin of initial evaluation for patients with suspected IEIs. This often involves quantitative adaptive immune evaluations such as flow for lymphocyte subsets and quantitative immunoglobulins, as well as qualitative evaluation by determining specific vaccine and other antigen responses to assess for potential T-cell, B-cell, and/or T-B communication defects leading to humoral immunodeficiency. More detailed characterization of lymphocyte subset numbers, activities, and responses to stimuli may also be performed if there is concern for cellular defects.

Clinical biomarker assays that provide information on immune activation states and adaptive-innate immune crosstalk have also become more available and commonly used with our deeper understanding of the immune pathways driving particular disease states. We now are able to assess levels of key cytokines (ie, interleukin [IL]-6, tumor necrosis factor alpha, interferon [IFN], and soluble IL-2Receptor [sIL-2R]) in the serum and select other bodily fluids that can inform about specific immune activation and polarization states, particularly in inflammatory settings. For example, both primary familial hemophagocytic lymphohistiocytosis (HLH) and macrophage activation syndrome, or HLH secondary to diverse rheumatologic, immune dysregulatory, or inflammatory etiologies, may have similar clinical manifestations.[5] To help distinguish between the disorders, the relative levels of biomarkers such as CXCL9 and IL-18 have been helpful tools, as the relative elevation of each may be different among the two disease states.[6,7] These not only help suggest potentially promising avenues of treatment but also inform diagnostic strategy. Although, as mentioned previously, no single assay should be interpreted in isolation, examining the combinations of elevated cytokines may inform the pathway(s) (ie, type I or II IFN, nuclear factor kappa B, inflammasome signaling) that may be dysregulated and thus suggest the genes to prioritize for analysis.

One caveat for all immunophenotyping, but particularly the timely capture and interpretation of serum cytokines in patients undergoing IEI workups, is the many potentially contributory and confounding variables that must be considered, including but not limited to acute illness, environmental triggers, and other medications. Thus, although we now have access to increasingly sensitive and specific clinical-grade assays for states such as type I IFN activation via IFN response gene signatures, all results must still be interpreted in the clinical context of the patient as they can also be increased in many physiologic states of stress and infection, as well as in non-Mendelian autoinflammatory and autoimmune conditions. As such, the diagnosis and evaluation of patients with suspected IEIs also often requires invocation of orthogonal methods such as molecular sequencing.

MOLECULAR TESTING

As for all genetic conditions, selection of genetic testing approach is predicated on multiple considerations, including the patient's clinical presentation and acuity, the suspected genetic differential and associated genetic architecture, and the potential impact on patient management. Realistically, socioeconomic and familial considerations also often play a role.

IEIs in particular are associated with a broad and unique repertoire of genetic paradigms that flaunt traditional genetic disease assumptions and thus may not always conform well to traditional genetic guidelines for variant triage and classification. Because many conditions feature incomplete penetrance and involve postreproductive selection, allele frequencies may be higher than expected for "rare" diseases, and degrees of evolutionary conservation may be lower than expected. Moreover, specific populations and individuals may often carry unique or private variants that may not be considered disease-causing on another haplotype background or in a different exposure environment. In addition, we know from painstaking studies that untranslated RNAs, noncoding mutations, silent/synonymous mutations (ie, leading to cryptic splicing), and copy number (CNV) and structural variants (SVs)[8] are all relevant concerns although poorly amenable to current variant detection and analysis strategies. Situations such as somatic mosaicism, uniparental disomy, sex-linked phenotypes, and locus sequence degeneracy further complicate testing choices. With few exceptions, the significant phenotypic heterogeneity among IEIs should lead to consideration of broad first-line molecular diagnostic testing involving simultaneous analysis of multiple genes whenever possible. Orthogonal testing for SVs and CNVs should also be considered, even in the absence of neurodevelopmental or congenital anomalies. Depending on the loci of interest or the intention of diagnosis versus screening, this can be performed using several approaches, with chromosomal microarrays and multiplex-ligation-dependent probe amplification being two of the more commonly seen methods.

However, this is already rapidly evolving with the emerging use of optical genome mapping, which promises to revolutionize the field of SV and CNV detection for IEIs.[9,10]

After a candidate variant is identified, one must then tackle the challenges of understanding how this variant may impact the function of the relevant gene product(s) and then how such a molecular impact relates to the patient's specific clinical findings. Many IEI genes (ie, *IL6ST, STATJ, IKZFJ*) are associated with multiple types of mutations with distinct inheritance patterns, pathogenic mechanisms, and associated clinical complications.[l] For example, loss of function (LOF) can be defined on a spectrum of nullomorphic to hypomorphic, but the clinical effects may not simply change in magnitude in correspondence with the degree of LOF—this is illustrated by hypomorphic chronic granulomatous disease (CGD)[11] and *RAGJ/2*[12] and heterozygous.

TACI/TNFRSFJ3B mutations[13] are associated with increased risk for autoimmunity as a consequence of hypomorphic activity rather than simply a less severe immunodeficiency.

Alternatively, a variant may lead to gain of function (GOF) in terms of downstream effects, but the actual lesion leads to a LOF of autoinhibitory activity—this is seen for several autoinflammatory conditions including the inflammasopathies.[14] In the case of patients with *PLCG2*-associated cold-induced urticaria, even GOF is not straightforward since the environmental temperature determines whether the mutation leads to GOF or LOF.[15] Moreover, multiple GOF mechanisms may exist for 1 gene—such as increased DNA-binding activity[16] versus increased protein levels[17] in the case of *IKZF1*. When a gene encodes a protein at the nexus of many signaling pathways, that is, *STAT3* and *USPJ8*, even LOF and GOF are not straightforward, and one must perform the studies needed to determine how individual pathways are affected in each cell type.[18,19] Dominant negative or other forms of destabilizing mutations are even more difficult to dissect, particularly for genes encoding key regulatory proteins such as transcription factors with multiple binding partners.[20] Similarly, one must be very careful about the functional assays chosen to assess alleles affecting proteins subjected to significant subcellular localization[21] or posttranslational regulation.[22]

Needless to say, mode of inheritance is also highly relevant to interpreting the mechanism of disease. It is significantly more common to see dominantly inherited missense alleles, such as those leading to GOF disease, arising *de novo*, while the presence of consanguinity or a known founder variant-associated ancestry often leads to suspicion for a recessive disease. Severe recessive forms of a condition may be elucidated first, only to be followed by the finding of additional patients with dominantly inherited form of the same condition, or vice versa.[23] When a single allele is found for a phenotype generally associated with biallelic disease, one must always ask, is a second lesion in *trans* truly not there or just insufficiently detected by the testing platform? In these situations, the availability of additional flow cytometry or other immunophenotypic studies may be a valuable sanity check. Finally, familial segregation studies must be interpreted with caution because of the rampant variable expressivity and incomplete penetrance seen for IEIs.

From both a research and clinical perspective, the increasingly widespread availability of novel genomics platforms has significantly advanced our understanding of the genetic underpinnings of IEIs. Clinical-grade NGS-based assays have become both time- and cost-effective, making them extremely attractive for helping to shorten diagnostic odysseys and reduce the need for more demanding or invasive tests. Most providers caring for patients with suspected IEIs have historically relied on targeted gene panels (TGPs). Most of these TGPs are now performed on an exome or genome backbone, and costs and turnaround times have become comparable. With the increasingly unwieldy pace and volume of IEI gene discovery, it is becoming more common to prefer whole-exome (WES) or even whole-genome sequencing (WGS) for firstline testing if available. This is particularly true for inpatients who are acutely ill or patients with poorly defined presentations with overlapping elements of immunodeficiency, immune dysregulation, and/or autoinflammation. One of the long-term advantages of broader testing is the ability to have the entire repertoire of variant calls for iterative reanalysis over time if the initial clinical analysis is negative, not to mention the ability to identify genetic conditions that may lead to secondary IEI phenotypes but would not be found on IEI-specific TGPs. However, with broader testing also comes the increased complexity of precounseling and postcounseling and ordering logistics, as well as increased risk for detection of more potentially irrelevant variants of uncertain significance. Thus, both pan-IEI and smaller more phenotype-specific TGPs (ie, for periodic fever syndromes) still remain in broad use by IEI providers who are not clinical geneticists. Regardless of who orders genetic testing, the complex considerations mentioned previously recommend a multidisciplinary team approach to genetic and diagnostic testing in general, including involvement of a clinical genetics practitioner with IEI familiarity—this is crucial for ensuring that clinically relevant genes of interest are being thoroughly interrogated and appropriately interpreted.

Specifically, emerging data for IEIs show that WES and WGS, particularly when a family-based trio approach is taken, can lead to improved diagnostic yield and reduced costs over other standard approaches if performed early in the diagnostic process.[7] Despite heterogeneity in IEI patient cohort selection, first-pass diagnostic yields rarely exceed 40%[24–26] unless enriched for highly selected subphenotypes or populations with significant endogamy. As for pan-IEI cohorts in general, currently reported diagnostic yields of comprehensive IEI- [27–29] or autoinflammatory disease-focused TGPs[30] also fall around 10% to 30%. From a research perspective, both WES and WGS may be helpful for identifying novel disease-associated genes and variants, as well as novel genotype-phenotype relationships. Widespread clinical use of WGS for IEI diagnosis currently remains limited although there is a general consensus that it may be more advantageous than WES for both upfront diagnosis and reanalysis by introducing less bias to and guaranteeing greater uniformity of coverage for variant detection.[31–33] However, both remain limited by the same mapping issues, not to mention reference genome limitations, inherent to current clinical NGS platforms in general. For phenotypes involving immune dysregulation and inflammation, somatic variation may be more of a concern, and the greater depth rather than breadth of coverage achieved by TGPs and WES may be preferred.[8] On the horizon are also third-generation long-read sequencing technologies that may prove to be game-changing for all classes of nucleic acid detection. However, even if we are able to robustly generate these data, there still remain the challenges of building the tools and infrastructure needed for storage, processing, and analysis.[34]

DISCUSSION

Despite the rapid advances in our understanding of IEI genetic and phenotypic landscapes, diagnosis continues to remain a challenge. As we have outlined previously, it is often difficult to categorize affected patients solely on the basis of genotype or phenotype, as there is significant heterogeneity to clinical presentations. A high index of suspicion must be maintained by providers in all fields, particularly where

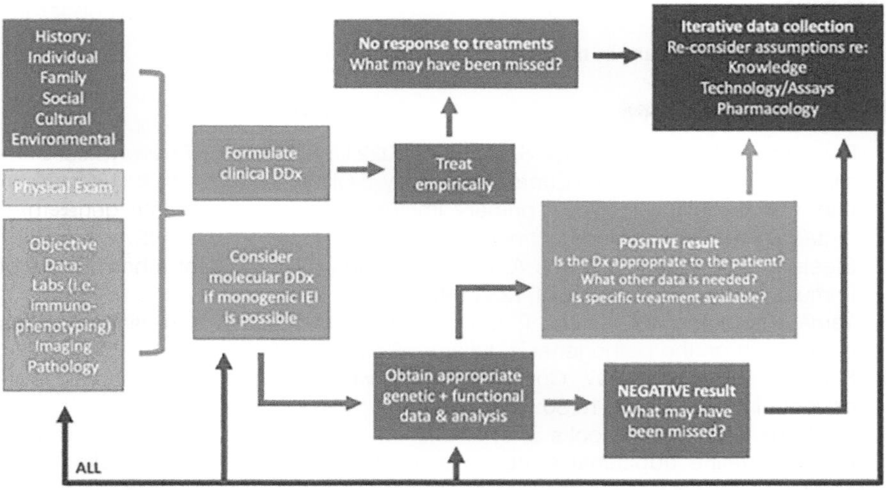

Fig. 2. IEI diagnosis is often an iterative process. In the absence of satisfactory diagnosis and treatment responses, assumptions about the nature of the clinical condition, its etiologies, and the strengths and limitations of the diagnostic assays and treatments used must be reconsidered. Additional data gathering is necessary even when a positive result is obtained because every individual's expression of a specific IEI can differ, even within families.

multisystem manifestations are present in the form of autoimmune, immune dysregulatory, autoinflammatory, immunodeficient, and/or additional atypical unexplained concerns.

Selecting diagnostic approaches remains a challenge in the workup of these patients.

This discussion has largely focused on genetic testing strategies, as the functional and immunophenotypic options for testing can be diverse and overwhelming to navigate for different clinical presentations. However, both approaches are equally important and should rarely be used alone for diagnosis (**Fig. 2**). Moreover, data from these studies should always be interpreted in the context of iterative and detailed clinical assessment, including observation of patient responses (or lack thereof) to certain treatments, which can prove highly valuable.

Looking forward, the emergence of many promising assay modalities and significant volumes of data generation raises additional challenges for the field in terms of how to pay for, store, integrate, and interpret all the multidimensional information in a clinically useful way. Finally, we are learning that immune diseases may arise from changes beyond those found in germline DNA,[4] from the growing repertoire of known disease-causing somatic mutations[35] and auto-antibodies[36] to the potential for epigenetic[37] or RNA-based mechanisms of disease.[38] Thus, additional strategies may need to be brought to bear for detection of these IEI "phenocopies."

CLINICS CARE POINTS

- There are now greater than 500 IEIs described, with newly monogenic disorders encompassing different cellular processes and phenotypes. Both immune phenotyping and molecular testing are required for suspected IEIs.

DISCLOSURE

S. Kaviany is a participant in the Gamifant (Sobi) speaker bureau.

REFERENCES

1. Bousfiha A, Moundir A, Tangye S, et al. The 2022 Update of IUIS Phenotypical Classification for Human Inborn Errors of Immunity. J Clin Immunol 2022;42:1508–20.
2. Itan Y, Casanova J-L. Novel primary immunodeficiency candidate genes predicted by the human gene connectome. Front Immunol 2015;6:142.
3. Staels F, Collignon T, Betrains A, et al. Monogenic Adult-Onset Inborn Errors of Immunity. Front Immunol 2021;12:753978.
4. Yamashita M, Inoue K, Okano T, et al. Inborn errors of immunity-recent advances in research on the pathogenesis. Inflamm Regen 2021;41:9.
5. Schulert GS, Canna SW. Convergent pathways of the hyperferritinemic syndromes. Int Immunol 2018;30:195–203.
6. de Jesus AA, Hou Y, Brooks S, et al. Distinct interferon signatures and cytokine patterns define additional systemic autoinflammatory diseases. J Clin Invest 2020;130:1669–82.
7. Weiss ES, Girard-Guyonvarc'h C, Holzinger D, et al. Interleukin-18 diagnostically distinguishes and pathogenically promotes human and murine macrophage activation syndrome. Blood 2018;131:1442–55.
8. Lee K, Abraham RS. Next-generation sequencing for inborn errors of immunity. Hum Immunol 2021;82:871–82.
9. Wan R, Schieck M, Caballero-Oteyza A, et al. Copy Number Analysis in a Large Cohort Suggestive of Inborn Errors of Immunity Indicates a Wide Spectrum of Relevant Chromosomal Losses and Gains. J Clin Immunol 2022;42:1083–92.
10. Sahajpal NS, Barseghyan H, Kolhe R, et al. Optical genome mapping identifies rare structural variations as predisposition factors associated with severe COVID-19. iScience 2022;25:103760.
11. De Ravin SS, Naumann N, Cowen EW, et al. Chronic granulomatous disease as a risk factor for autoimmune disease. J Allergy Clin Immunol 2008;122:1097–103.
12. Chen K, Wu W, Mathew D, et al. Autoimmunity due to RAG deficiency and estimated disease incidence in RAG1/2 mutations. J Allergy Clin Immunol 2014; 133:880–2.e10.
13. Romberg N, Chamberlain N, Saadoun D, et al. CVID-associated TACI mutations affect autoreactive B cell selection and activation. J Clin Invest 2013;123:4283–93.
14. Aksentijevich I, Schnappauf O. Molecular mechanisms of phenotypic variability in monogenic autoinflammatory diseases. Nat Rev Rheumatol 2021;17:405–25.
15. Milner JD. PLAID: a Syndrome of Complex Patterns of Disease and Unique Phenotypes. J Clin Immunol 2015;35:527–30.
16. Hoshino A, Boutboul D, Zhang Y, et al. Gain-of-function IKZF1 variants in humans cause immune dysregulation associated with abnormal T/B cell late differentiation. Sci Immunol 2022;7:eabi7160.
17. Brodie SA, Khincha PP, Giri N, et al. Pathogenic germline IKZF1 variant alters hematopoietic gene expression profiles. Cold Spring Harb Mol Case Stud 2021;7: a006015.
18. Lodi L, Faletti LE, Maccari ME, et al. STAT3-confusion-of-function: Beyond the loss and gain dualism. J Allergy Clin Immunol 2022;150:1237–41.e3.
19. Martin-Fernandez M, Buta S, Voyer TL, et al. A partial form of inherited human USP18 deficiency underlies infection and inflammation. J Exp Med 2022;219: e20211273.

20. Kuehn HS, Nunes-Santos CJ, Rosenzweig SD. Germline IKZF1 mutations and their impact on immunity: IKAROS-associated diseases and pathophysiology. Expert Rev Clin Immunol 2021;17:407–16.
21. Gamez-Dfaz L, Seidel MG. Different Apples, Same Tree: Visualizing Current Biological and Clinical Insights into CTLA-4 Insufficiency and LRBA and DEF6 Deficiencies. Front Pediatr 2021;9:662645.
22. Beck DB, Werner A, Kastner DL, et al. Disorders of ubiquitylation: unchained inflammation. Nat Rev Rheumatol 2022;18:435–47.
23. Wan R, Fänder J, Zakaraia I, et al. Phenotypic spectrum in recessive STING-associated vasculopathy with onset in infancy: Four novel cases and analysis of previously reported cases. Front Immunol 2022;13:1029423.
24. Stranneheim H, Lagerstedt-Robinson K, Magnusson M, et al. Integration of whole genome sequencing into a healthcare setting: high diagnostic rates across multiple clinical entities in 3219 rare disease patients. Genome Med 2021;13:40.
25. Similuk MN, Yan J, Ghosh R, et al. Clinical exome sequencing of 1000 families with complex immune phenotypes: Toward comprehensive genomic evaluations. J Allergy Clin Immunol 2022;150(4):947–54.
26. Hebert A, Simons A, Schuurs-Hoeijmakers JHM, et al. Trio-based whole exome sequencing in patients with suspected sporadic inborn errors of immunity: A retrospective cohort study. Elife 2022;11:e78469.
27. Engelbrecht C, Urban M, Schoeman M, et al. Clinical Utility of Whole Exome Sequencing and Targeted Panels for the Identification of Inborn Errors of Immunity in a Resource-Constrained Setting. Front Immunol 2021;12:665621.
28. Yska H.A.F., Elsink K., Kuijpers T.W., et al., Diagnostic Yield of Next Generation Sequencing in Genetically Undiagnosed Patients with Primary Immunodeficiencies: a Systematic Review, *J Clin Immunol*, 39, 2019, 577–591.
29. Vorsteveld EE, Hoischen A, van der Made CI. Next-Generation Sequencing in the Field of Primary Immunodeficiencies: Current Yield, Challenges, and Future Perspectives. Clin Rev Allergy Immunol 2021;61:212–25.
30. Omoyinmi E, Standing A, Keylock A, et al. Clinical impact of a targeted next-generation sequencing gene panel for autoinflammation and vasculitis. PLoS One 2017;12:e0181874.
31. Meyts I, Bosch B, Bolze A, et al. Exome and genome sequencing for inborn errors of immunity. J Allergy Clin Immunol 2016;138:957–69.
32. Costain G., Jobling R., Walker S., et al., Periodic reanalysis of whole-genome sequencing data enhances the diagnostic advantage over standard clinical genetic testing, *Eur J Hum Genet*, 26, 2018, 740–744.
33. Lionel A.C., Costain G., Monfared N., et al., Improved diagnostic yield compared with targeted gene sequencing panels suggests a role for whole-genome sequencing as a first-tier genetic test, *Genet Med*, 20, 2018, 435–443.
34. Wang Y, Zhao Y, Bollas A, et al. Nanopore sequencing technology, bioinformatics and applications. Nat Biotechnol 2021;39:1348–65.
35. Beck DB, Ferrada MA, Sikora KA, et al. Somatic Mutations in UBA1 and Severe Adult-Onset Autoinflammatory Disease. N Engl J Med 2020;383:2628–38.
36. Cheng A, Holland SM. Anticytokine autoantibodies: Autoimmunity trespassing on antimicrobial immunity. J Allergy Clin Immunol 2022;149:24–8.
37. Romano R., Cillo F., Moracas C., et al., Epigenetic Alterations in Inborn Errors of Immunity, *J Clin Med Res*, 11 (5), 2022, 1261.
38. Rassoulzadegan M, Cuzin F. From paramutation to human disease: RNA-mediated heredity. Semin Cell Dev Biol 2015;44:47–50.

Type I Interferonopathies

A Clinical Review

Christine S. Wang, MD, MSCS

KEYWORDS

- Type I interferonopathy • Aicardi-goutières syndrome • Monogenic lupus
- Inborn errors of immunity • Interferonopathies

KEY POINTS

- Monogenic Type I interferonopathies are increasingly described in the medical literature. Early multi-organ dysfunction and systemic inflammation, particularly with a TORCH-like phenotype or early onset of Systemic Lupus Erythematosus or lupus-like disease, especially with severe features not responding to conventional immunotherapies, should prompt concern for an interferonopathy.
- Severe chilblains, particularly with extensive ulceration or digital amputation, early onset interstitial lung disease, early onset glomerulonephritis with lupus-like phenotype, or intracranial calcifications with leukodystrophy should raise concern for a Type I interferonopathy.
- Increased risk for infections can occur with multiple Type I interferonopathies, and concurrent infections do not exclude a Type I interferonopathy.
- A high index of suspicion should be maintained in adolescents and young adults or individuals without elevated interferon gene signatures but with concerning clinical phenotypes secondary to heterogeneity in symptom onset and severity.

BACKGROUND

Inborn errors of immunity comprise a large group of disorders caused by damaging genetic variants that affect innate and adaptive immune function resulting in autoinflammation, autoimmunity, and/or immune dysregulation. A subgroup of these disorders, termed "Type I interferonopathies", occur secondary to mutations in genes leading to the dysregulation of Type I interferon signaling, which are normally activated as part of the innate immune response to predominantly viral but also bacterial antigens. Understanding the molecular defects causing monogenic Type I interferonopathies have expanded our understanding of complex autoimmune diseases such as Systemic Lupus Erythematosus (SLE) and Dermatomyositis, where many affected

Department of Pediatric Rheumatology, C.S. Mott Children's Hospital, University of Michigan, 1500 East Medical Center Drive SPC 5718, Ann Arbor, MI 48109, USA
E-mail address: chrswang@med.umich.edu

Rheum Dis Clin N Am 49 (2023) 741–756
https://doi.org/10.1016/j.rdc.2023.06.002
rheumatic.theclinics.com
0889-857X/23/

individuals demonstrate an increased Type I interferon gene signature (IGS). The objective of this review is to summarize clinical phenotypes of monogenic Type I interferonopathies to aid clinicians in identifying patients who require evaluation. Early diagnosis and treatment are invaluable as most affected individuals have severe clinical manifestations and increased mortality. In-depth review of the molecular mechanisms underlying Type I interferonopathies is beyond the scope of this review but are reviewed in these cited articles.[1,2]

WHEN TO CONSIDER AN INTERFERONOPATHY

While Type I interferonopathies can have heterogeneous phenotypes, the majority present early in life with multi-organ derangement and persistent systemic inflammation. Infections can be co-occurring and does not exclude diagnosis. Clinicians should consider Type I interferonopathies in young patients, especially in the neonatal period, with severe multi-system dysfunction and systemic inflammation that cannot be explained by infectious causes alone. Patients who present with a TORCH syndrome, commonly characterized by the neonatal development of intra-cranial calcifications, hepatosplenomegaly, fever, petechiae or purpura, and cytopenias, but with negative infectious testing should raise concern for a Type I interferonopathy. Type I interferonopathy should also be considered in patients with early onset lupus-like phenotypes, especially in those with severe manifestations that have been refractory to standard treatments. Clinical manifestations that should raise index of suspicion with associated disorders are summarized in **Box 1**. Common symptom of concern includes unexplained intracranial calcifications, interstitial lung disease, severe chilblains, and neutrophilic dermatosis (**Fig. 1**). Lab abnormalities are common including systemic inflammation and autoantibodies (see **Box 1**). Although affected individuals often display an elevated Type I IGS, there are exceptions to this rule,[3] and a normal IGS does not exclude an interferonopathy. Definitive diagnosis via genetic sequencing demonstrating a pathogenic mutation in a disease-causing gene is essential.

CLINICAL SYNDROME(S) AND ASSOCIATED MOLECULAR DEFECTS

Clinical phenotypes and associated molecular aberrations (**Fig. 2**) are discussed later in discussion.

AICARDI-GOUTIÈRES SYNDROME

Patient with AGS exhibit variable phenotypes but commonly presents with neurologic impairment secondary to leukodystrophy, intracranial calcifications, and cerebral atrophy.[4] Other manifestations include chilblains, which is reported in ~40% of patients,[5] glaucoma,[6] hepatosplenomegaly, and cerebral vascular involvement resulting in stroke.[7] Laboratory abnormalities can include systemic inflammation including an elevated IGS, elevated liver enzymes, thrombocytopenia, and CSF pleocytosis.[4]

Seven genes involved in intracellular nucleic acid metabolism have been implicated in causing AGS with variable modes of inheritance (**Table 1**). AGS has two timeframes of clinical presentation, neonatal-onset AGS and late-onset or atypical AGS. The neonatal form presents at birth or in the first few weeks of life with fever, poor feeding, irritability, and seizures are reported in up to 50% of affected neonates.[5] There is typically an acute encephalopathic phase followed by the stabilization of neurologic symptoms.[8] Brain imaging abnormalities can support the diagnosis. As 20% of cases present in the neonatal period, AGS can be confused with TORCH infections, which

Box 1
Common clinical and lab abnormalities clinical symptoms

Clinical symptoms:

General:
- Multi-organ involvement, recurrent fever, early age of onset, failure to thrive, developmental delay
- Pseudo-TORCH phenotype: Aicardi-Goutières Syndrome (AGS), UPS18 deficiency, STAT2 gain-of-function

Cutaneous:
- Raynaud phenomena/Chilblains: Familial chilblains lupus, AGS, STING-associated Vasculopathy with Onset in Infancy (SAVI)
- Neutrophilic dermatosis: Proteasome-Associated Autoinflammatory Syndromes (PRAAS)/ Chronic Atypical Neutrophilic Dermatosis with Lipodystrophy and Elevated temperature (CANDLE), PRAID
- Lipodystrophy/Panniculitis: PRAAS/CANDLE

Gastrointestinal:
- Chronic diarrhea: Tricho-hepato-enteric syndrome (THES), X-linked Reticulate Pigmentary Disorder (XLPRD)
- Enterocolitis: XLPRD

Hematologic:
- Autoimmune cytopenia
- Lymphoproliferative disorder: Loss-of-function PRKCD, Autoimmune lymphoproliferative disorder (ALPs)

Musculoskeletal:
- Arthritis: COPA, AGS5, CANDLE
- Skeletal abnormalities: Spondyloenchondrodysplasia with immune dysregulation (SPENCD), Singleton-Merten Syndrome (SMS)

Neurologic:
- Intracranial calcifications: AGS, ISG15 deficiency, UPS18 deficiency, STAT2 Gain-of-Function, CANDLE
- Cerebral atrophy: AGS
- Leukodystrophy: AGS
- Seizure: AGS, ISG15 deficiency, UPS18 deficiency
- Stroke: AGS5

Ophthalmologic
- Glaucoma: AGS, SMS

Pulmonary:
- Interstitial lung disease: SAVI, COPA
- Diffuse alveolar hemorrhage: COPA (more common), SAVI (reported in a few patients), DNASEL3 loss-of-function (rare)

Renal:
- Glomerulonephritis: Monogenic lupus

Lab abnormalities
- Chronic systemic inflammation with disproportionally elevated sedimentation rate compared to C-reactive protein
- CSF pleocytosis
- Elevated CSF neopterin
- Elevated IGS
- Autoantibodies such as double-stranded DNA (dsDNA) and anti-neutrophil cytoplasmic antibodies (ANCA)

present similarly. The early-onset form of AGS is more frequently associated with defects in *TREX1*, *RNASEH2A*, and *RNASEH2C*.

Late-onset or atypical AGS poses a greater diagnostic challenge as symptoms typically occur after several months of seemingly normal infantile development. Clinical symptoms can include spasticity and weakness, decline in head circumference

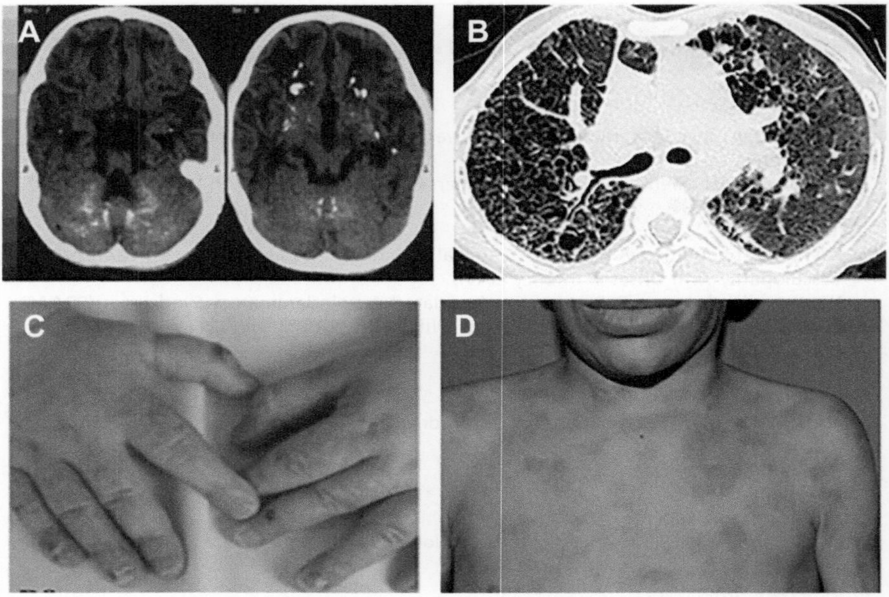

Fig. 1. Common clinical manifestations of Type I interferonopathy. (*A*). Intracranial CT demonstrating intracranial calcifications (*B*). Interstitial lung disease with diffuse ground glass opacities and fibrosis (*C*). Chilblains with ulceration (*D*). Annular neutrophilic plaques with lipodystrophy. (A): From Goutières F. Aicardi-Goutières syndrome. Brain Dev. 2005;27(3):201-206. (B and C): From Frémond ML, Hadchouel A, Berteloot L, et al. Overview of STING-Associated Vasculopathy with Onset in Infancy (SAVI) Among 21 Patients. J Allergy Clin Immunol Pract. 2021;9(2):803-818.e11.(D). From Dávila-Seijo P, Hernández-Martín A, Torrelo A. Autoinflammatory syndromes for the dermatologist. Clin Dermatol. 2014;32(4):488-501.

growth, developmental delay or regression accompanied by systemic features of inflammation such as fever.[9] However, cases of normal intellectual function[10] and normal brain imaging with milder phenotypes, especially with AGS Type 2,[11] have been reported. Late-onset AGS is more frequently associated with defects in *RNASEH2B*, *SAMHD1*, *ADAR,* and *IFIH1*.

MONOGENIC LUPUS AND LUPUS-LIKE DISEASE

Systemic Lupus Erythematosus (SLE) is a complex heterogenous multisystem autoimmune disease characterized by the production of autoantibodies targeting nuclear antigens.[12] Several monogenic mutations have been described to cause early-onset SLE, fulfilling classification criteria from the American College of Rheumatology (ACR) for SLE,[13] or lupus-like phenotypes (**Table 2**). Mechanistically genetic alterations can affect complement regulation, nucleic acid clearance and sensing, self-tolerance, and/or regulation of Type I interferon signaling. Monogenic lupus should be considered in early-onset SLE, especially in individuals 5 years or younger, or in individuals with severe disease manifestations that are resistant to standard SLE therapies.

Complement Deficiencies

Deficiencies in C1q, C1r, C1s, C2, or C4 protein function have been associated with developing a lupus-like phenotype as well as recurrent infections. C1q deficiency is

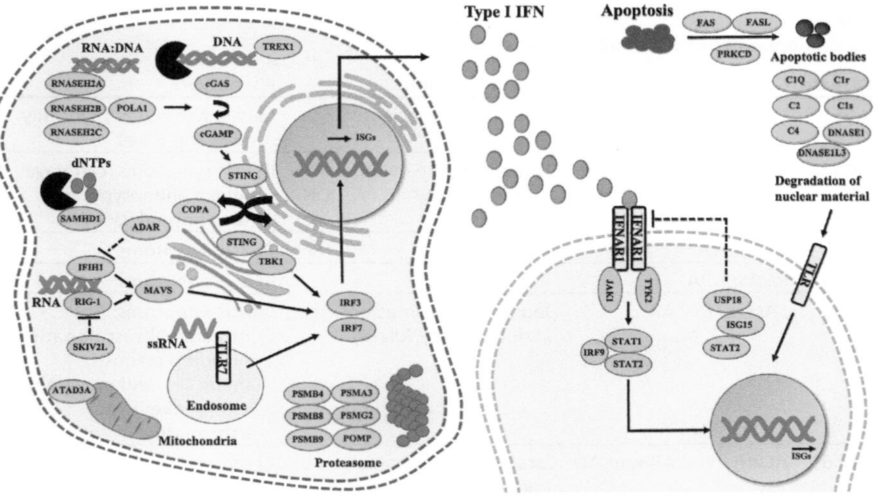

Fig. 2. Monogenic mutations resulting in the dysregulation of Type I production. Colored in orange are select proteins mutated in type I interferonopathies. cGAMP, cyclic guanosine monophosphate–adenosine monophosphate; cGAS, cyclic GMP-AMP synthase; IFN, interferon; IFNAR, interferon-α receptor; IRF, interferon regulatory factor; ISG, interferon stimulator genes; JAK, janus kinase; MAVS, mitochondrial antiviral-signaling protein; RIG-I, retinoic acid-inducible gene 1; STAT, signal transducer and activator of transcription; TBK1, TANK-binding kinase 1; TLR, toll-like receptor; TYK, tyrosine kinase.

most strongly linked with the development of SLE or lupus-like syndrome with ~90% of individuals developing clinical symptoms.[14,15] Photosensitivity and cutaneous symptoms including discoid rash are most common and glomerulonephritis, central nervous system, and oral ulcer involvement can be observed.[15,16] Defects in *C1s* and/or *C1r* cause clinical manifestations in approximately 65% of affected individuals. Signs include severe skin manifestations and lupus nephritis occurring in ~40% of cases. *C1s/C1r* deficiency is also associated with increased infections and many affected individuals die at a young age secondary to infection.[17] The most common complement deficiency in Western Europeans is *C2*, though lupus occurs in only 10% to 30% with C2 deficiency.[14] Individuals with C2 deficiency typically present with milder symptoms including cutaneous lupus, arthritis, and photosensitivity.[18] C4 deficiency is uncommon, but approximately 75% of affected individuals will develop symptoms. As there are multiple loci to the C4 gene, a lower C4 gene copy number also increases the risk for SLE.[19] Severe photosensitivity and glomerulonephritis are commonly seen in C4 deficiency.

Nucleic Acid Clearance/Nucleic Acid Sensing

Mutations in *DNASE1* and *DNASE1L3*, which encode endonucleases, cause decreased degradation of DNA.[20–22] Two patients have been described with *DNASE1* mutations who had SLE with high titer IgG nucleosomal and dsDNA antibodies and Sjogren's syndrome.[22] Loss of function mutations in *DNASE1L3* cause childhood-onset SLE with lupus nephritis and positive anti-neutrophil cytoplasmic (ANCA) antibodies.[21] Other manifestations include hypocomplementemic urticarial vasculitis[23] and rarely alveolar hemorrhages and inflammatory bowel disease.[24] Biallelic mutations in *DNASE2*, which encodes a lysosomal endonuclease, also causes an SLE-

Table 1
Clinical phenotypes of Aicardi-Goutières syndrome

Disease	Gene	Inheritance	Protein Function	Phenotype
AGS1	*TREX-1*	AR and AD	3′-5′ DNA exonuclease	Classic symptoms[a]; typically neonatal onset
AGS2	*RNASEH2B*	AR	Subunits of the complex that degrades RNA in RNA:DNA hybrids	Classic symptoms; can have milder phenotype, may have normal IGS
AGS3	*RNASEH2C*			Classic symptoms
AGS4	*RNASEH2A*			Classic symptoms
AGS5	*SAMHD1*	AR	Degrades deoxynucleoside triphosphate (dNTP)	Classic symptoms; intracranial vasculopathy including stenosis, aneurysm, and moyamoya[7] with stroke; joint arthropathy[87]
AGS6	*ADAR*	AR and AD	Catalyze the deamination of adenosine to inosine in double-stranded RNA	Classic symptoms; dyschromatosis symmetrica hereditaria[88]; cardiac valve disease[89]; bilateral striatal necrosis[90]
ASG7	*IFIH1*	AD	Encodes MDA5, a cytosolic receptor for double-stranded RNA	Classic symptoms but can have later onset, milder phenotype or asymptomatic[91]

Abbreviations: AD, autosomal dominant; AGS, Aicardi-Goutières syndrome; AR, autosomal recessive; IGS, interferon gene signature.
[a] Intracranial calcification, cerebral atrophy, white matter lesions.

like phenotype though patients did not fulfill full ACR SLE criteria. All had onset of neonatal pancytopenia, hepatosplenomegaly, and eventual liver fibrosis, and later onset of recurrent fevers and membranoproliferative glomerulonephritis. All had elevation of dsDNA antibodies.[25]

Mutations in *TREX1,* which encodes an exonuclease, and *SAMHD1*, which regulates the level of cytosolic deoxynucleotides, can cause familial chilblains lupus (FCL).[26–28] FCL demonstrates autosomal dominant inheritance and is a form of cutaneous lupus erythematosus presenting in early childhood with painful skin lesions in acral regions exacerbated by cold exposure.

Defects in *IFIH1*, a cytosolic nucleic acid sensor, have been identified in patients with AGS, but has also been described to cause early onset-SLE, IgA deficiency, and lower limb spasticity.[29]

A gain-of-function mutation in *TLR7,* which encodes a nucleic acid sensing intracellular receptor, has been described to cause an SLE phenotype.[30] The mutation causes aberrant B-cell survival and increased follicular and extrafollicular helper T-cells. Clinically, the individual developed early-onset SLE with autoimmune cytopenia and subsequently developed renal disease, arthralgias, and hemichorea.[30]

Apoptosis/Self-Tolerance

Mutations in *PRKCD*, encoding protein kinase δ, cause defective B-cell apoptosis and increased immature B-cell proliferation. The clinical phenotype encompasses

Table 2
Monogenic lupus and lupus-like phenotypes

Gene	Inheritance	Protein Function	Phenotype
C1QA, C1QB, C1QC	AR	Complement regulation	SLE, GN, discoid rash, oral ulcers, CNS involvement
C1r/C1s	AR	Complement regulation	SLE, cutaneous lupus, GN, severe infections
C2	AR	Complement regulation	SLE, cutaneous lupus, arthritis, milder phenotype with less renal involvement
C4A, C4B	AR	Complement regulation	SLE, photosensitivity, cutaneous lupus, GN
DNASE1	AD	Nucleic acid clearance	SLE, Sjogren's syndrome
DNASE1L3	AR	Nucleic acid clearance	SLE, GN, hypocomplementemic urticarial vasculitis, pulmonary hemorrhage, inflammatory bowel disease
DNASE2	AR	Nucleic acid clearance	Neonatal pancytopenia, hepatosplenomegaly, liver fibrosis, membranoproliferative GN
SAMHD1	AD	Nucleic acid clearance	Familial chilblain lupus, AGS (AR)
TREX1	AD	Nucleic acid clearance	Familial chilblain lupus, AGS (AR)
IFIHI	AD	Nucleic acid sensing	SLE with IgA deficiency and spasticity, AGS
TLR7	AD	Nucleic acid sensing	SLE with autoimmune cytopenia, renal disease, arthralgia
PRKCD	AR	Apoptosis regulation/self-tolerance	SLE, cutaneous lupus, GN, lymphoproliferative disease, recurrent infections
TNFRSF6	AD	Apoptosis	ALPS, cytopenia
FASLG	AD	Apoptosis	ALPS, SLE
ACP5	AR	Regulation of osteopontin	SLE, cutaneous lupus, GN, autoimmune cytopenia, skeletal dysplasia, cerebral calcifications, spasticity, recurrent infections

Abbreviations: AD, autosomal dominant; AGS, Aicardi-Goutières syndrome; ALPS, autoimmune lymphoproliferative syndrome; AR, autosomal recessive; CNS, central nervous system; GN, glomerulonephritis; SLE, systemic lupus erythematosus.

cutaneous lupus, glomerulonephritis and lymphoproliferative disease.[31,32] Patients also have recurrent infections reminiscent of chronic granulomatous disease.[33]

Mutations in *TNFRSF6* encoding Fas and *FASLG* encoding Fas ligand leads to ineffective apoptosis resulting in increased auto-reactive T-cell causing autoimmune lymphoproliferative syndrome (ALPS).[34,35] Mutation in *FASLG* also causes an SLE-like phenotype with cutaneous rash, cytopenias and glomerulonephritis.[36]

Disruption of Type I Interferon Signaling

Mutations of the tartrate-resistant acid phosphatase gene (*ACP5*) cause spondyloenchondrodysplasia with immune dysregulation(SPENCD).[37] Defective *ACP5* causes decreased inactivation of osteopontin, disrupting Type I interferon production.[38] Affected individuals can display autoimmunity with up to 50% fulfilling SLE criteria. Clinical symptoms include cutaneous rash, glomerulonephritis, anti-phospholipid syndrome, and/or autoimmune cytopenias.[39–41] Other described features include Sjogren's syndrome, Raynaud's phenomenon, vitiligo, and hypothyroidism. The defining feature of SPENCD is skeletal dysplasia with short stature, platyspondyly, and enchondromas. Neurologic manifestations can include cerebral calcifications and spasticity. Recurrent infections also occur.

STIMULATOR OF INTERFERON GENES-ASSOCIATED VASCULOPATHY WITH ONSET IN INFANCY

SAVI is characterized by early onset systemic inflammation, small vessel vasculopathy resulting in cutaneous disease, and interstitial lung disease secondary to autosomal dominant gain-of-function mutations in *TMEM173*.[42] *TMEM173* encodes for stimulator of interferon genes (STING), a key adaptor protein important in interferon β production. Gain-of-function mutations in STING lead to increased interferon production, and SAVI patients have a prominent IGS.[43]

Symptom onset is classically in the first year of life (~70–75%),[44,45] though commencement in adolescence and adulthood have been reported. Skin and lung involvement are the most common clinical features. Skin manifestations include vasculopathic lesions that are most prominent in acral areas. Severe Raynaud phenomenon leading to chronic ulceration and tissue damage causing digital gangrene with autoamputation have been reported.[46–48] Nasal septal perforation, periungual erythema, nail dystrophy, livedo reticularis, and telangiectasia are also possible features. Cutaneous symptoms are notably exacerbated by cold exposure.

Lung involvement with early interstitial lung disease (ILD) and subsequent fibrosis leads to significant morbidity and mortality.[49] Symptoms can be insidious but may include dyspnea, tachypnea, cough, and hypoxia. Chest CT and pulmonary function tests are recommended to screen for ILD.[50] Alveolar hemorrhage and hilar and paratracheal adenopathy have also been reported.[42,51] SAVI and COPA syndrome are the main interferonopathies that present with predominant lung involvement.

Other clinical features include musculoskeletal manifestations with arthralgia, arthritis and myositis, failure to thrive, and less commonly basal ganglia calcifications, pericarditis, hepatitis, glaucoma, glomerulonephritis, and thyroiditis.[45]

COATOMER PROTEIN A SYNDROME

COPA syndrome is an autosomal dominant condition with variable expressivity resulting from defects in coatomer protein A (*COPA*), causing aberrant intracellular trafficking resulting in endoplasmic reticulum stress.[52] Most individuals display clinical symptoms prior to 5 years of age but rarely can present as adults. Pulmonary disease is ubiquitous with the two most common manifestations being diffuse alveolar hemorrhage and ILD.[53] Unexplained pulmonary hemorrhage, especially in a young child, should prompt consideration for COPA. Inflammatory arthritis, which is typically polyarticular, is also common. Glomerulonephritis also occurs in a subset of individuals.

PROTEASOME-ASSOCIATED AUTOINFLAMMATORY SYNDROMES

Proteasomes are complexes that degrade unwanted proteins. Mutations in proteasome-related proteins cause the upregulation of the interferon pathway, and cause PRAAS/Chronic Atypical Neutrophilic Dermatosis with Lipodystrophy and Elevated temperature (CANDLE).[54–56] Mutations in *PSMB4*, *PSMB8*, *PSMB9*, *PSMA3, PSMG2*, and *POMP* have been described with PRAAS.[54,57] The clinical spectrum encompasses early-onset fever, neutrophilic skin disease, pernio, panniculitis and lipodystrophy, muscle wasting, and joint contractures.[58] Other features can include intracranial calcifications, cytopenias, hepatosplenomegaly and recurrent infections.

Mutations in *POMP* have also been described in POMP-related autoinflammation and immune dysregulation disease (PRAID), which is a distinct interferonopathy from CANDLE, though there is significant clinical overlap.[59,60] Individuals with PRAID present with early onset neutrophilic skin disease, febrile episodes, and chronic inflammation, but have not been described to date as having significant lipodystrophy. Vasculitic rashes can occur with PRAID.[59] Individuals with PRAID also have more severe infections compared to patients with CANDLE.[59,60]

SINGLETON-MERTEN SYNDROME

SMS is an autosomal dominant disorder caused by gain-of-function mutations in *IFIH1* or *DDX58,* which are genes affecting nucleic acid sensing.[61–63] Typical SMS is associated with *IFIH1* mutations and present with abnormal dentition, early-onset aortic and valvular calcifications, and skeletal abnormalities (acro-osteolysis, osteopenia), and can also cause glaucoma, muscle weakness, joint laxity, tendon rupture, and psoriasis.[61,64] Atypical SMS is described with *DDX58* mutations resulting in milder phenotypes without dental abnormalities and tendon rupture,[63] but a recent publication reported that *DDX58* mutations can also present as typical SMS, so the phenotype is heterogenous.[62]

ISG15 DEFICIENCY

ISG15 deficiency is an autosomal recessive disorder that results in autoinflammation and immunodeficiency with susceptibility to mycobacterial infections.[65,66] Mutations in *ISG15* cause loss of stabilization of the USP18 protein, which is a negative regulator of interferon α/β receptor signaling.[67,68] Clinically affected individuals often present with central nervous system symptoms (brain calcifications and seizure),[68] necrotizing skin ulceration,[69] and mycobacterial disease.[66]

USP18 DEFICIENCY

USP18 deficiency is an autosomal recessive disorder secondary to mutations in *USP18.* USP18, stabilized by ISG15, normally down-regulates the signaling of Type I interferons and loss-of-function mutations result in the activation of Type 1 interferon.[70] Clinically affected individuals present with severe symptoms in late gestation to early infancy with a pseudo-TORCH phenotype including intracranial calcifications and hemorrhage, seizure, respiratory insufficiency, liver dysfunction and thrombocytopenia.[70,71]

STAT2 GAIN-OF-FUNCTION

Homozygous missense variants in *STAT2* disrupt STAT2 interaction with USP18.[72,73] Clinical symptoms are similar to USP18 deficiency with early onset multi-organ dysfunction including intracranial calcifications and hemorrhage, recurrent fever, respiratory insufficiency, hepatosplenomegaly, thrombocytopenia, and proteinuria.[72,74]

TRICHO-HEPATO-ENTERIC SYNDROME (THES)

THES is an autosomal recessive disorder secondary to defects in *SKIV2L* or *TTC37*, two genes involved in aberrant mRNA decay. SKIV2L also limits the activation of RIG-I receptors, which is a pattern recognition receptor responsible for stimulating Type I interferon activation. Increased Type I interferon has been reported with mutations in SKIV2L but not TTC37.[75] Clinically, individuals always present with hair abnormalities including wooly, brittle and scant hair, intractable diarrhea starting in infancy, and facial dysmorphism including coarse facial features, broad forehead, and broad nasal root.[76,77] Other manifestations can include skin abnormalities such as café-au-lait spots, liver disease, mild intellectual disability, growth failure, immunodeficiency with hypogammaglobulinemia, and increased predisposition to infections such as Epstein-Barr virus.[76–78]

ATAD3A DEFICIENCY

Mutations in *ATAD3A* result in mitochondrial dysfunction and increased leakage of mitochondrial DNA into the cytosol resulting in Type I interferon induction.[79,80] Clinically affected individuals present with neurologic abnormalities including developmental delay, hypotonia, spasticity, and optic atrophy, though one patient has been described with normal intellectual function.[80] Systemic sclerosis has been reported in one individual.[80]

X-LINKED RETICULATE PIGMENTARY DISORDER

XLRPD is an x-linked recessive disorder due to mutations in *POLA1* resulting in loss-of-function. *POLA1* is required for the synthesis of cytosolic RNA:DNA, which modulates interferon activation.[81] Affected individuals present with skin manifestations including early-onset diffuse skin hyperpigmentation with reticulate pattern, recurrent lung infections, distinct facial features with frontally upswept hair and flared eyebrows and chronic diarrhea and enterocolitis.[81,82] Other features include hypohydrosis, urethral strictures, and corneal scarring.[81]

CURRENT THERAPIES

Type I interferonopathies are often resistant to conventional immunosuppressive therapies, but corticosteroids remain a mainstay of therapy. In recent years there have been promising studies using JAK-inhibitors to treat Type I interferonopathies.[83,84] Monoclonal antibodies targeting the type I interferon receptor (anifrolumab) and interferon-alpha (sifalimumab) may also have potential therapeutic benefits.[85] STING inhibitors are also under development.[86]

SUMMARY

Monogenic Type I interferonopathies represent a growing group of inborn errors of immunity that result from damaging genetic mutations that lead to increased Type I interferon activation. Advances in genetic sequencing have expanded the ability to diagnosis patients with concerning clinical phenotypes sooner. As these diseases often present early in life, pediatric providers must be aware of concerning symptoms for an interferonopathy, as early diagnosis and treatment is key to preventing irreversible organ damage and mortality.

CLINICS CARE POINTS

- Early identification of affected individuals through genetic testing is essential to direct appropriate treatment and improve long term outcomes.
- Corticosteriods remain a widely used therapy, but targeted treaments such as JAK inhibitors show promise.

DISCLOSURE

The author has no conflicts of interest related to this work.

REFERENCES

1. Crow YJ, Stetson DB. The type I interferonopathies: 10 years on. Nat Rev Immunol 2022;22(8):471–83.
2. d'Angelo DM, Di Filippo P, Breda L, et al. Type I Interferonopathies in Children: An Overview. Front Pediatr 2021;9:631329.
3. Garau J, Cavallera V, Valente M, et al. Molecular Genetics and Interferon Signature in the Italian Aicardi Goutieres Syndrome Cohort: Report of 12 New Cases and Literature Review. J Clin Med 2019;8(5):750.
4. Crow YJ, Manel N. Aicardi-Goutieres syndrome and the type I interferonopathies. Nat Rev Immunol 2015;15(7):429–40.
5. Rice G, Patrick T, Parmar R, et al. Clinical and molecular phenotype of Aicardi-Goutieres syndrome. Am J Hum Genet 2007;81(4):713–25.
6. Orcesi S, La Piana R, Fazzi E. Aicardi-Goutieres syndrome. Br Med Bull 2009;89:183–201.
7. Thiele H, du Moulin M, Barczyk K, et al. Cerebral arterial stenoses and stroke: novel features of Aicardi-Goutieres syndrome caused by the Arg164X mutation in SAMHD1 are associated with altered cytokine expression. Hum Mutat 2010;31(11):E1836–50.
8. Crow YJ, Chase DS, Lowenstein Schmidt J, et al. Characterization of human disease phenotypes associated with mutations in TREX1, RNASEH2A, RNASEH2B, RNASEH2C, SAMHD1, ADAR, and IFIH1. Am J Med Genet 2015;167A(2):296–312.
9. Di Donato G, d'Angelo DM, Breda L, et al. Monogenic Autoinflammatory Diseases: State of the Art and Future Perspectives. Int J Mol Sci 2021;22(12):6360.
10. McEntagart M, Kamel H, Lebon P, et al. Aicardi-Goutieres syndrome: an expanding phenotype. Neuropediatrics 1998;29(3):163–7.
11. Svingen L, Goheen M, Godfrey R, et al. Late diagnosis and atypical brain imaging of Aicardi-Goutieres syndrome: are we failing to diagnose Aicardi-Goutieres syndrome-2? Dev Med Child Neurol 2017;59(12):1307–11.

12. Elkon KB, Stone VV. Type I interferon and systemic lupus erythematosus. J Interferon Cytokine Res 2011;31(11):803–12.
13. Hochberg MC. Updating the American College of Rheumatology revised criteria for the classification of systemic lupus erythematosus. Arthritis Rheum 1997; 40(9):1725.
14. Macedo AC, Isaac L. Systemic Lupus Erythematosus and Deficiencies of Early Components of the Complement Classical Pathway. Front Immunol 2016;7:55.
15. Garau J, Charras A, Varesio C, et al. Altered DNA methylation and gene expression predict disease severity in patients with Aicardi-Goutieres syndrome. Clin Immunol 2023;249:109299.
16. Stegert M, Bock M, Trendelenburg M. Clinical presentation of human C1q deficiency: How much of a lupus? Mol Immunol 2015;67(1):3–11.
17. Lintner KE, Wu YL, Yang Y, et al. Early Components of the Complement Classical Activation Pathway in Human Systemic Autoimmune Diseases. Front Immunol 2016;7:36.
18. Jonsson G, Sjoholm AG, Truedsson L, et al. Rheumatological manifestations, organ damage and autoimmunity in hereditary C2 deficiency. Rheumatology 2007; 46(7):1133–9.
19. Pereira KM, Faria AG, Liphaus BL, et al. Low C4, C4A and C4B gene copy numbers are stronger risk factors for juvenile-onset than for adult-onset systemic lupus erythematosus. Rheumatology 2016;55(5):869–73.
20. Leffler J, Ciacma K, Gullstrand B, et al. A subset of patients with systemic lupus erythematosus fails to degrade DNA from multiple clinically relevant sources. Arthritis Res Ther 2015;17(1):205.
21. Al-Mayouf SM, Sunker A, Abdwani R, et al. Loss-of-function variant in DNASE1L3 causes a familial form of systemic lupus erythematosus. Nat Genet 2011;43(12): 1186–8.
22. Yasutomo K, Horiuchi T, Kagami S, et al. Mutation of DNASE1 in people with systemic lupus erythematosus. Nat Genet 2001;28(4):313–4.
23. Ozcakar ZB, Foster J 2nd, Diaz-Horta O, et al. DNASE1L3 mutations in hypocomplementemic urticarial vasculitis syndrome. Arthritis Rheum 2013;65(8):2183–9.
24. Tusseau M, Lovsin E, Samaille C, et al. DNASE1L3 deficiency, new phenotypes, and evidence for a transient type I IFN signaling. J Clin Immunol 2022;42(6): 1310–20.
25. Rodero MP, Tesser A, Bartok E, et al. Type I interferon-mediated autoinflammation due to DNase II deficiency. Nat Commun 2017;8(1):2176.
26. Ravenscroft JC, Suri M, Rice GI, et al. Autosomal dominant inheritance of a heterozygous mutation in SAMHD1 causing familial chilblain lupus. Am J Med Genet 2011;155A(1):235–7.
27. Gunther C, Berndt N, Wolf C, et al. Familial chilblain lupus due to a novel mutation in the exonuclease III domain of 3' repair exonuclease 1 (TREX1). JAMA Dermatol 2015;151(4):426–31.
28. Linggonegoro DW, Song H, Jones KM, et al. Familial chilblain lupus in a child with heterozygous mutation in SAMHD1 and normal interferon signature. Br J Dermatol 2021;185(3):650–2.
29. Van Eyck L, De Somer L, Pombal D, et al. Brief Report: IFIH1 Mutation Causes Systemic Lupus Erythematosus With Selective IgA Deficiency. Arthritis Rheumatol 2015;67(6):1592–7.
30. Brown GJ, Canete PF, Wang H, et al. TLR7 gain-of-function genetic variation causes human lupus. Nature 2022;605(7909):349–56.

31. Kuehn HS, Niemela JE, Rangel-Santos A, et al. Loss-of-function of the protein kinase C delta (PKCdelta) causes a B-cell lymphoproliferative syndrome in humans. Blood 2013;121(16):3117–25.
32. Belot A, Kasher PR, Trotter EW, et al. Protein kinase cdelta deficiency causes mendelian systemic lupus erythematosus with B cell-defective apoptosis and hyperproliferation. Arthritis Rheum 2013;65(8):2161–71.
33. Neehus AL, Moriya K, Nieto-Patlan A, et al. Impaired respiratory burst contributes to infections in PKCdelta-deficient patients. J Exp Med 2021;218(9):e20210501.
34. Consonni F, Gambineri E, Favre C. ALPS, FAS, and beyond: from inborn errors of immunity to acquired immunodeficiencies. Ann Hematol 2022;101(3):469–84.
35. Holzelova E, Vonarbourg C, Stolzenberg MC, et al. Autoimmune lymphoproliferative syndrome with somatic Fas mutations. N Engl J Med 2004;351(14):1409–18.
36. Wu J, Wilson J, He J, et al. Fas ligand mutation in a patient with systemic lupus erythematosus and lymphoproliferative disease. J Clin Invest 1996;98(5): 1107–13.
37. Renella R, Schaefer E, LeMerrer M, et al. Spondyloenchondrodysplasia with spasticity, cerebral calcifications, and immune dysregulation: clinical and radiographic delineation of a pleiotropic disorder. Am J Med Genet 2006;140(6): 541–50.
38. Wong CK, Lit LC, Tam LS, et al. Elevation of plasma osteopontin concentration is correlated with disease activity in patients with systemic lupus erythematosus. Rheumatology 2005;44(5):602–6.
39. Lausch E, Janecke A, Bros M, et al. Genetic deficiency of tartrate-resistant acid phosphatase associated with skeletal dysplasia, cerebral calcifications and autoimmunity. Nat Genet 2011;43(2):132–7.
40. Briggs TA, Rice GI, Daly S, et al. Tartrate-resistant acid phosphatase deficiency causes a bone dysplasia with autoimmunity and a type I interferon expression signature. Nat Genet 2011;43(2):127–31.
41. An J, Briggs TA, Dumax-Vorzet A, et al. Tartrate-Resistant Acid Phosphatase Deficiency in the Predisposition to Systemic Lupus Erythematosus. Arthritis Rheumatol 2017;69(1):131–42.
42. Liu Y, Jesus AA, Marrero B, et al. Activated STING in a vascular and pulmonary syndrome. N Engl J Med 2014;371(6):507–18.
43. Kim H, de Jesus AA, Brooks SR, et al. Development of a Validated Interferon Score Using NanoString Technology. J Interferon Cytokine Res 2018;38(4): 171–85.
44. Dai Y, Liu X, Zhao Z, et al. Stimulator of Interferon Genes-Associated Vasculopathy With Onset in Infancy: A Systematic Review of Case Reports. Front Pediatr 2020;8:577918.
45. Fremond ML, Hadchouel A, Berteloot L, et al. Overview of STING-Associated Vasculopathy with Onset in Infancy (SAVI) Among 21 Patients. J Allergy Clin Immunol Pract 2021;9(2):803–818 e811.
46. Lin B, Torreggiani S, Kahle D, et al. Case Report: Novel SAVI-Causing Variants in STING1 Expand the Clinical Disease Spectrum and Suggest a Refined Model of STING Activation. Front Immunol 2021;12:636225.
47. Chia J, Eroglu FK, Ozen S, et al. Failure to thrive, interstitial lung disease, and progressive digital necrosis with onset in infancy. J Am Acad Dermatol 2016;74(1): 186–9.
48. Munoz J, Rodiere M, Jeremiah N, et al. Stimulator of Interferon Genes-Associated Vasculopathy With Onset in Infancy: A Mimic of Childhood Granulomatosis With Polyangiitis. JAMA Dermatol 2015;151(8):872–7.

49. David C, Fremond ML. Lung Inflammation in STING-Associated Vasculopathy with Onset in Infancy (SAVI). Cells 2022;11(3):318.
50. Cetin Gedik K, Lamot L, Romano M, et al. The 2021 European Alliance of Associations for Rheumatology/American College of Rheumatology Points to Consider for Diagnosis and Management of Autoinflammatory Type I Interferonopathies: CANDLE/PRAAS, SAVI, and AGS. Arthritis Rheumatol 2022;74(5):735–51.
51. Tang X, Xu H, Zhou C, et al. STING-Associated Vasculopathy with Onset in Infancy in Three Children with New Clinical Aspect and Unsatisfactory Therapeutic Responses to Tofacitinib. J Clin Immunol 2020;40(1):114–22.
52. Vece TJ, Watkin LB, Nicholas S, et al. Copa Syndrome: a Novel Autosomal Dominant Immune Dysregulatory Disease. J Clin Immunol 2016;36(4):377–87.
53. Tsui JL, Estrada OA, Deng Z, et al. Analysis of pulmonary features and treatment approaches in the COPA syndrome. ERJ Open Res 2018;4(2):00017–2018.
54. Liu Y, Ramot Y, Torrelo A, et al. Mutations in proteasome subunit beta type 8 cause chronic atypical neutrophilic dermatosis with lipodystrophy and elevated temperature with evidence of genetic and phenotypic heterogeneity. Arthritis Rheum 2012;64(3):895–907.
55. Arima K, Kinoshita A, Mishima H, et al. Proteasome assembly defect due to a proteasome subunit beta type 8 (PSMB8) mutation causes the autoinflammatory disorder, Nakajo-Nishimura syndrome. Proc Natl Acad Sci U S A 2011;108(36):14914–9.
56. Agarwal AK, Xing C, DeMartino GN, et al. PSMB8 encoding the beta5i proteasome subunit is mutated in joint contractures, muscle atrophy, microcytic anemia, and panniculitis-induced lipodystrophy syndrome. Am J Hum Genet 2010;87(6):866–72.
57. Brehm A, Liu Y, Sheikh A, et al. Additive loss-of-function proteasome subunit mutations in CANDLE/PRAAS patients promote type I IFN production. J Clin Invest 2015;125(11):4196–211.
58. Torrelo A. CANDLE Syndrome As a Paradigm of Proteasome-Related Autoinflammation. Front Immunol 2017;8:927.
59. Poli MC, Ebstein F, Nicholas SK, et al. Heterozygous Truncating Variants in POMP Escape Nonsense-Mediated Decay and Cause a Unique Immune Dysregulatory Syndrome. Am J Hum Genet 2018;102(6):1126–42.
60. Meinhardt A, Ramos PC, Dohmen RJ, et al. Curative Treatment of POMP-Related Autoinflammation and Immune Dysregulation (PRAID) by Hematopoietic Stem Cell Transplantation. J Clin Immunol 2021;41(7):1664–7.
61. Rutsch F, MacDougall M, Lu C, et al. A specific IFIH1 gain-of-function mutation causes Singleton-Merten syndrome. Am J Hum Genet 2015;96(2):275–82.
62. Ferreira CR, Crow YJ, Gahl WA, et al. DDX58 and Classic Singleton-Merten Syndrome. J Clin Immunol 2019;39(1):75–80.
63. Jang MA, Kim EK, Now H, et al. Mutations in DDX58, which encodes RIG-I, cause atypical Singleton-Merten syndrome. Am J Hum Genet 2015;96(2):266–74.
64. Feigenbaum A, Muller C, Yale C, et al. Singleton-Merten syndrome: an autosomal dominant disorder with variable expression. Am J Med Genet 2013;161A(2):360–70.
65. Waqas SF, Sohail A, Nguyen AHH, et al. ISG15 deficiency features a complex cellular phenotype that responds to treatment with itaconate and derivatives. Clin Transl Med 2022;12(7):e931.
66. Bogunovic D, Byun M, Durfee LA, et al. Mycobacterial disease and impaired IFN-gamma immunity in humans with inherited ISG15 deficiency. Science 2012;337(6102):1684–8.

67. Perng YC, Lenschow DJ. ISG15 in antiviral immunity and beyond. Nat Rev Microbiol 2018;16(7):423–39.
68. Zhang X, Bogunovic D, Payelle-Brogard B, et al. Human intracellular ISG15 prevents interferon-alpha/beta over-amplification and auto-inflammation. Nature 2015;517(7532):89–93.
69. Martin-Fernandez M, Bravo Garcia-Morato M, Gruber C, et al. Systemic Type I IFN Inflammation in Human ISG15 Deficiency Leads to Necrotizing Skin Lesions. Cell Rep 2020;31(6):107633.
70. Meuwissen ME, Schot R, Buta S, et al. Human USP18 deficiency underlies type 1 interferonopathy leading to severe pseudo-TORCH syndrome. J Exp Med 2016; 213(7):1163–74.
71. Alsohime F, Martin-Fernandez M, Temsah MH, et al. JAK Inhibitor Therapy in a Child with Inherited USP18 Deficiency. N Engl J Med 2020;382(3):256–65.
72. Duncan CJA, Thompson BJ, Chen R, et al. Severe type I interferonopathy and unrestrained interferon signaling due to a homozygous germline mutation in STAT2. Sci Immunol 2019;4(42):eaav7501.
73. Arimoto KI, Lochte S, Stoner SA, et al. STAT2 is an essential adaptor in USP18-mediated suppression of type I interferon signaling. Nat Struct Mol Biol 2017; 24(3):279–89.
74. Gruber C, Martin-Fernandez M, Ailal F, et al. Homozygous STAT2 gain-of-function mutation by loss of USP18 activity in a patient with type I interferonopathy. J Exp Med 2020;217(5):e20192319.
75. Eckard SC, Rice GI, Fabre A, et al. The SKIV2L RNA exosome limits activation of the RIG-I-like receptors. Nat Immunol 2014;15(9):839–45.
76. Vely F, Barlogis V, Marinier E, et al. Combined Immunodeficiency in Patients With Trichohepatoenteric Syndrome. Front Immunol 2018;9:1036.
77. Fabre A, Martinez-Vinson C, Goulet O, et al. Syndromic diarrhea/Tricho-hepato-enteric syndrome. Orphanet J Rare Dis 2013;8:5.
78. Fabre A, Breton A, Coste ME, et al. Syndromic (phenotypic) diarrhoea of infancy/tricho-hepato-enteric syndrome. Arch Dis Child 2014;99(1):35–8.
79. Lepelley A, Wai T, Crow YJ. Mitochondrial Nucleic Acid as a Driver of Pathogenic Type I Interferon Induction in Mendelian Disease. Front Immunol 2021;12:729763.
80. Lepelley A, Della Mina E, Van Nieuwenhove E, et al. Enhanced cGAS-STING-dependent interferon signaling associated with mutations in ATAD3A. J Exp Med 2021;218(10):e20201560.
81. Starokadomskyy P, Gemelli T, Rios JJ, et al. DNA polymerase-alpha regulates the activation of type I interferons through cytosolic RNA:DNA synthesis. Nat Immunol 2016;17(5):495–504.
82. Starokadomskyy P, Escala Perez-Reyes A, Burstein E. Immune Dysfunction in Mendelian Disorders of POLA1 Deficiency. J Clin Immunol 2021;41(2):285–93.
83. Sanchez GAM, Reinhardt A, Ramsey S, et al. JAK1/2 inhibition with baricitinib in the treatment of autoinflammatory interferonopathies. J Clin Invest 2018;128(7): 3041–52.
84. Mura E, Masnada S, Antonello C, et al. Ruxolitinib in Aicardi-Goutieres syndrome. Metab Brain Dis 2021;36(5):859–63.
85. Sim TM, Ong SJ, Mak A, et al. Type I Interferons in Systemic Lupus Erythematosus: A Journey from Bench to Bedside. Int J Mol Sci 2022;23(5):2505.
86. Guerini D. STING Agonists/Antagonists: Their Potential as Therapeutics and Future Developments. Cells 2022;11(7):1159.
87. White TE, Brandariz-Nunez A, Martinez-Lopez A, et al. A SAMHD1 mutation associated with Aicardi-Goutieres syndrome uncouples the ability of SAMHD1 to

restrict HIV-1 from its ability to downmodulate type I interferon in humans. Hum Mutat 2017;38(6):658–68.
88. Liu L, Zhang L, Huang P, et al. Case Report: Aicardi-Goutieres Syndrome Type 6 and Dyschromatosis Symmetrica Hereditaria With Congenital Heart Disease and Mitral Valve Calcification - Phenotypic Variants Caused by Adenosine Deaminase Acting on the RNA 1 Gene Homozygous Mutations. Front Pediatr 2022;10: 852903.
89. Crow Y, Keshavan N, Barbet JP, et al. Cardiac valve involvement in ADAR-related type I interferonopathy. J Med Genet 2020;57(7):475–8.
90. Piekutowska-Abramczuk D, Mierzewska H, Bekiesinska-Figatowska M, et al. Bilateral striatal necrosis caused by ADAR mutations in two siblings with dystonia and freckles-like skin changes that should be differentiated from Leigh syndrome. Folia Neuropathol 2016;54(4):405–9.
91. Rice GI, Park S, Gavazzi F, et al. Genetic and phenotypic spectrum associated with IFIH1 gain-of-function. Hum Mutat 2020;41(4):837–49.

Suppressor of Cytokine Signaling 1 Haploinsufficiency

A New Driver of Autoimmunity and Immunodysregulation

Meng Liu, MD[a,b], Evan Hsu[a], Yan Du, MD, PhD[a,c],
Pui Y. Lee, MD, PhD[a,*]

KEYWORDS

• SOCS1 • SOCS1 haploinsufficiency • Autoimmunity • Autoimmune disease

KEY POINTS

- Suppressor of cytokine signaling 1 (SOCS1) functions as a negative regulator of cytokine signaling by inhibiting the activation of Janus kinases downstream of cytokine receptors.
- Socs1 deficiency in mice causes a fatal inflammatory disease mediated by lymphocytes and interferon gamma.
- SOCS1 haploinsufficiency in humans causes autoimmunity and immunodysregulation with multiorgan system manifestations.

INTRODUCTION

Suppressor of cytokine signaling (SOCS) proteins are pivotal intracellular modulators that negatively regulate cytokines signaling, mainly by targeting tyrosine kinases. During the past 2 decades, 8 members of SOCS proteins have been identified: SOCS1 to SOCS7 and cytokine-inducible Src homology 2 (SH2)-containing protein (CIS).[1–5] The structures of SOCS protein family members are highly conserved; each has a variable N-terminal region, a central SH2 domain, and a C-terminal SOCS box.[6]

SOCS1 is among the most extensively studied members of the SOCS family. A role of SOCS1 has been described in different diseases, including malignancies,

[a] Division of Immunology, Boston Children's Hospital and Harvard Medical School, Boston, MA, USA; [b] Department of Rheumatology and Immunology, Guangdong Second Provincial General Hospital, Guangzhou, Guangdong, China; [c] Department of Rheumatology, The Second Affiliated Hospital of Zhejiang University School of Medicine, Hangzhou, Zhejiang, China
* Corresponding author. Boston Children's Hospital, 1 Blackfan Circle, Karp RB10th Floor, Boston, MA 02115.
E-mail address: pui.lee@childrens.harvard.edu

Rheum Dis Clin N Am 49 (2023) 757–772
https://doi.org/10.1016/j.rdc.2023.06.003 rheumatic.theclinics.com
0889-857X/23/

autoimmune disorders, and infections.[6–13] Notably, SOCS1 (and SOCS3) possesses a kinase inhibitory region (KIR) located upstream of the SH2 domain. The KIR motif and SH2 domain bind to Janus kinases (JAK) with high affinity to inhibit substrate phosphorylation.[14–16] SOCS1 peptide mimetics containing the KIR sequence have shown therapeutic efficacy in experimental models of autoimmune disorders.[17]

The *SOCS1* gene in humans and rodents are highly conserved. More than 2 decades ago, SOCS1 deficiency in mice was found to cause a lethal inflammatory disease driven by lymphocytes and interferon gamma (IFN-γ). A human autoimmune disease caused by monoallelic pathogenic variants in SOCS1, termed SOCS1 haploinsufficiency, was described only 3 years ago.[18] To date, 18 symptomatic patients with SOCS1 haploinsufficiency have been described in the literature. These patients display diverse manifestations of autoimmunity and immune dysregulation in multiorgan systems.[18–23]

In this review, the authors discuss the biology of SOCS1 and lessons from murine models of Socs1 deficiency. As SOCS1 haploinsufficiency is a relatively new monogenic disease, the authors provide an overview of the genetics, phenotypic spectrum, and treatment of this condition and discuss approaches for diagnostic evaluation.

AN OVERVIEW OF SUPPRESSOR OF CYTOKINE SIGNALING 1 BIOLOGY

A Historical Perspective on the Discovery of Suppressor of Cytokine Signaling 1

The *SOCS1* gene was discovered independently by 3 groups using different methods in 1997.[2–4] Starr and colleagues used retrovirus encoding a complementary DNA (cDNA) library to infect the murine monocytic leukemic M1 cell line, which yielded a clone termed 4A2 that was resistant to interleukin-6 (IL-6). Sequencing of the cDNA stably inserted in the genome of 4A2 led to the identification of the *SOCS1* gene that encoded a protein with 212 amino acids.[2] The sequence of SOCS1 seemed highly conserved in humans, mice, and rats with 95% to 99% homology.[2] In parallel, Endo and colleagues isolated a new SH2-domain–containing protein, called JAK-binding protein (JAB), using a yeast two-hybrid system. JAB interacted with the JAK homology domain 1 (JH1) domain of JAK1, JAK2 and JAK3 and suppressed the tyrosine-kinase activity and subsequent activation of signal transducer and activator transcription (STAT) proteins.[3] Naka and colleagues described a new gene named STAT-induced STAT inhibitor-1 (SSI-1) using a monoclonal antibody against the SH2 domain of STAT3. SSI-1 did not compete directly with STAT3 but instead inhibited upstream JAK kinases to reduce STAT3 activity.[4] These groups published their findings simultaneously, and *SOCS1*, *JAB*, and *SSI-1* encoded the same protein based on their cDNA sequence.

Notably, Starr and colleagues also cloned *SOCS2* and *SOCS3* in the same study that described *SOCS1*.[2] Based on the structural similarities to the known SOCS proteins, Hilton and colleagues identified 4 new SOCS family members (SOCS4–SOCS7) in 1998 based on the conserved sequence of SOCS box near the C terminal region.[5]

Functions of Suppressor of Cytokine Signaling 1

As a negative regulator of cytokines signaling, SOCS1 expression can be induced by numerous cytokines including IL-4, IL-6, IL-2, IFN-α/β/γ, leukemia-inhibitory factor, and granulocyte colony-stimulating factor. The SOCS1 protein then acts to prevent overactivation of these cytokine pathways to maintain immune homeostasis.[4,24–27] SOCS1 regulates cytokine signaling through several structural domains: (1) the unique KIR motif interacts with the catalytic groove of JAK tyrosine kinases, acting as a nonphosphorylatable pseudosubstrate to block access by other substrates[16,17]; (2) the

SH2 domain binds to the activation loop of JAKs and prevents phosphorylation[16]; (3) the SOCS box recruits an E3 ubiquitin ligase complex, which contains Elongins B and C, RING box protein 2, and Cullin-5, to promote the ubiquitination and degradation of target protein complex (**Fig. 1**A).[28–31] A recent study demonstrated that disruption of either the KIR motif or the SH2 domain is sufficient to cause the profound phenotype of Socs1-deficient mice.[32]

The JAK-STAT pathways mediate the signaling of more than 50 cytokines and growth factors. These pathways play diverse roles in immune cell activation, proliferation, and differentiation. There are 4 JAKs in humans: JAK1, JAK2, JAK3, and tyrosine kinase 2 (TYK2). A recent study demonstrated that SOCS1 has the highest affinity for JAK1 and JAK2. Weaker binding was detected between SOCS1 and TYK2, whereas no interaction was found for JAK3.[33] The best characterized role of SOCS1 is the negative regulation of IFN signaling (**Fig. 1**B). Interferons are antiviral cytokines, and all 3 types of interferons mediate their effects through JAK-STAT: type I (IFN-α/β) and type III IFN (IFN-λ) utilize JAK1 and TYK2 to activate STAT1/STAT2 heterodimers, whereas type II IFN (IFN-γ) signaling requires JAK1 and JAK2 to activate STAT1 homodimers.[34] The ability to inhibit JAKs licenses SOCS1 to function as a central regulator of IFN signaling.

The roles of SOCS1 are diverse and implicate other key immune mediators, including Toll-like receptor (TLR), nuclear factor (NF)-κB, mitogen-activated protein kinase/p38 signaling, and NLRP3 inflammasome.[35–38] However, the mechanism of SOCS1-mediated suppression of these pathways is less established, and some studies have not found direct participation of SOCS1 in TLR and NF-κB signaling.[39,40]

Relationship with Other Suppressor of Cytokine Signaling Family Members

The functional specificity of SOCS proteins is largely determined by the SH2 domain, which interacts with and suppresses the activity of tyrosine kinases. SOCS1 and

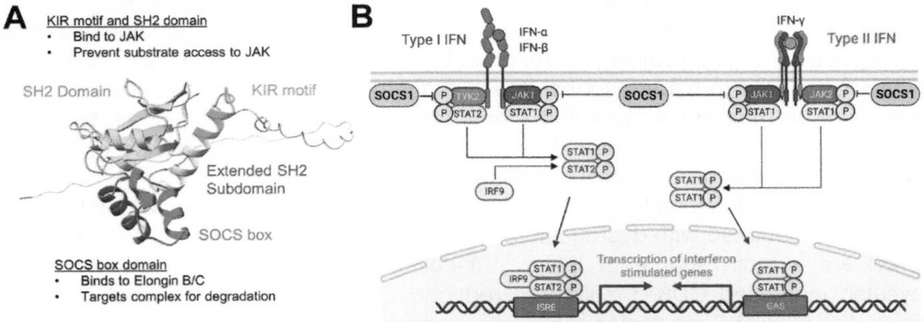

Fig. 1. SOCS1 structure and function. (*A*) The predicted structure of SOCS1 modeled using AlphaFold and generated using UCSF ChimeraX.[31] Structural components are highlighted by the following color scheme: start codon (*blue*), KIR domain (*green*), extended SH2 subdomain (*beige*), SH2 domain (*orange*), and SOCS box (*red*). (*B*) Interferon signaling and the role of SOCS1. Both type I and type II IFN receptors activate JAK-STAT pathways to induce the transcription of IFN-stimulated genes. SOCS1 inhibits the phosphorylation of JAK1, JAK2, and TYK2. GAS, gamma-activated sequence; IFN, interferon; IRF9, interferon regulatory factor 9; ISRE, interferon-stimulated response element; JAK, Janus kinases; KIR, kinase inhibitory region; SH2, Src homology; SOCS, suppressor of cytokine signaling; STAT, signal transducers and activators of transcription; TYK2, tyrosine kinase 2. (Created with BioRender.com.)

SOCS3 are closely related, as they share 37% amino acid homology in the SH2 domain. Other pairings based on evolutionary conservation include CIS and SOCS2 (45% homology), SOCS4 and SOCS5 (88% homology), and SOCS6 and SOCS7 (54% homology).[41]

The similarities between SOCS1 and SOCS3 are further highlighted by the presence of the KIR motif, which is not found in other SOCS family members. However, SOCS1 and SOCS3 have nonredundant effects on target signaling pathways despite of their structural homology. SOCS3 can simultaneously bind to a phosphorylated cytokine receptor by the SH2 domain and to the JAK2 kinase domain by the KIR motif.[42] The mechanism was demonstrated for the negative regulation the IL-6 family cytokines.[43] This feature was also illustrated by the disruption of SOCS3 function in the absence of the target cytokine receptor, whereas SOCS1 can still suppress JAK signaling without the receptor.[14] Compared with *Socs1*$^{-/-}$ mice, *Socs1*$^{-/-}$ and *Socs3*$^{-/-}$ double-deficient mice showed earlier blockade of T-cell development and exacerbated inflammation, which provides additional support for the nonredundant functions of SOCS1 and SOCS3.

Both SOCS1 and CIS are involved in the regulation of IL-2 signaling. CIS interacts with IL-2Rβ subunit to reduce IL-2–mediated STAT5 phosphorylation in CD4^{+} T cells.[44] With equivalent expression levels, SOCS1 possesses greater affinity to IL-2Rβ compared to CIS in vitro.[45] The functions of SOCS2 and SOCS4 to SOCS7 are less explored. Further investigations are needed to determine the functional relationships of SOCS1 with other members of SOCS family.

SUPPRESSOR OF CYTOKINE SIGNALING 1 DEFICIENCY IN MICE

Long before the discovery of humans with pathogenic variants in *SOCS1*, murine models have demonstrated the critical importance of SOCS1 in vivo. In 1998, 2 studies reported that *Socs1*$^{-/-}$ mice show early lethality (within 3 weeks of birth), with fatty degeneration and necrosis of the liver cells, macrophage infiltration of multiple organs, and hematopoietic abnormalities.[46,47] Increased apoptosis of lymphocytes was found in the thymus, spleen, bone marrow, and peripheral blood, but the pathogenesis was unclear. Alexander and colleagues reported that the *Socs1*$^{-/-}$ mice display multiorgan inflammation due to hyperresponsiveness to IFN-γ. Survival was restored when the animals were treated with anti-IFN-γ antibody or bred to a Ifng$^{-/-}$ strain to create Socs1$^{-/-}$Ifng$^{-/-}$dual deficiency. This study emphasized the importance of SOCS1 as a negative regulator of IFN-γ signaling.[48]

Marine and colleagues further discovered that the perinatal lethality of the *Socs1*$^{-/-}$ mice is associated with dysregulated differentiation and function of T lymphocytes, which are a main source of IFN-γ.[49] T-cell profiling of *Socs1*$^{-/-}$ *IFN-γ*$^{-/-}$mice revealed increased CD8^{+}T cells and reduced CD4/CD8 ratio.[50,51] Apart from the IFN-γ, the lack of Socs-1 also resulted in augmented IL-4 signaling, which licenses the activation of natural killer (NK) T cells that contribute to the mortality of the *Socs1*$^{-/-}$ mice.[52] The neonatal fatality of *Socs1*$^{-/-}$ mice can be rescued by the deficiency of lymphocytes (Rag2$^{-/-}$), deletion of STAT1 or STAT6, or depletion of NKT cells.[49,52] As IFN-γ and IL-4 are the signature cytokines produced by Th1 and Th2 cells, respectively, Fujimoto and colleagues showed that freshly isolated *Socs1*$^{-/-}$ CD4^{+}T cells produced more INF-γ and IL-4 than controls when stimulated with anti-CD3, suggesting that SOCS1 insufficiency skews T cell polarization toward both Th1 and Th2.[53] Moreover, *Socs1*$^{-/-}$ CD4^{+} T cells displayed sustained IL-12–induced STAT4 and IL-4–induced STAT6 activation to sustain enhanced T cell polarization.[53]

HAPLOINSUFFICIENCY OF SUPPRESSOR OF CYTOKINE SIGNALING 1

The knock-out animal models collectively revealed a critical role of SOCS1 in maintaining immune homeostasis, as Socs1-deficient mice spontaneously develop early-onset fatal inflammatory disease without any exogenous trigger. Given the severity of the phenotype in mice and the degree of homology between murine and human SOCS1, a complete deficiency of SOCS1 is unlikely to be survivable in humans. Interestingly, Fujimoto and colleagues found that although partial restoration of Socs1 expression in *Socs1*$^{-/-}$ mice rescued them from early fatality, those mice developed features of systemic lupus erythematosus (SLE) including anti-DNA autoantibodies and glomerulonephritis.[54] The investigators further showed that heterozygous deficiency of Socs1 in female mice is associated with the development of autoimmunity due to aberrant $CD4^+$ T-cell function.[54] This study provided the first evidence for a gene dosage effect of *Socs1* and that SOCS1 haploinsufficiency may cause pathologic consequences.[54]

The 2 index cases of human SOCS1 haploinsufficiency were described by Thaventhiran and colleagues in 2020.[18] The investigators performed whole-genome sequencing (WGS) on 1318 patients with primary immunodeficiency and identified multiple pathogenic or likely pathogenic variants including SOCS1.[18] Several months later, Lee and colleagues reported 2 unrelated patients with SOCS1 haploinsufficiency, and one of these patients developed multisystem inflammatory syndrome in children, a cytokine storm highlighted by overproduction of IFN-γ.[19] In parallel, Hadjadj and colleagues described 10 patients and 5 carriers in Europe with diverse genotype and clinical manifestations.[20] Michniacki and colleagues established a case of SOCS1 haploinsufficiency due to complete deletion of *SOCS1* gene on one allele.[22] Most recently, Hale and colleagues described 2 patients with a previously reported *SOCS1* variant.[23] In this section, the authors discuss the phenotypes, mutations, treatment, and functional studies of SOCS1 haploinsufficiency in humans. They refer readers to available reviews on the involvement of SOCS1 in other human diseases.[12,55,56]

Pathogenic Suppressor of Cytokine Signaling 1 Variants

SOCS1 is encoded by a single exon on chromosome 16 in the human genome. SOCS1 haploinsufficiency is caused by monoallelic pathogenic variants that disrupt either the expression or the function of SOCS1. **Fig. 2** depicts the *SOCS1* variants from the known cases of SOCS1 haploinsufficiency. The index cases were discovered by WGS, whereas most subsequent cases were found by whole-exome sequencing (WES).

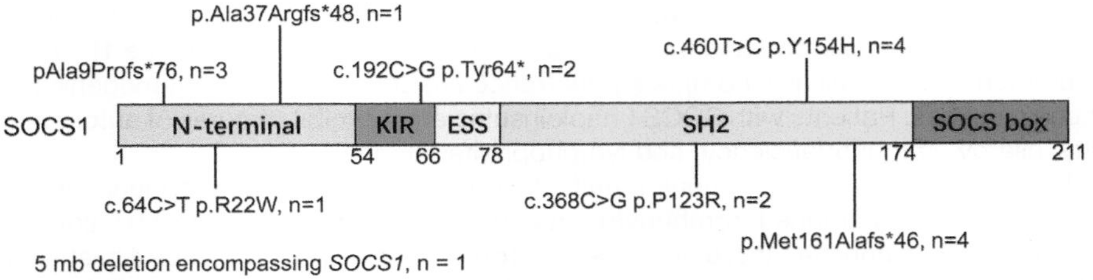

Fig. 2. Variants associated with SOCS1 haploinsufficiency. SOCS1 variants and their locations according to the structural domains. The number of known symptomatic cases associated with each variant is displayed. KIR, kinase inhibitory region; SH2, Src homology 2; SOCS, suppressor of cytokine signaling. (Subpanel on protein structure generated with UCSF Chimera, developed by the Division of Immunology, Boston Children's Hospital and Harvard Medical School, Boston, MA, USA.)

One case with a large deletion that included the entire *SOCS1* sequence was found by chromosomal microarray. At the time of preparing this review, *SOCS1* is not yet included in commercially available next-generation sequencing (NGS) panels for inborn errors of immunity, primary immunodeficiency, or autoinflammatory syndromes.

The pathogenic variants in the known cases include de novo mutations (n = 5) and variants inherited in an autosomal dominant manner. Most of these disease-associated variants are insertions/deletions with frameshift or nonsense variants that are predicted to cause loss of function (LOF). Four unrelated cases were found to have insertion variants (c.476_480insGCCGC or c.480_481insGCGGC), both of which result in frameshift and early termination (p.M161fs*46).[18,20,23] The next most common LOF variant is a frameshift variant caused by c.24del (p.Ala9Profs*76) found in 3 individuals.[19,20] As mentioned earlier, one patient was found to have complete deletion of a *SOCS1* allele due to a 5 megabase deletion on chromosome 16.[22] Among the 5 patients with de novo variants, all 5 possessed LOF variants.[18,19,22,23] Seven symptomatic patients, all in the European cohort described by Hadjadj and colleagues, were found to have missense variants.[20] These variants were located upstream of the KIR sequence (c.64C>T, p.Arg22Trp) or within the SH2 domain (c.368C>G; p.P123 R and c.460T>C; p.Y154H). Four symptomatic individuals with the p.Y154H variant were found in the same kindred.[20] Functional studies demonstrated that these missense variants strongly impaired the suppressive function of SOCS1 with similar efficacy compared with the p.Ala9Profs*76 LOF variant.[20]

It is important to note that not all individuals with deleterious *SOCS1* variants are symptomatic. Hadjadj and colleagues found pathogenic variants of *SOCS1* in 5 healthy carriers from screening family members of affected individuals. The father of one of the probands reported by Lee and colleagues was also an asymptomatic carrier.[19,20] Interestingly, all 6 of these asymptomatic individuals were males, whereas 11/18 symptomatic patients were females. Although interpretation is limited by the small sample size, these patterns are in line with the higher prevalence of autoimmune diseases in females and also congruent with the development of an SLE-like disease in female but not male *Socs1*$^{+/-}$ mice.

Collectively, these genetic findings suggest that SOCS1 haploinsufficiency is a monogenic disease with autosomal dominant inheritance and incomplete penetrance. Inference of a genotype to phenotype correlation is not plausible at this time given the limited number of cases in the literature and the highly variable clinical manifestations and disease severity.

Clinical Spectrum

Even with the limited number of cases in the literature, the clinical spectrum of SOCS1 haploinsufficiency is broad and the disease severity is highly variable (**Table 1**). These characteristics as well as incomplete penetrance are common among monogenic immune diseases. Patients with SOCS1 haploinsufficiency exhibit features of autoimmunity, allergy, immunodeficiency, and lymphoproliferation (**Fig. 3**).

The most common autoimmune manifestation of SOCS1 haploinsufficiency is immune cytopenia. Immune thrombocytopenia (ITP) and Evans syndrome (ITP, autoimmune hemolytic anemia, and/or immune neutropenia) have been described in at least 11 patients (61%), often as the presenting feature.[19–22] Two patients were diagnosed with SLE with glomerulonephritis.[20] Other organ-specific features of autoimmunity include arthritis, spondyloarthritis/enthesitis, psoriasis, uveitis, hepatitis, pancreatitis, and thyroiditis.[20]

SOCS1 haploinsufficiency is associated with features of allergy, possibly related to the usage of JAKs by Th2 cytokines. Atopic eczema, allergic rhinoconjunctivitis,

Table 1
Genotype and phenotype of patients with *SOCS1* haploinsufficiency

Case	Genotype	Sex	Age at Onset	Clinical Phenotype	Treatment	Ref
A1	c.480_481insGCGGC p.M161fs*46	F	8 y	Recurrent bacterial infections, CVID, ITP, granulomatous uveitis, hepatitis, GLILD, splenomegaly	IVIG, GC, anti-D immunoglobulin, RTX	Thaventhiran et al,[18] 2020; Körholz et al,[21] 2021
A2	c.192C>G P. Tyr64*	F	5 y	Pneumonia with empyema, dental abscesses, local HSV infection, shingles, ES, alopecia areata, eczema, rhinoconjunctivitis, asthma, HSM, hyper IgE-like syndrome	GC, IVIG, Romiplostim	Thaventhiran et al,[18] 2020; Körholz et al,[21] 2021
A3	c.192C>G P. Tyr64*	M	7 y	Viral infections, Hashimoto thyroiditis, rhinoconjunctivitis, asthma, EAA, splenomegaly, pernicious anemia	GC, levothyroxine, vitamin B12	Thaventhiran et al,[18] 2020; Körholz et al,[21] 2021
B1	c.106del p. A37fs*48	M	5 mo	ES	GC, MMF	Lee et al,[19] 2020
B2	c.24del p. A9fs*76	M	14 y	ES, MIS-C, SARS-Cov-2 infection	MMF, Eltrombopag, GC, IVIG, FFP	Lee et al,[19] 2020
C1	c.368C>G p. P123R	F	2 y	Severe ITP	GC, IVIG, TPOr agonist, MMF	Hadjadj et al,[20] 2020
C2	c.368C>G p. P123 R	F	6 y	ITP, thyroiditis, polyarthritis	GC, Hormonal replacement	Hadjadj et al,[20] 2020
C3	c.24delA p. A9fs*76	F	5 y	ES, adenopathy, splenomegaly, bronchopulmonary infection	GC, IVIG, Rapa	Hadjadj et al,[20] 2020
C4	c.24delA p. A9fs*76	M	3 y	Celiac disease, psoriasis, Hodgkin lymphoma	Topical therapy	Hadjadj et al,[20] 2020

(*continued on next page*)

Table 1
(continued)

Case	Genotype	Sex	Age at Onset	Clinical Phenotype	Treatment	Ref
C5	c.476_480dupGCCGC p.M161fs*46	F	3 y	ES, adenopathy, HSM	GC, MMF	Hadjadj et al,[20] 2020
C6	c.64C>T p. R22W	M	16 y	SLE: glomerulonephritis	GC, MMF, HCQ	Hadjadj et al,[20] 2020
C7	c.460T>C p. Y154H	F	9 y	SLE: polyarthritis, glomerulonephritis	GC, MTX, HCQ, CTX, MMF, baricitinib	Hadjadj et al,[20] 2020
C8	c.460 T > C p. Y154H	F	16 y	ITP	GC, IVIG, HCQ, AZA, RTX, splenectomy	Hadjadj et al,[20] 2020
C9	c.460T>C p. Y154H	M	15 y	Psoriasis	Topical treatment	Hadjadj et al,[20] 2020
C10	c.460T>C p. Y154H	F	44 y	Psoriasis, SpA, autoimmune hepatitis, pancreatitis	GC, HCQ, MTX, TNFi	Hadjadj et al,[20] 2020
D1	5 mb deletion that includes *SOCS1*	F	5 y	Enthesitis, arthralgias, eosinophilia	GC, IVIG, RTX, TPOr agonist, romiplostim, tofacitinib	Michniacki et al,[22] 2022
E1	c.480_481insGCGGC p.M161fs*46	F	7 y	ALPS, HPS, ACR, severe pneumonia, fungemia	IVIG, G-CSF, Rapa, liver transplant	Hale et al,[23] 2023
E2	c.480_481insGCGGC p.M161fs*46	M	5 y	Recurrent fever, hepatitis, eczema, allergic rhinitis, HSM, LAD	None	Hale et al,[23] 2023

Abbreviations: ACR, acute cellular rejection; ALPS, autoimmune lymphoproliferative syndrome; AZA, azathioprine; CTX, cyclophosphamide; CVID, common variable immunodeficiency; EAA, eosinophilic allergic alveolitis; ES, Evans syndrome; FFP, fresh frozen plasma; GC, glucocorticoids; G-CSF, granulocyte colony-stimulating factor; GLILD, granulomatous lymphocytic interstitial lung disease; HCQ, hydroxychloroquine; HPS, hepatopulmonary syndrome; HSM, hepatosplenomegaly; HSV, herpes simplex virus; ITP, immune thrombocytopenia; IVIG, intravenous immunoglobulin; LAD, lymphadenopathy; MIS-C, multisystem inflammatory syndrome in children; MMF, mycophenolate mofetil; MTX, methotrexate; Rapa, rapamycin (sirolimus); RTX, rituximab; SARS-Cov-2, severe acute respiratory syndrome coronavirus 2; SLE, systemic lupus erythematosus; SOCS1, suppressor of cytokine signaling1; SpA, spondyloarthritis; TNFi, tumor necrosis factor inhibitor; TPO agonist, thrombopoietin receptor.

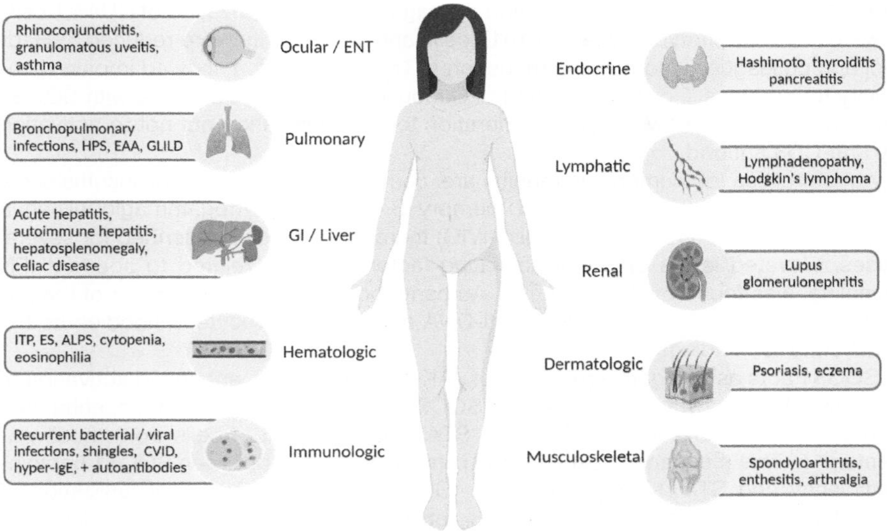

Fig. 3. Clinical manifestations of SOCS1 haploinsufficiency. A summary of clinical features reported in the 18 published cases of SOCS1 haploinsufficiency. ALPS, autoimmune lymphoproliferative syndrome; CIVD, common variable immunodeficiency; EAA, eosinophilic allergic alveolitis; ENT, ear, nose, and throat; ES, Evans syndrome; GI, gastrointestinal; GLILD, granulomatous lymphocytic interstitial lung disease; HPS, hepatopulmonary syndrome; ITP, immune thrombocytopenia. (Created with BioRender.com.)

allergic asthma, and eosinophilic allergic alveolitis have been described in a few patients.[21] The 2 index cases reported by Thaventhiran and colleagues exhibited severe immunodeficiency with recurrent bacterial and viral infections.[18] One of the patients was diagnosed with common variable immunodeficiency, and the same individual later developed granulomatous lymphocytic interstitial lung disease.[18] Although lymphopenia and hypogammaglobulinemia are noted in patients with SOCS1 haploinsufficiency, severe infections are less commonly described in subsequent case series.[18]

Consistent with the aberrant lymphocyte proliferation and activation seen in the experimental models of Socs1 deficiency, features of lymphoproliferation including lymphadenopathy, splenomegaly, and hepatosplenomegaly have been noted in some patients with SOCS1 haploinsufficiency. One patient was diagnosed with autoimmune lymphoproliferative syndrome and another case was diagnosed with Hodgkin lymphoma.[20,23] Other nonspecific features associated with SOCS1 haploinsufficiency include recurrent fever, fatigue, macular rash, recurrent epistaxis and bruising, recurrent emesis, and diarrhea. The most recent case report described a patient with severe noncirrhotic portal hypertension leading to hepatopulmonary syndrome.[23]

The clinical spectrum of SOCS1 haploinsufficiency will continue to expand, as more cases are described. It is notable that a substantial fraction of individuals with this condition may be asymptomatic. Disease onset in patients with SOCS1 haploinsufficiency may require a second hit, possibly by infectious triggers.[19]

Immunologic Abnormalities

Studies on *Socs1*$^{+/-}$ mice have implicated CD4^{+} T lymphocytes, B lymphocytes, and regulatory T (Treg) lymphocytes in the development of autoimmunity.[50–53] CD8^{+} T cell, CD4^{+} T cell, and NK cell counts are variable among the available studies on human

SOCS1 haploinsufficiency. Körholz and colleagues noted polarization of $CD4^+$ T cells toward a Th1 phenotype, whereas Th17 cells and Treg counts were reduced.[21] Hadjadj and colleagues also noted a reduction in Treg cells, which showed impaired capacity to suppress T-cell proliferation.[20] Curiously, T cells from patients with SOCS1 haploinsufficiency showed hyperproliferation to IL-2 stimulation but not to activation by anti-CD3 antibody.[20]

Abnormalities of humoral immunity are common in SOCS1 haploinsufficiency. Impaired development of switched memory B cells and hypogammaglobulinemia requiring intravenous immunoglobulin (IVIG) therapy have been described for several cases. Elevated levels of B-cell–activating factor, possibly related to aberrant IFN signaling, was found by 2 studies.[20,22] Autoantibodies are present in most of the patients, with antinuclear antibodies, anti-DNA and anti-erythrocyte antibodies as the most common findings.[20,21]

SOCS1 acts as a negative regulator of JAKs, and therefore, enhanced activation of the JAK-STAT pathway is expected for SOCS1 haploinsufficiency. Indeed, enhanced and prolonged activation of JAK1 and STAT1 is observed in cells from these patients.[19–22] This mechanism explains the clinical similarities between SOCS1 haploinsufficiency and STAT1 gain of function (GOF). Corresponding to the utilization of STAT1 by interferons, increased expression of IFN-stimulated genes regulated by type I and type II IFN is featured in SOCS1 haploinsufficiency. However, interferons are not the only dysregulated cytokines in this disease. Profiling of proinflammatory markers in the peripheral blood showed increased levels of many cytokines and chemokines in patients with SOCS1 haploinsufficiency.[20,22] The cytokine derangements recapitulate the patterns seen in patients with STAT1-GOF and STAT3-GOF.[20]

The focal adhesion kinase 1-protein kinase B-ribosomal protein S6 kinase pathway is hyperactivated in peripheral blood mononuclear cells (PBMCs) from patients and also in healthy $CD4^+$ T cells after SOCS1 knockdown. Furthermore, monocytes from patients with SOCS1 haploinsufficiency are also hyperresponsive to stimulation by TLR ligands and IFN-γ.[21] Such chronic immune activation may also contribute to the elevated expression of proapoptotic genes and decreased expression of antiapoptotic genes.[19]

Treatment Experience

As with most monogenic immune diseases, various treatment approaches have been tried by clinicians long before the causative gene is identified.[57] The diverse clinical manifestations in patients with *SOCS1* haploinsufficiency translate into variable use of immunomodulatory agents. The use of glucocorticoids, IVIG, disease-modifying antirheumatic drugs (DMARDs), and biologics has been described in the different reports.[19–23] The treatment plan is tailored to the patient's disease manifestations. For patients with ITP or Evans syndrome, treatment approach typically consists of corticosteroids, IVIG, rituximab, and/or thrombopoietin receptor agonists. DMARDs such as mycophenolate mofetil (MMF), hydroxychloroquine, methotrexate, and azathioprine are sometimes given to patients with autoimmune manifestations. Supportive treatment with antimicrobials and IVIG is often prescribed for patients with immunodeficiency. To the authors' knowledge, none of the published cases of SOCS1 haploinsufficiency has undergone hematopoietic stem cell transplant.

The potent inhibitory effects of SOCS1 on JAK activation and IFN signaling make JAK inhibitors an intriguing treatment option for patients with SOCS1 haploinsufficiency. The first-generation JAK inhibitors include baricitinib, ruxolitinib, and tofacitinib. All 3 medications have been used to treat monogenic autoinflammatory diseases caused by aberrant IFN production or IFN signaling.[57] Because SOCS1 functions as endogenous JAK inhibitor, it seems logical that insufficient levels of SOCS1 can be compensated by pharmacologic inhibition of JAKs. This view is supported by in vitro studies on cells from patients with SOCS1 haploinsufficiency that showed attenuation of IFN-γ–induced STAT1 phosphorylation, CXCL9 production, IL-2–induced STAT5 phosphorylation, and excessive T-cell proliferation by the JAK1/2 inhibitor ruxolitinib.[20]

Data on the clinical efficacy of JAK inhibitors in patients with *SOCS1* haploinsufficiency are highlighted in 2 cases.[20,22] The first patient presented with SLE (polyarthritis and glomerulonephritis) initially responded to MMF but switched to the JAK1/2 inhibitor baricitinib due to intolerance to MMF.[20] Baricitinib was well tolerated with a starting dose of 2 mg daily followed by an increase to 2 mg twice daily.[20] This patient exhibited a reduction in anti-DNA autoantibody titers and dampened IFN-γ–induced phosphorylation of STAT1 after 3 months of therapy.[20] The second case was a 5-year-old girl with complete loss of an *SOCS1* allele due to a large deletion.[22] She developed diffuse enthesitis and refractory cytopenia that did not improve completely with methylprednisolone pulses, IVIG, rituximab, and romiplostim.[22] Given the experience with tofacitinib (a JAK1/3 inhibitor) for juvenile idiopathic arthritis, she was treated with tofacitinib 4 mg twice daily.[22,58] Her enthesitis resolved, and her platelet counts have remained in the normal range on tofacitinib monotherapy.[22] Moreover, the IFN signature in PBMC and heightened response to type I and type II IFN normalized after treatment initiation.[22] In both cases, treatment with JAK inhibitors seems to be safe, although long-term data and experience from additional patients are needed to further assess the therapeutic potentials of JAK inhibition.

Methods for the Evaluation of Suppressor of Cytokine Signaling 1 Haploinsufficiency

SOCS1 haploinsufficiency is a relatively new autoimmune disease, and little guidance is available for its diagnostic evaluation. For an individual or kindred with clinical features suggestive of SOCS1 haploinsufficiency, genetic evaluation by targeted sequencing of the *SOCS1* gene, WES, or WGS should be considered based on availability. The diagnosis is supported by the presence of a predicted LOF *SOCS1* variant (ie, indels with frameshift or nonsense variant), a chromosomal alteration (ie, deletion) that disrupts SOCS1, or a missense variant previously associated with SOCS1 haploinsufficiency.

Functional evaluation of novel *SOCS1* variants, typically on a research basis, can provide complementary data to illustrate the loss of protein function. Exogenous expression of mutant *SOCS1* in cell lines can determine protein stability and the capacity to suppress JAK activation. The latter can be assayed by IFN-induced phosphorylation of STAT1 or using a reporter system for IFN-induced transcriptional activity (ie, luciferase driven by the IFN stimulation response element or gamma activation sequence). The functional impact of a novel *SOCS1* variant can be established by creating patient-derived cell lines or by gene editing of a target cell line. Complementary studies can also be performed using primary cells. The IFN transcriptomic signature can be examined in PBMC, and IFN-induced phosphorylation of STAT1 can be performed on monocytes. However, the IFN signature and hyperresponsiveness to IFN stimulation are not specific to the diagnosis of SOCS1 haploinsufficiency.

FUTURE STUDIES

With increased awareness of SOCS1 haploinsufficiency, it is anticipated that SOCS1 will be incorporated into commercial NGS panels for evaluation of inborn errors of immunity and targeted sequencing will also become increasingly available. More patients will be discovered, likely including many that have been diagnosed with various autoimmune diseases.

Data on SOCS1 haploinsufficiency from different parts of the world will allow construction of a more comprehensive genotype and phenotype spectrum. We will learn about the nature history of the disease and the relative efficacy of treatment options. These data will inform the development of clinical trials for affected individuals and help formulate approaches to manage asymptomatic carriers. Moreover, immunophenotyping studies will help us understand the relationship between SOCS1 haploinsufficiency and other monogenic immunodysregulatory/autoimmune diseases.

Although not yet used in humans, peptides based on the KIR motif of SOCS1 (termed SOCS1 mimetics) can inhibit JAK activation and have been shown to ameliorate disease in several animal models.[17,59–61] Whether these peptides can effectively replace the hemizygous loss of endogenous SOCS1 and their relative safety and efficacy compared with JAK inhibitors are intriguing topics for future research.

SUMMARY

Cytokines play a critical role in preparing our immune response to invading pathogens. However, a system to regulate the inflammatory effects of cytokines is equally important to prevent collateral damage. SOCS1 is a key regulator of the JAK-STAT pathway that prevents excessive signaling of interferons and other cytokines. Based on animal models and the early studies of human SOCS1 haploinsufficiency, SOCS1 serves as an essential guardian that fine-tunes the balance between immunity and autoimmunity. Future studies will help us better understand the phenotypic heterogeneity of SOCS1 haploinsufficiency and provide more effective personalized therapeutic approaches.

CLINICS CARE POINTS

- SOCS1 haploinsufficiency is caused by monoallelic LOF variants that disrupt the expression and/or function of SOCS1.
- SOCS1 haploinsufficiency should be consider in unusual cases of autoimmunity and immunodysregulation with multiorgan manifestations.
- JAK inhibition may be a promising approach for the treatment of SOCS1 haploinsufficiency.

DISCLOSURE

The authors have declared no conflict of interest.

REFERENCES

1. Yoshimura A, Ohkubo T, Kiguchi T, et al. A novel cytokine-inducible gene CIS encodes an SH2-containing protein that binds to tyrosine-phosphorylated interleukin 3 and erythropoietin receptors. EMBO J 1995;14(12):2816–26.
2. Starr R, Willson TA, Viney EM, et al. A family of cytokine-inducible inhibitors of signalling. Nature 1997;387(6636):917–21.
3. Endo TA, Masuhara M, Yokouchi M, et al. A new protein containing an SH2 domain that inhibits JAK kinases. Nature 1997;387(6636):921–4.

4. Naka T, Narazaki M, Hirata M, et al. Structure and function of a new STAT-induced STAT inhibitor. Nature 1997;387(6636):924–9.
5. Hilton DJ, Richardson RT, Alexander WS, et al. Twenty proteins containing a C-terminal SOCS box form five structural classes. Proc Natl Acad Sci U S A 1998; 95(1):114–9.
6. Low ZY, Wen Yip AJ, Chow VTK, et al. The Suppressor of Cytokine Signalling family of proteins and their potential impact on COVID-19 disease progression. Rev Med Virol 2022;32(3):e2300.
7. Alston CI, Dix RD. SOCS and Herpesviruses, With Emphasis on Cytomegalovirus Retinitis. Front Immunol 2019;10:732.
8. Johnson HM, Lewin AS, Ahmed CM. SOCS, Intrinsic Virulence Factors, and Treatment of COVID-19. Front Immunol 2020;11:582102.
9. Masuzaki R, Kanda T, Sasaki R, et al. Suppressors of Cytokine Signaling and Hepatocellular Carcinoma. Cancers 2022;14(10). https://doi.org/10.3390/cancers14102549.
10. Dai L, Li Z, Liang W, et al. SOCS proteins and their roles in the development of glioblastoma. Oncol Lett 2022;23(1):5.
11. Sobah ML, Liongue C, Ward AC. SOCS Proteins in Immunity, Inflammatory Diseases, and Immune-Related Cancer. Front Med 2021;8:727987.
12. Sharma J, Larkin J 3rd. Therapeutic Implication of SOCS1 Modulation in the Treatment of Autoimmunity and Cancer. Front Pharmacol 2019;10:324.
13. Wang H, Wang J, Xia Y. Defective Suppressor of Cytokine Signaling 1 Signaling Contributes to the Pathogenesis of Systemic Lupus Erythematosus. Front Immunol 2017;8:1292.
14. Nicholson SE, Willson TA, Farley A, et al. Mutational analyses of the SOCS proteins suggest a dual domain requirement but distinct mechanisms for inhibition of LIF and IL-6 signal transduction. EMBO J 1999;18(2):375–85.
15. Sasaki A, Yasukawa H, Suzuki A, et al. Cytokine-inducible SH2 protein-3 (CIS3/SOCS3) inhibits Janus tyrosine kinase by binding through the N-terminal kinase inhibitory region as well as SH2 domain. Gene Cell 1999;4(6):339–51.
16. Yasukawa H, Misawa H, Sakamoto H, et al. The JAK-binding protein JAB inhibits Janus tyrosine kinase activity through binding in the activation loop. EMBO J 1999;18(5):1309–20.
17. Ahmed CM, Larkin J 3rd, Johnson HM. SOCS1 Mimetics and Antagonists: A Complementary Approach to Positive and Negative Regulation of Immune Function. Front Immunol 2015;6:183.
18. Thaventhiran JED, Lango Allen H, Burren OS, et al. Whole-genome sequencing of a sporadic primary immunodeficiency cohort. Nature 2020;583(7814):90–5.
19. Lee PY, Platt CD, Weeks S, et al. Immune dysregulation and multisystem inflammatory syndrome in children (MIS-C) in individuals with haploinsufficiency of SOCS1. J Allergy Clin Immunol 2020;146(5):1194–200.e1.
20. Hadjadj J, Castro CN, Tusseau M, et al. Early-onset autoimmunity associated with SOCS1 haploinsufficiency. Nat Commun 2020;11(1):5341.
21. Körholz J, Gabrielyan A, Sowerby JM, et al. One Gene, Many Facets: Multiple Immune Pathway Dysregulation in SOCS1 Haploinsufficiency. Front Immunol 2021; 12:680334.
22. Michniacki TF, Walkovich K, DeMeyer L, et al. SOCS1 Haploinsufficiency Presenting as Severe Enthesitis, Bone Marrow Hypocellularity, and Refractory Thrombocytopenia in a Pediatric Patient with Subsequent Response to JAK Inhibition. J Clin Immunol 2022;42(8):1766–77.

23. Hale RC, Owen N, Yuan B, et al. Phenotypic Variability of SOCS1 Haploinsufficiency. J Clin Immunol 2023. https://doi.org/10.1007/s10875-023-01460-4.
24. Sporri B, Kovanen PE, Sasaki A, et al. JAB/SOCS1/SSI-1 is an interleukin-2-induced inhibitor of IL-2 signaling. Blood 2001;97(1):221–6.
25. Starr R, Fuchsberger M, Lau LS, et al. SOCS-1 binding to tyrosine 441 of IFN-gamma receptor subunit 1 contributes to the attenuation of IFN-gamma signaling in vivo. J Immunol 2009;183(7):4537–44.
26. Song MM, Shuai K. The suppressor of cytokine signaling (SOCS) 1 and SOCS3 but not SOCS2 proteins inhibit interferon-mediated antiviral and antiproliferative activities. J Biol Chem 1998;273(52):35056–62.
27. Crespo A, Filla MB, Russell SW, et al. Indirect induction of suppressor of cytokine signalling-1 in macrophages stimulated with bacterial lipopolysaccharide: partial role of autocrine/paracrine interferon-alpha/beta. Biochem J 2000;349(Pt 1):99–104.
28. Zhang JG, Farley A, Nicholson SE, et al. The conserved SOCS box motif in suppressors of cytokine signaling binds to elongins B and C and may couple bound proteins to proteasomal degradation. Proc Natl Acad Sci U S A 1999;96(5):2071–6.
29. Kamura T, Maenaka K, Kotoshiba S, et al. VHL-box and SOCS-box domains determine binding specificity for Cul2-Rbx1 and Cul5-Rbx2 modules of ubiquitin ligases. Genes Dev 2004;18(24):3055–65.
30. Bullock AN, Debreczeni JE, Edwards AM, et al. Crystal structure of the SOCS2-elongin C-elongin B complex defines a prototypical SOCS box ubiquitin ligase. Proc Natl Acad Sci U S A 2006;103(20):7637–42.
31. Jumper J, Evans R, Pritzel A, et al. Highly accurate protein structure prediction with AlphaFold. Nature 2021;596(7873):583–9.
32. Doggett K, Keating N, Dehkhoda F, et al. The SOCS1 KIR and SH2 domain are both required for suppression of cytokine signaling in vivo. Cytokine 2023;165:156167.
33. Liau NPD, Laktyushin A, Lucet IS, et al. The molecular basis of JAK/STAT inhibition by SOCS1. Nat Commun 2018;9(1):1558.
34. Schneider WM, Chevillotte MD, Rice CM. Interferon-stimulated genes: a complex web of host defenses. Annu Rev Immunol 2014;32:513–45.
35. Zhang L, Xu C, Chen X, et al. SOCS-1 Suppresses Inflammation Through Inhibition of NALP3 Inflammasome Formation in Smoke Inhalation-Induced Acute Lung Injury. Inflammation 2018;41(4):1557–67.
36. Mansell A, Smith R, Doyle SL, et al. Suppressor of cytokine signaling 1 negatively regulates Toll-like receptor signaling by mediating Mal degradation. Nat Immunol 2006;7(2):148–55.
37. Baetz A, Frey M, Heeg K, et al. Suppressor of cytokine signaling (SOCS) proteins indirectly regulate toll-like receptor signaling in innate immune cells. J Biol Chem 2004;279(52):54708–15.
38. Ryo A, Suizu F, Yoshida Y, et al. Regulation of NF-kappaB signaling by Pin1-dependent prolyl isomerization and ubiquitin-mediated proteolysis of p65/RelA. Mol Cell 2003;12(6):1413–26.
39. Gingras S, Parganas E, de Pauw A, et al. Re-examination of the role of suppressor of cytokine signaling 1 (SOCS1) in the regulation of toll-like receptor signaling. J Biol Chem 2004;279(52):54702–7.
40. Prele CM, Woodward EA, Bisley J, et al. SOCS1 regulates the IFN but not NFkappaB pathway in TLR-stimulated human monocytes and macrophages. J Immunol 2008;181(11):8018–26.

41. Linossi EM, Calleja DJ, Nicholson SE. Understanding SOCS protein specificity. Growth Factors 2018;36(3–4):104–17.
42. Kershaw NJ, Murphy JM, Liau NP, et al. SOCS3 binds specific receptor-JAK complexes to control cytokine signaling by direct kinase inhibition. Nat Struct Mol Biol 2013;20(4):469–76.
43. Babon JJ, Varghese LN, Nicola NA. Inhibition of IL-6 family cytokines by SOCS3. Semin Immunol 2014;26(1):13–9.
44. Aman MJ, Migone TS, Sasaki A, et al. CIS associates with the interleukin-2 receptor beta chain and inhibits interleukin-2-dependent signaling. J Biol Chem 1999; 274(42):30266–72.
45. Liau NPD, Babon JJ. Expression and Purification of JAK1 and SOCS1 for Structural and Biochemical Studies. Methods Mol Biol 2018;1725:267–80.
46. Naka T, Matsumoto T, Narazaki M, et al. Accelerated apoptosis of lymphocytes by augmented induction of Bax in SSI-1 (STAT-induced STAT inhibitor-1) deficient mice. Proc Natl Acad Sci U S A 1998;95(26):15577–82.
47. Starr R, Metcalf D, Elefanty AG, et al. Liver degeneration and lymphoid deficiencies in mice lacking suppressor of cytokine signaling-1. Proc Natl Acad Sci U S A 1998;95(24):14395–9.
48. Alexander WS, Starr R, Fenner JE, et al. SOCS1 is a critical inhibitor of interferon gamma signaling and prevents the potentially fatal neonatal actions of this cytokine. Cell 1999;98(5):597–608.
49. Marine JC, Topham DJ, McKay C, et al. SOCS1 deficiency causes a lymphocyte-dependent perinatal lethality. Cell 1999;98(5):609–16.
50. Cornish AL, Davey GM, Metcalf D, et al. Suppressor of cytokine signaling-1 has IFN-gamma-independent actions in T cell homeostasis. J Immunol 2003;170(2): 878–86.
51. Ilangumaran S, Ramanathan S, La Rose J, et al. Suppressor of cytokine signaling 1 regulates IL-15 receptor signaling in CD8+CD44high memory T lymphocytes. J Immunol 2003;171(5):2435–45.
52. Naka T, Tsutsui H, Fujimoto M, et al. SOCS-1/SSI-1-deficient NKT cells participate in severe hepatitis through dysregulated cross-talk inhibition of IFN-gamma and IL-4 signaling in vivo. Immunity 2001;14(5):535–45.
53. Fujimoto M, Tsutsui H, Yumikura-Futatsugi S, et al. A regulatory role for suppressor of cytokine signaling-1 in T(h) polarization in vivo. Int Immunol 2002;14(11): 1343–50.
54. Fujimoto M, Tsutsui H, Xinshou O, et al. Inadequate induction of suppressor of cytokine signaling-1 causes systemic autoimmune diseases. Int Immunol 2004; 16(2):303–14.
55. Trengove MC, Ward AC. SOCS proteins in development and disease. Am J Clin Exp Immunol 2013;2(1):1–29.
56. Fujimoto M, Naka T. SOCS1, a Negative Regulator of Cytokine Signals and TLR Responses, in Human Liver Diseases. Gastroenterol Res Pract 2010;2010. https://doi.org/10.1155/2010/470468.
57. Du Y, Liu M, Nigrovic PA, et al. Biologics and JAK inhibitors for the treatment of monogenic systemic autoinflammatory diseases in children. J Allergy Clin Immunol 2023;151(3):607–18.
58. Ruperto N, Brunner HI, Synoverska O, et al. Tofacitinib in juvenile idiopathic arthritis: a double-blind, placebo-controlled, withdrawal phase 3 randomised trial. Lancet 2021;398(10315):1984–96.

59. La Manna S, Lopez-Sanz L, Bernal S, et al. Cyclic mimetics of kinase-inhibitory region of Suppressors of Cytokine Signaling 1: Progress toward novel anti-inflammatory therapeutics. Eur J Med Chem 2021;221:113547.
60. La Manna S, Fortuna S, Leone M, et al. Ad-hoc modifications of cyclic mimetics of SOCS1 protein: Structural and functional insights. Eur J Med Chem 2022;243: 114781.
61. He C, Yu CR, Mattapallil MJ, et al. SOCS1 Mimetic Peptide Suppresses Chronic Intraocular Inflammatory Disease (Uveitis). Mediators Inflamm 2016;2016: 2939370.

Deficiency of Adenosine Deaminase 2

Clinical Manifestations, Diagnosis, and Treatment

Andrew Grim, MD[a], Keila R. Veiga, MD[b,1], Nadine Saad, MD[a,*,1]

KEYWORDS

- Adenosine deaminase 2 • DADA2 • Autoinflammatory • Immunodeficiency
- Neutropenia • Polyarteritis nodosa (PAN) • Stroke • Vasculitis

KEY POINTS

- Deficiency of adenosine deaminase 2 (DADA2) is a monogenic autoinflammatory disease caused by biallelic mutation in the ADA2 gene, which is necessary for purine synthesis.
- The clinical features may vary by individual but are characterized by vasculopathy, hematologic abnormalities, and immunodeficiencies.
- The most common vascular features are cutaneous, such as livedoid rash and polyarteritis-like lesions, and early-onset stroke.
- The treatment of choice for vasculitis and inflammatory disease is tumor necrosis factor alpha inhibitors. Hematopoietic stem cell transplant is reserved for refractory or severe hematologic disease.

INTRODUCTION

Deficiency of adenosine deaminase 2 (DADA2) is an autoinflammatory disorder occurring due to the absent or diminished activity of ADA2, an isoenzyme of adenosine deaminase (ADA).[1–3] Deficiency of ADA1, the other isoenzyme of ADA, is responsible for lymphopenia and 10% to 20% of severe combined immunodeficiency (SCID) cases.[4–6] It has only been in the past decade that a clinical disorder related to ADA2 has been described.[1,2]

The authors declare they have no financial interests.
[a] Division of Pediatric Rheumatology, Department of Pediatrics, Michigan Medicine, 1500 East Medical Center Drive, Ann Arbor, MI 48109, USA; [b] Division of Pediatric Rheumatology, Department of Pediatrics, New York Medical College/Maria Fareri Children's Hospital, 100 Woods Road, Valhalla, NY 10595, USA
[1] These authors share senior authorship.
* Corresponding author.
E-mail address: nmsaad@med.umich.edu

Rheum Dis Clin N Am 49 (2023) 773–787
https://doi.org/10.1016/j.rdc.2023.06.004
rheumatic.theclinics.com

The first reports of DADA2 were published in 2014 through 2 independent groups. Zhou and colleagues identified 3 unrelated children with multiorgan involvement, including intermittent fevers, recurrent lacunar strokes, livedoid rash, hepatosplenomegaly, and hypogammaglobulinemia. Through whole-exome sequencing, damaging homozygous missense mutations in the *CECR1* (Cat Eye Syndrome Chromosome Region 1) gene, which encodes ADA2, were identified as a common link between these individuals. In addition, these patients had significantly diminished ADA2 activity in plasma compared with unaffected individuals.[1]

Simultaneously, Elkan and colleagues identified 19 patients with features of polyarteritis nodosa. Consistent with the findings of Zhou and colleagues, *CECR1* was identified as a candidate gene, and these individuals had lower ADA2 plasma levels. The investigators postulated an autosomal recessive mode of inheritance.[2]

As our understanding of DADA2 has progressed, other manifestations have been identified including hematologic abnormalities and immune dysregulation.[1–3,7] The aim of this review is to inform the clinician about the clinical manifestations, diagnosis, and treatment of DADA2.

PATHOGENESIS

To better understand the pathogenesis of DADA2, it is important to review the normal function of ADA. ADA is one of the essential enzymes in the salvage pathway of purine biosynthesis.[6,8] Purines are essential to human biology.[6,8–10] They have a variety of important functions, including the generation of DNA and RNA, providing cellular energy and intracellular signaling, and serving as cofactors for other enzymes.[6,9,10] Purines are generated by de novo purine biosynthesis or through the purine salvage pathway.[6,10]

ADA catalyzes deamination of adenosine and 2′-deoxyadenosine into inosine and deoxyinosine, respectively, in the salvage pathway of purine biosynthesis (**Fig. 1**).[6,7] ADA has 2 isoforms: ADA1 and ADA2. **Table 1** provides a comparison of ADA1 and ADA2.[3] ADA1 is present in all human tissues and in erythrocytes, as well as in small quantities in the circulating plasma.[11] ADA2 is highly expressed in immune cells.[7]

ADA1 plays an important role in T-cell proliferation, highlighting its role in the development of autosomal recessive forms of SCID.[3,4] ADA2 plays a role throughout both the innate and adaptive immune pathways, with a complex overlap between both pathways. **Fig. 2** highlights this interaction. The loss of ADA2 leads to decreased conversion of adenosine to inosine. Adenosine consequently has multiple effects on different areas of the immune system.

One mechanism is through the polarization of proinflammatory M1 macrophages. In vitro assays in patients with DADA2 show macrophage polarization toward M1 macrophages and decreased antiinflammatory M2 macrophages.[1,12] In DADA2, there is a decrease in memory T cells and upregulation of the Janus kinase-signal transducer and activator of transcription-interferon (JAK-STAT-IFN) pathways, leading to increased type 1 interferon signaling.[12–18] IFN-γ contributes to the polarization of M1 macrophages. M1 macrophages secrete tumor necrosis factor alpha (TNF-α) that both decreases the amount of regulatory T cells and contributes to neutrophil extracellular traps (NETs) formation.

Another pathological mechanism in DADA2 is the accumulation of adenosine, which leads to chronic neutrophilic activation and NETosis dysregulation with spontaneous NETs formation and a further positive feedback look with continued polarization of M1 macrophages.[16,19] The cascade of proinflammatory cytokines, including IFN-γ, culminates in endothelial damage and vasculopathy.[7]

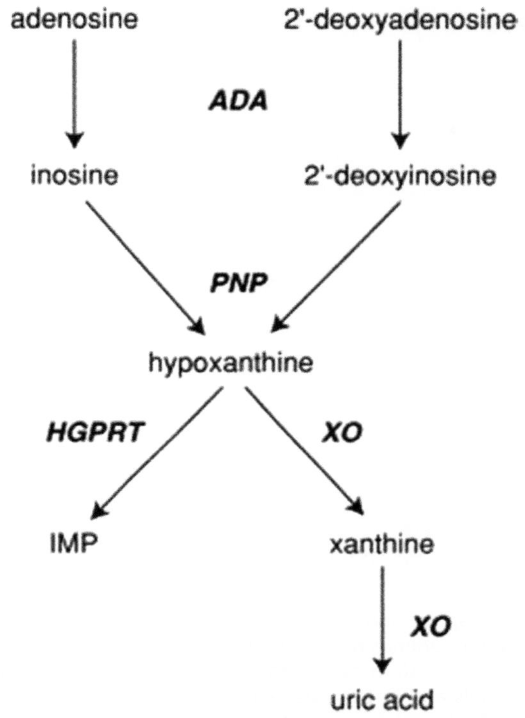

Fig. 1. Adenosine deaminase catalyzes deamination of adenosine and 2′-deoxyadenosine as part of the purine salvage pathway. (*From* Blackburn MR, Kellems RE. Adenosine deaminase deficiency: metabolic basis of immune deficiency and pulmonary inflammation. *Adv Immunol.* 2005;86:1-41.)

In addition, accumulation of adenosine and TNF-α results in impaired B-cell proliferation; this is a result of impaired secretion of IL-21, which is critical for B-cell function, as well as altered expression of CD40L by T cells,[7,20] and this leads to a lower production of immunoglobulins.[7]

Table 1
Comparison of adenosine deaminase 1 and adenosine deaminase 2

Characteristics of ADA1 and ADA2		
	ADA1	ADA2
Gene	*ADA*	*ADA2*
Chromosome	20q13.2	22q11.1
Expression	Ubiquitous	Myeloid cells, lymphocytes, lung, bone marrow, spleen, thymus
Protein structure	41-kDa monomer	59-kDa monomer-homodimer
Function	Adenosine deaminase	Adenosine deaminase, regulation of cell proliferation and differentiation
Clinical phenotype when deficient	T-B-NK-SCID	Deficiency of ADA2

Modified from Meyts I, Aksentijevich I. Deficiency of Adenosine Deaminase 2 (DADA2): Updates on the Phenotype, Genetics, Pathogenesis, and Treatment. *J Clin Immunol.* 2018;38(5):569-578.

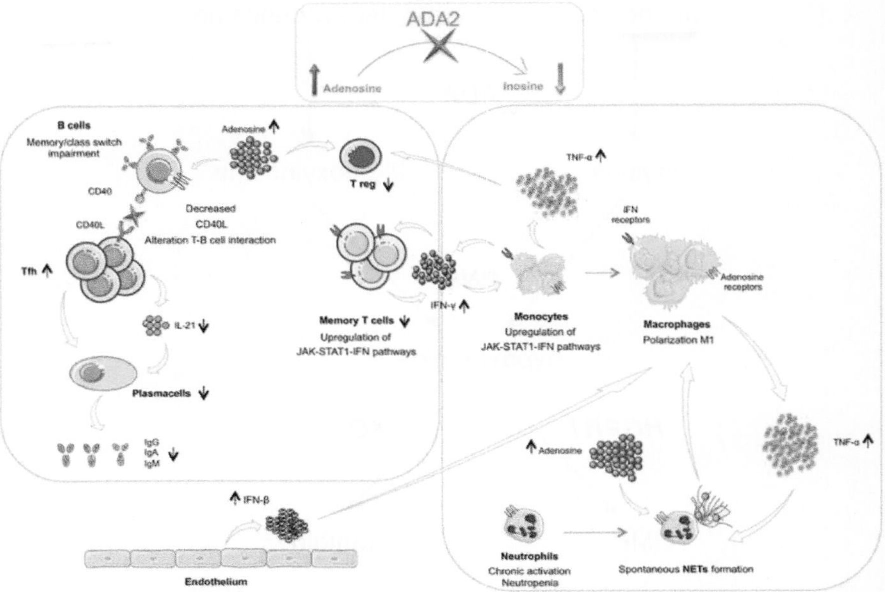

Fig. 2. Overlap of the adaptive and innate immune system in DADA2. Deficiency of ADA2 leads to an accumulation of adenosine. As shown in the left panel, increased levels of adenosine alter T- and B-cell interactions by decreasing CD40L expressed on T cells. This results in generation of plasma cells and in turn, decreased secretion of immunoglobulins. In addition, increased levels of adenosine act on T cells. Lower levels of regulatory and memory T cells lead to upregulation of the JAK-STAT-IFN pathways. As shown in the panel on the right, increased IFN-γ leads to polarization of macrophages to inflammatory type M1 macrophages. In addition, increased adenosine leads to spontaneous NETs formation. This also leads to polarization of type M1 macrophages. The cascade of proinflammatory cytokines from the upregulated JAK-STAT-IFN pathway culminates in endothelial damage. (*Adapted from* Signa S, Bertoni A, Penco F, et al. Adenosine Deaminase 2 Deficiency (DADA2): A Crosstalk Between Innate and Adaptive Immunity. *Front Immunol.* 2022;13:935957.)

Research is ongoing to elucidate other functions of ADA2 beyond its enzymatic activity. ADA2 has been described as part of a family of adenosine-derived growth factors essential for tissue development in insects.[21,22] This role as a growth factor is best described in the *Drosophila* fly model.[23,24] Knock-out of the corresponding gene results in abnormal larval development.[23] Structural studies of the ADA2 from human plasma suggest that the unique N-terminal domain of ADA2 proteins is involved in enzyme binding to cell surface receptors and may be responsible for the receptor-mediated growth factor activity.[11,25]

Another active area of research is the mediation of monocyte-T cell interactions by ADA2.[26,27] Zavialov and colleagues[27] have shown that monocytes undergoing differentiation into dendritic cells and macrophages secrete ADA2. In addition, their experiments suggest that ADA2 is capable of binding to T cells. In their studies, T cells that were not enriched with ADA2 did not proliferate, but when ADA2 was added, they saw a proliferation of CD4+ T cells. The investigators also hypothesize that monocytes that secrete ADA2, and the dendritic cells and macrophages that they differentiate into that also produce ADA2, are required to induce CD4+ T-cell proliferation. They found that ADA2 alone did not induce T-cell proliferation; however, there was a response when increasing numbers of monocytes were added. In addition, when T cells were experimentally separated from monocytes by a pore membrane, T cells were unable to proliferate. These studies suggest that not only does ADA2 have growth factor abilities but physical interaction of monocytes with T cells is also necessary.[27]

GENETICS

The *CECR1* gene is located on chromosome 22q11.1 and encodes the ADA2 protein.[1] DADA2 is caused by biallelic mutations in the ADA2 gene and is inherited in an autosomal recessive pattern. The initial seminal studies[1,2] reported that most patients had compound heterozygous; however, a recent review notes more than half (58.4%) are homozygous for *CECR1* mutations.[28] The latter study emphasized the inherited nature of DADA2.

Mutations causing DADA2 can be located over the entire coding region of the *CECR1* gene.[29] As of March 2023, 104 disease-causing (pathogenic or likely pathogenic) mutations have been reported in the Infevers database.[30] Seventy-nine percent of the mutations were substitutions, 17% were deletions, and the remaining were duplications or delins (deletion/insertions). A further 41 variants are reported in Infevers that are either benign, variants of unknown significance or not classified.[30]

Caorsi and colleagues[31] reported 3 patients with a phenotype consistent with DADA2 and low ADA2 enzymatic activity with either only one or no mutations in the ADA2 gene; this suggests there are mutations affecting regulatory noncoding sequences or genomic deletions. Identifying these types of mutations is out of the scope of commercially available genetic testing.

Pathogenic mutations for DADA2 have variability in occurrence based on geographic location. The 2 most common pathogenic mutations are p.Gly47Arg (G47R) and p.Arg169Gln (R169Q). G47R mutations are more commonly found in Turkish, Israeli, and South Asian populations, whereas the R169Q mutation is more common in European populations.[2,32–35] Jee and colleagues used the Genome Aggregation Database to estimate a carrier frequency of 1 in 236 and a prevalence rate of about 1 in 220,000. They found that the rates were highest in the Finnish population, with a carrier frequency of 1 in 160 and prevalence of 1 in 103,000.[36]

Determining correlations between the genotype and phenotype is an active area of interest. A 2020 study by Lee and colleagues analyzing the genotype-phenotype correlation in 152 patients demonstrated that mutations causing complete or almost complete loss of ADA2 activity were associated with severe hematologic manifestations: pure red blood cell aplasia (PRCA) and bone marrow failure. Mutations leading to partially retained ADA2 activity (at least 3%) were associated with predominantly vasculitis symptom.[37] Ozen and colleagues[32] inferred that the location of the mutation may play a role in the phenotype after analyzing 24 patients, 14 with a polyarteritis nodosa (PAN)-like phenotype, 9 with Diamond-Blackfan anemia (DBA) type features, and 1 with immunodeficiency. In contrast to Lee's study, all had similar ADA2 activity levels. Patients with a DBA/immunodeficiency phenotype had mutations in the dimerization domain, whereas patients with a PAN-like phenotype had mutations in the catalytic domain.[32] In a series of 9 patients with an identical homozygous R169Q mutation, Van Montfrans and colleagues found a widely varying phenotypic presentation, although they did note that ADA2 enzyme activity was higher in those presenting with primarily with cutaneous symptoms.[35] It is likely that genetics, epigenetics, and environmental factors all play a role in disease phenotype.

DIAGNOSIS

The diagnosis of DADA2 requires a high index of suspicion, as there are no formal diagnostic criteria available. Confounding the diagnosis of DADA2 is the wide range of symptoms and varying severity.

All individuals with DADA2 that have so far been described have low (<5% of normal) or undetectable ADA2 catalytic activity,[38] suggesting it may be preferred to perform ADA2 activity as the initial evaluation, followed by genetic testing for confirmation of the diagnosis. Determining ADA2 enzyme activity has been traditionally performed in 1 of 2 ways. In the deaminase reaction, adenosine is converted to inosine with ammonia released as a byproduct. Spectrophotometric assays to detect ammonia can indicate enzymatic activity of ADA2. Detecting the products of this reaction (inosine and, further downstream, hypoxanthine) can be performed with high-performance liquid chromatography assays.[28] Both methods are currently only available on a research basis.

Genetic testing for DADA2 mutations is possible but can have limitations. Small deletions or duplications may be missed by commercially available or standard genetic sequencing (Sanger sequencing, next-generation sequencing–based targeted panels, or exome sequencing).[29] For the detection of small genomic deletions, duplications, or single-exon copy-number variants (>50 base pairs), multiplex ligation-dependent probe amplification analysis can be used. However, this is not currently part of routine testing for DADA2.[29] Furthermore, some patients have been described with a single or no mutation, with a low or minimal ADA2 enzymatic activity level supportive of the diagnosis.[31]

In a patient with suggestive clinical and laboratory findings of DADA2, performing both the ADA2 catalytic activity level and genetic testing can be helpful in making the diagnosis.[29] In patients with symptoms to suggest an autoinflammatory syndrome, but without symptoms more commonly seen in DADA2, it may be prudent to initially perform genetic testing to assess for a wider range of genetic mutations to explain the symptoms. After confirming a diagnosis of DADA2, testing family members (such as parents and siblings) and prenatal testing should strongly be considered.

PRESENTATION

Fig. 3 provides a summarized overview of clinical manifestations of DADA2.

VASCULITIS/VASCULOPATHY

The most frequent phenotypic presentations reported in DADA2 are vascular. The 2 seminal papers describing DADA2 by Zhou and colleagues and Erkan and colleagues describe DADA2 mutations and reduced ADA2 activity in patients with early-onset strokes and vasculopathy and in patients who were previously diagnosed with PAN, respectively.[1,2] Cutaneous and neurologic vascular involvement is most commonly observed, with involvement of other systems including gastrointestinal, renal, cardiac, and pulmonary reported less frequently.[1,2,31,39,40]

Cutaneous

The most common cutaneous manifestations reported are a livedoid rash or livedo racemosa.[1,2,31,40] Barron and colleagues reported in an observational study of 60 patients with DADA2 that 74% had livedo racemosa, and this was followed by a PAN-like presentation and subcutaneous nodules in 57%, Raynaud phenomena in 22%, verrucous warts in 19%, and ulcerations in 5%.[40] This distribution of cutaneous findings is

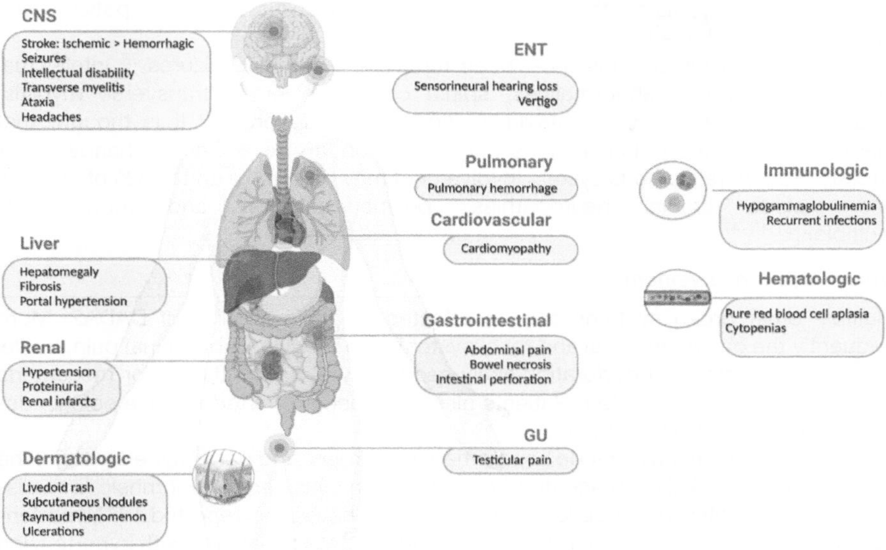

Fig. 3. Clinical manifestations of DADA2. DADA2 affects multiple organ symptoms. Most common manifestations are neurologic, hematologic, cutaneous, and immunologic. This figure highlights other potential manifestations of DADA2. (Created with BioRender.com.)

consistent with previous reports.[1,2,31,39] Several series have reported histopathologic features consistent with vasculitis including fibrinoid necrosis of vessel walls, lymphovascular occlusion in medium vessels with inflammatory infiltrates and intravascular thrombi, and dense chronic inflammation surrounding affected blood vessels.[40–42]

Neurologic

Involvement of the central nervous system (CNS), particularly early-onset strokes, was identified in early reports of DADA2.[1] CNS involvement is estimated to occur in 50% to 77% of patients. Strokes remain the most common neurologic manifestation, and ischemic strokes are more common than hemorrhagic. Ischemic strokes are more commonly lacunar, whereas hemorrhagic strokes tend to be parenchymal, although they have also been seen in subarachnoid space.[43] Hemorrhagic strokes often occur in the setting of past ischemic strokes.

An intrinsic coagulopathy is not common in patients with DADA2, so it is thought that anticoagulation and antiplatelet medication use in patients with previous ischemic strokes may play a role in the development of future hemorrhagic strokes. Barron and colleagues did report one patient who presented with a hemorrhagic stroke without any history of ischemic stroke or use of medication raising a suspicion for a possible intrinsic endothelial dysfunction in patients with DADA2.[40,44] Strokes most often occur when a patient is in a period of active inflammation and are more common in younger patients.[40]

Neuroimaging in patients may show evidence of ischemic strokes, hemorrhagic strokes, and, less commonly, spinal infarcts, posterior reversible encephalopathy syndrome (PRES), and aneurysms.[43] In a series of 12 patients with vascular type DADA2, 1 patient had MRA findings notable for intracranial aneurysms.[43] In the series by Barron and colleagues,[40] 18 of 60 individuals had neuroimaging performed and had no evidence of aneurysms or other signs of intracranial vasculitis, although 2 patients with hypertension did have PRES.

Other CNS manifestations have been reported, including seizures,[39] intellectual disability, behavioral abnormalities, spinal cord involvement/transverse myelitis, sensorineural hearing loss,[40] ataxia, vertigo, and headaches.[35] It is thought that many of these CNS manifestations may be secondary to ischemic changes after strokes. Peripheral nervous system involvement may be seen in up to 53% of patients and include cranial neuropathies, polyneuropathies, and mononeuritis multiplex.[31,45–47]

Other Organ Involvement

Multiple other organ systems can be affected by the vasculitis of DADA2. More frequently the gastrointestinal and renal systems are involved. Abdominal pain, bowel necrosis, and intestinal perforation likely secondary to vasculitis and/or mesenteric ischemia have been reported. Patients also have been reported to have splenic defects suggestive of prior infarcts.[39,40,32]

Liver involvement may include hepatomegaly, fibrosis, and portal hypertension. The liver involvement likely represents both vascular involvement and intrinsic liver disease.[40] Pancreatitis and infarctions of the pancreas have been reported.[1,39] Hypertension, proteinuria, and renal infarcts are all reported.[40] Many patients with hypertension may have a diagnosis of PAN before genetic testing confirming a *CECR1* mutation. Testicular involvement has been reported with several patients describing testicular pain, which is a symptom classically found in PAN.[48] There have been 3 reported cases of cardiomyopathy in DADA2[40,49] and 2 reported cases of pulmonary hemorrhage.[39,50]

HEMATOLOGIC

Hematologic disorders associated with DADA2 tend to occur early in life. Typical hematologic abnormalities include lymphopenia, neutropenia, PRCA, thrombocytopenia, and pancytopenia.[40] Coombs-positive autoimmune hemolytic anemia has also been reported.[32] Cytopenia may be the initial presentation, occurring in 50% of patients.[51] Lymphocytopenia was the first documented cytopenia and is commonly seen in all clinical DADA2 phenotypes.[52] Bone marrow biopsy typically demonstrates hypoplasia of the affected lineages, suggesting a defect in cell production.[38]

Anemia can be found in greater than 50% of cases extending beyond what would be considered anemia of chronic disease and is often multifactorial.[38,52] Severe refractory anemia resembling DBA and PRCA have been reported in 10% of patients.[52] Patients with DBA-like anemia have subtle or no dysmorphic features and more lymphoproliferation and immunological abnormalities.[52] Genetic evaluation, typically by whole-exome sequencing, show biallelic *CECR1* mutations, whereas DBA-associated mutations in ribosomal proteins genes and *GATA-1* are absent.[3]

IMMUNODEFICIENCY

DADA2 was initially recognized due to its inflammatory phenotype, but initial reports by Zhou and colleagues[1] demonstrated hypogammaglobulinemia with consistently low immunoglobulin M (IgM) levels in a subset of 5 patients. DADA2 is associated with a milder immunodeficiency compared with ADA1 deficiency. Humoral deficiency is the most common, specifically low IgM levels.[52] Across studies that quantified immunoglobulins, low IgG and or IgM levels have been reported in 67% of patients with DADA2.[38]

Immunodeficiency is a consequence of both T- and B-cell dysregulation. Schena and colleagues investigated B- and T-cell phenotypes and immune responses in 14 patients with DADA2. They found a decrease in memory B cells, specifically switched memory B cells, as well as a decrease in CD4/8 memory T cells. The frequency of circulating T follicular helper cells was increased, but they had impairment in IL-21 production potentially contributing to an impaired B-cell help[20]; this could explain the B-cell dysregulation in DADA2 with an intrinsic defect in both B cells as well as T cells, leading to impaired antibody production.[52]

Immunodeficiency can range from mild, which is more common in vascular predominant disease, to severe, for which hematologic predominant disease is a risk factor.[53] Recurrent infections were reported in only 16% of patients, the most common being bacterial infections. Viral infections, particularly herpes virus, have also been reported, suggesting not only B cells are affected.[52,54] Barron and colleagues[40] reported verrucous warts in 19% of patients; the warts were not thought to be due to vasculopathy/vasculitis and instead due to immunodeficiency as described in a case series of 2 patients with cutaneous warts and DADA2.[55]

Schepp and colleagues[54] identified 9 patients with DADA2 presenting with combined variable immunodeficiency disease and onset of immunodeficiency before 10 years of age after presenting with recurrent sinopulmonary infections. Caorsi and colleagues,[31] in a cohort of 48 patients, documented low IgG levels in 3 patients; none reported recurrent infections.

Lymphoproliferation can occur in DADA2, with general lymphadenopathy reported in 10% and splenomegaly in 30%.[51] Autoimmune lymphoproliferative syndrome, clonal lymphoproliferation, T large granular lymphocytosis, and lymphoma have been described.[56] A patient with DADA2 and multicentric Castleman disease has also been reported, responding to inhibition of IL-6.[10] In rare instances, patients with DADA2 have presented with hemophagocytic lymphohistiocytosis.[56]

TREATMENT

Treatment of DADA2 deficiency can be challenging, and case mortality is estimated to be around 8%, mostly related to vasculopathy-associated complications and infections.[40]

Several medications have been used in the treatment of DADA2 deficiency, including nonsteroidal antiinflammatory drugs (NSAIDs), corticosteroids, azathioprine, cyclosporine, cyclophosphamide, methotrexate, mycophenolate mofetil, thalidomide, and TNF inhibitors. Anticoagulation and antiplatelet therapies, including aspirin, clopidogrel, heparin, and warfarin, are commonly prescribed in patients with DADA2 with a history of stroke.[40]

The classic immunosuppressive drugs are not considered long-term treatment of DADA2 due to the lack of efficacy for certain manifestations of the disease such as cytopenias. There is also the risk of toxicity with long-term use of these medications.[40] In a cohort of 48 patients with DADA2 deficiency, all patients showed a partial response to NSAIDs and complete response to high-dose steroids with relapse on tapering. Cerebral strokes and intestinal invagination typically occurred at the time of steroid tapering.[31]

TNF inhibitors have been the most successful in controlling clinical manifestations associated with DADA2 compared with other biologics, specifically inflammatory phenotypes.[40] Their use was offered in these patients once perivascular TNF was found in skin biopsies of patients with DADA2.[40] Deuitch demonstrated increased inflammatory signals and overproduction of cytokines mediated by IFN and nuclear factor kappa B pathways. Treatment with TNF inhibition led to reduction in inflammation, rescued the skewed differentiation toward the proinflammatory M1 macrophage subset, and restored integrity of endothelial cells in blood vessels.[12]

Etanercept (ETN) is the initial therapy in the majority due to ease of use. In a longitudinal cohort, several patients were transitioned from ETN to an anti-TNFα monoclonal antibody due to optic neuritis as well as nonneurologic complications.[40]

TNF inhibition has shown to be effective in reduction of stroke occurrence, decrease in inflammatory burden (erythrocyte sedimentation rate and C-reactive protein) as well as improvement in complete blood count parameters.[40] Improvement in hepatic manifestations has also been demonstrated. Patients with hematologic and immune dysregulation may have persistent disease despite TNF inhibition. For instance, patients with pure red cell aplasia typically remain transfusion dependent while on TNF therapy. In addition, patients with hypogammaglobulinemia also continued to demonstrate low IgG levels while on anti-TNF therapy.[40]

Özen and colleagues aimed to investigate the characteristics and ADA2 enzymatic activities of patients with DADA2. In their cohort of patients with polyarteritis nodosa-like phenotype, all patients were refractory to corticosteroids, with all patients responding to TNF inhibition with ETN except for one patient who died shortly after diagnosis. In the DBA-like phenotype, 44% (4 out of 9) responded to corticosteroid treatment, with 2 patients who were subsequently treated with hematopoietic stem cell transplantation (HSCT) and are now in remission. In this cohort, none of the patients with DBA-like features were treated with ETN, which suggests it is not a treatment of choice for patients with a DBA-like phenotype.[32]

In terms of biological therapies, anti-IL-1 therapy has had conflicting results. Poor responses to anakinra have been reported.[57,58] However, one patient has been reported to have a good outcome with anakinra,[35] whereas another with renal amyloidosis in DADA2 was successfully treated with canakinumab.[59] Anti-IL-6 treatment has been used in a patient with Castleman disease found to have elevated IL-6 levels but resulted in relapses with stroke in others.[51] For some patients, the cost of life-long biological therapy, specifically TNF inhibition, may not be feasible.[40]

Yin and colleagues[60] described a 3-year-old boy diagnosed with DADA2 after presenting with fever, elevated acute phase reactants, lymphadenopathy as well as severe asymptomatic hypertension with initial improvement when treated with thalidomide. Thalidomide has been found to be an effective and less expensive treatment in some patients, with studies showing its ability to inhibit the actions of TNF-α.[61] Caorsi and colleagues[31] noted a complete response in 6 patients in their cohort treated with thalidomide, although the drug was later withdrawn due to neurologic toxicity in 3 patients.

For patients suffering from refractory cytopenia, vasculopathy, or immunodeficiency, HSCT is now considered a viable treatment option. Escherich and colleagues[62] described the case of a 2-year-old girl who developed severe anemia in the first few weeks of life requiring frequent transfusions. She was ultimately found to have low ADA2 enzyme activity. Further workup demonstrated a reduced number of memory B cells. She was initially treated with TNF blockade as well as steroids with persistent disease. She was ultimately treated with HSCT. It is often the severity of anemia or pancytopenia that drives the need of curative treatment with HSCT.[56,57,62]

Barron and colleagues[40] conducted a retrospective study on the outcome of HSCT in patients with DADA2, demonstrating that it was an effective treatment of DADA2 reversing refractory cytopenia, vasculopathy, and immunodeficiency with a definitive cure with greater than 95% survival. Complications related to HSCT include graft versus host disease, infection, and Lennox-Gastaut–like epilepsy.[40]

For patients with severe neutropenia or pancytopenia where transplant is not an option, investigation is ongoing with carefully chosen targeted therapies such as aggressive T-cell suppression to improve their cytopenias.[40] Research into gene therapy for DADA2 is also ongoing.[40]

SUMMARY

Since the initial reports in 2014, DADA2 has been identified as a monogenic autoinflammatory disease caused by biallelic mutations in the *CECR1* gene. ADA is essential for human biology and plays a role in the synthesis of DNA and RNA. Mutations in ADA lead to toxic accumulations of precursors of inosine and 2′-deoxyinosine. The intricacy of the pathogenesis of DADA2 is under investigation. A complex overlap between both the innate and adaptive immune system, and the upregulation of proinflammatory cytokines and IFN-γ gives rise to the endothelial damage and vasculopathy of DADA2.

Although DADA2 has a variable presentation, features of vasculitis and vasculopathy, particularly early-onset strokes and cutaneous vasculitis, should alert the physician to this diagnosis. Additional features such as cytopenias, hypogammaglobulinemia, and lymphoproliferative disease are diagnostic clues. The diagnosis of DADA2 is made through a combination of measuring ADA2 enzyme activity and genetic testing. TNF-α inhibitors are commonly used for predominant vascular symptoms. Hematopoietic stem cell transplant may be needed in refractory disease or disease with severe hematologic manifestations.

CLINICS CARE POINTS

- DADA2 is a monogenic autoinflammatory disease caused by biallelic mutation in the *CECR1* gene.
- Clinical features are characterized by vasculopathy, hematologic abnormalities, and immunodeficiencies.
- The most common vascular features are cutaneous, such as livedoid rash and polyarteritis-like lesions, and early-onset stroke.
- The treatment of choice for vasculitis and inflammatory disease is TNF-α inhibitors. HSCT is reserved for refractory or severe hematologic disease.

REFERENCES

1. Zhou Q, Yang D, Ombrello AK, et al. Early-onset stroke and vasculopathy associated with mutations in ADA2. N Engl J Med 2014;370(10):911–20.
2. Navon Elkan P, Pierce SB, Segel R, et al. Mutant adenosine deaminase 2 in a polyarteritis nodosa vasculopathy. N Engl J Med 2014;370(10):921–31.
3. Meyts I, Aksentijevich I. Deficiency of adenosine deaminase 2 (DADA2): updates on the phenotype, genetics, pathogenesis, and treatment. J Clin Immunol 2018;38(5):569–78.
4. Bradford KL, Moretti FA, Carbonaro-Sarracino DA, et al. Adenosine deaminase (ADA)-deficient severe combined immune deficiency (SCID): molecular pathogenesis and clinical manifestations. J Clin Immunol 2017;37(7):626–37.
5. Kwan A, Abraham RS, Currier R, et al. Newborn screening for severe combined immunodeficiency in 11 screening programs in the United States. JAMA 2014;

312(7):729–38, published correction appears in JAMA. 2014 Nov 26;312(20): 2169. Bonagura, Vincent R [Added].
6. Blackburn MR, Kellems RE. Adenosine deaminase deficiency: metabolic basis of immune deficiency and pulmonary inflammation. Adv Immunol 2005;86:1–41.
7. Signa S, Bertoni A, Penco F, et al. Adenosine deaminase 2 deficiency (DADA2): a crosstalk between innate and adaptive immunity. Front Immunol 2022;13:935957.
8. Flinn AM, Gennery AR. Adenosine deaminase deficiency: a review. Orphanet J Rare Dis 2018;13(1):65.
9. Pareek V, Pedley AM, Benkovic SJ. Human de novo purine biosynthesis. Crit Rev Biochem Mol Biol 2021 Feb;56(1):1–16.
10. Pedley AM, Benkovic SJ. A new view into the regulation of purine metabolism: the purinosome. Trends Biochem Sci 2017 Feb;42(2):141–54.
11. Zavialov AV, Engström A. Human ADA2 belongs to a new family of growth factors with adenosine deaminase activity. Biochem J 2005;391(Pt 1):51–7.
12. Deuitch NT, Yang D, Lee PY, et al. TNF inhibition in vasculitis management in adenosine deaminase 2 deficiency (DADA2). J Allergy Clin Immunol 2022; 149(5):1812–6.e6.
13. Yap JY, Moens L, Lin MW, et al. Intrinsic defects in B cell development and differentiation, T cell exhaustion and altered unconventional T cell generation characterize human adenosine deaminase type 2 deficiency. J Clin Immunol 2021;41(8): 1915–35.
14. Nihira H, Izawa K, Ito M, et al. Detailed analysis of Japanese patients with adenosine deaminase 2 deficiency reveals characteristic elevation of type II interferon signature and STAT1 hyperactivation. J Allergy Clin Immunol 2021;148(2): 550–62.
15. Insalaco A, Moneta GM, Pardeo M, et al. Variable clinical phenotypes and relation of interferon signature with disease activity in ADA2 deficiency. J Rheumatol 2019;46(5):523–6.
16. Belot A, Wassmer E, Twilt M, et al. Mutations in CECR1 associated with a neutrophil signature in peripheral blood. Pediatr Rheumatol Online J 2014;12:44.
17. Skrabl-Baumgartner A, Plecko B, Schmidt WM, et al. Autoimmune phenotype with type I interferon signature in two brothers with ADA2 deficiency carrying a novel CECR1 mutation. Pediatr Rheumatol Online J 2017;15(1):67.
18. Watanabe N, Gao S, Wu Z, et al. Analysis of deficiency of adenosine deaminase 2 pathogenesis based on single-cell RNA sequencing of monocytes. J Leukoc Biol 2021;110(3):409–24.
19. Carmona-Rivera C, Khaznadar SS, Shwin KW, et al. Deficiency of adenosine deaminase 2 triggers adenosine-mediated NETosis and TNF production in patients with DADA2. Blood 2019;134(4):395–406.
20. Schena F, Penco F, Volpi S, et al. Dysregulation in B-cell responses and T follicular helper cell function in ADA2 deficiency patients. Eur J Immunol 2021;51(1): 206–19.
21. Maier SA, Podemski L, Graham SW, et al. Characterization of the adenosine deaminase-related growth factor (ADGF) gene family in Drosophila. Gene 2001;280(1–2):27–36.
22. Charlab R, Valenzuela JG, Andersen J, et al. The invertebrate growth factor/ CECR1 subfamily of adenosine deaminase proteins. Gene 2001;267(1):13–22.
23. Dolezal T, Dolezelova E, Zurovec M, et al. A role for adenosine deaminase in Drosophila larval development. PLoS Biol 2005;3(7):e201.

24. Zurovec M, Dolezal T, Gazi M, et al. Adenosine deaminase-related growth factors stimulate cell proliferation in Drosophila by depleting extracellular adenosine. Proc Natl Acad Sci U S A 2002;99(7):4403–8.
25. Zavialov AV, Yu X, Spillmann D, et al. Structural basis for the growth factor activity of human adenosine deaminase ADA2. J Biol Chem 2010;285(16):12367–77.
26. Kaljas Y, Liu C, Skaldin M, et al. Human adenosine deaminases ADA1 and ADA2 bind to different subsets of immune cells. Cell Mol Life Sci 2017;74(3):555–70.
27. Zavialov AV, Gracia E, Glaichenhaus N, et al. Human adenosine deaminase 2 induces differentiation of monocytes into macrophages and stimulates proliferation of T helper cells and macrophages. J Leukoc Biol 2010;88(2):279–90.
28. Huang Z, Li T, Nigrovic PA, et al. Polyarteritis nodosa and deficiency of adenosine deaminase 2 - Shared genealogy, generations apart. Clin Immunol 2020;215: 108411.
29. Schnappauf O, Zhou Q, Moura NS, et al. Deficiency of adenosine deaminase 2 (DADA2): hidden variants, reduced penetrance, and unusual inheritance. J Clin Immunol 2020;40(6):917–26.
30. Infevers: an online database for autoinflammatory mutations. Copyright. Available at: https://infevers.umai-montpellier.fr/. Accessed: March 2023.
31. Caorsi R, Penco F, Grossi A, et al. ADA2 deficiency (DADA2) as an unrecognised cause of early onset polyarteritis nodosa and stroke: a multicentre national study. Ann Rheum Dis 2017;76(10):1648–56, published correction appears in Ann Rheum Dis. 2019 Jul;78(7):e73.
32. Özen S, Batu ED, Taşkıran EZ, et al. A monogenic disease with a variety of phenotypes: deficiency of adenosine deaminase 2. J Rheumatol 2020;47(1):117–25.
33. Kisla Ekinci RM, Balci S, Hershfield M, et al. Deficiency of adenosine deaminase 2: a case series revealing clinical manifestations, genotypes and treatment outcomes from Turkey. Rheumatology 2020;59(1):254–6.
34. Caorsi R, Penco F, Schena F, et al. Monogenic polyarteritis: the lesson of ADA2 deficiency. Pediatr Rheumatol Online J 2016;14(1):51.
35. Van Montfrans JM, Hartman EA, Braun KP, et al. Phenotypic variability in patients with ADA2 deficiency due to identical homozygous R169Q mutations. Rheumatology 2016;55(5):902–10.
36. Jee H, Huang Z, Baxter S, et al. Comprehensive analysis of ADA2 genetic variants and estimation of carrier frequency driven by a function-based approach. J Allergy Clin Immunol 2022;149(1):379–87.
37. Lee PY, Kellner ES, Huang Y, et al. Genotype and functional correlates of disease phenotype in deficiency of adenosine deaminase 2 (DADA2). J Allergy Clin Immunol 2020;145(6):1664–72.e10.
38. Lee PY. Vasculopathy, immunodeficiency, and bone marrow failure: the intriguing syndrome caused by deficiency of adenosine deaminase 2. Front Pediatr 2018; 6:282.
39. Sharma A, Naidu G, Sharma V, et al. Deficiency of adenosine deaminase 2 in adults and children: experience from India. Arthritis Rheumatol 2021;73(2): 276–85.
40. Barron KS, Aksentijevich I, Deuitch NT, et al. The spectrum of the deficiency of adenosine deaminase 2: an observational analysis of a 60 patient cohort. Front Immunol 2022;12:811473.
41. Gonzalez Santiago TM, Zavialov A, Saarela J, et al. Dermatologic features of ADA2 deficiency in cutaneous polyarteritis nodosa. JAMA Dermatol 2015; 151(11):1230–4, published correction appears in JAMA Dermatol. 2016 Sep

1;152(9):1065] [published correction appears in JAMA Dermatol. 2016 Sep 1;152(9):1065.
42. Chasset F, Fayand A, Moguelet P, et al. Clinical and pathological dermatological features of deficiency of adenosine deaminase 2: a multicenter, retrospective, observational study. J Am Acad Dermatol 2020;83(6):1794–8.
43. Geraldo AF, Caorsi R, Tortora D, et al. Widening the neuroimaging features of adenosine deaminase 2 deficiency. AJNR Am J Neuroradiol 2021;42(5):975–9.
44. Lee PY, Huang Y, Zhou Q, et al. Disrupted N-linked glycosylation as a disease mechanism in deficiency of ADA2. J Allergy Clin Immunol 2018;142(4):1363–5.e8.
45. Gibson KM, Morishita KA, Dancey P, et al. Identification of novel adenosine deaminase 2 gene variants and varied clinical phenotype in pediatric vasculitis. Arthritis Rheumatol 2019;71(10):1747–55.
46. Sozeri B, Ercan G, Dogan OA, et al. The same mutation in a family with adenosine deaminase 2 deficiency. Rheumatol Int 2021;41(1):227–33.
47. Liebowitz J, Hellmann DB, Schnappauf O. Thirty years of followup in 3 patients with familial polyarteritis nodosa due to adenosine deaminase 2 deficiency. J Rheumatol 2019;46(8):1059–60.
48. Clarke K, Campbell C, Omoyinmi E, et al. Testicular ischemia in deficiency of adenosine deaminase 2 (DADA2). Pediatr Rheumatol Online J 2019;17(1):39.
49. Tanatar A, Karadağ ŞG, Sözeri B, et al. ADA2 deficiency: case series of five patients with varying phenotypes. J Clin Immunol 2020;40(2):253–8.
50. Bulut E, Erden A, Karadag O, et al. Deficiency of adenosine deaminase 2; special focus on central nervous system imaging. J Neuroradiol 2019;46(3):193–8.
51. Moens L, Hershfield M, Arts K, et al. Human adenosine deaminase 2 deficiency: a multi-faceted inborn error of immunity. Immunol Rev 2019;287(1):62–72.
52. Pinto B, Deo P, Sharma S, et al. Expanding spectrum of DADA2: a review of phenotypes, genetics, pathogenesis and treatment. Clin Rheumatol 2021;40(10):3883–96.
53. Kendall JL, Springer JM. The many faces of a monogenic autoinflammatory disease: adenosine deaminase 2 deficiency. Curr Rheumatol Rep 2020;22(10):64.
54. Schepp J, Proietti M, Frede N, et al. Screening of 181 patients with antibody deficiency for deficiency of adenosine deaminase 2 sheds new light on the disease in adulthood. Arthritis Rheumatol 2017;69(8):1689–700.
55. Arts K, Bergerson JRE, Ombrello AK, et al. Warts and DADA2: a mere coincidence? J Clin Immunol 2018;38(8):836–43.
56. Hashem H, Dimitrova D, Meyts I. Allogeneic hematopoietic cell transplantation for patients with deficiency of adenosine deaminase 2 (DADA2): approaches, obstacles and special considerations. Front Immunol 2022;13:932385.
57. Hashem H, Bucciol G, Ozen S, et al. Hematopoietic cell transplantation cures adenosine deaminase 2 deficiency: report on 30 patients. J Clin Immunol 2021;41(7):1633–47, published correction appears in J Clin Immunol. 2022 Oct;42(7):1580-1581.
58. Garg N, Kasapcopur O, Foster J 2nd, et al. Novel adenosine deaminase 2 mutations in a child with a fatal vasculopathy. Eur J Pediatr 2014;173(6):827–30.
59. Kisla Ekinci RM, Balci S, Bisgin A, et al. Renal amyloidosis in deficiency of adenosine deaminase 2: successful experience with canakinumab. Pediatrics 2018;142(5):e20180948.
60. Yin J, Fan X, Ma J, et al. ADA2 deficiency (DADA2) misdiagnosed as systemic onset juvenile idiopathic arthritis in a child carrying a novel compound heterozygous ADA2 mutation: a case report. Transl Pediatr 2023;12(1):97–103.

61. Moreira AL, Sampaio EP, Zmuidzinas A, et al. Thalidomide exerts its inhibitory action on tumor necrosis factor alpha by enhancing mRNA degradation. J Exp Med 1993;177(6):1675–80.
62. Escherich C, Bötticher B, Harmsen S, et al. The growing spectrum of DADA2 manifestations-diagnostic and therapeutic challenges revisited. Front Pediatr 2022;10:885893.

COPA Syndrome from Diagnosis to Treatment

A Clinician's Guide

Noa Simchoni, MD, PhD[a], Tiphanie P. Vogel, MD, PhD[b], Anthony K. Shum, MD[a,c,*]

KEYWORDS

• COPA syndrome • Autoantibody • Interstitial lung disease • Alveolar hemorrhage • Arthritis • Nephritis • Child • Infant

KEY POINTS

- COPA syndrome is a rare autosomal dominant disorder characterized by high autoantibody levels and interstitial lung disease in the presence or absence of inflammatory arthritis and renal disease.
- Prominent pulmonary manifestations of COPA syndrome include cough, tachypnea/exercise intolerance, alveolar hemorrhage (which can be insidious), respiratory failure, and interstitial lung disease characterized by cysts, centrilobular nodules, and/or pulmonary fibrosis.
- Arthritis in COPA syndrome is indistinguishable from rheumatoid arthritis or juvenile arthritis.
- Immune suppression is critical for patients with COPA syndrome.
- JAK inhibitors may be an option to slow progression of ILD, the most common cause of death for patients with COPA syndrome and typically the most refractory aspect of disease.

INTRODUCTION

Rare genetic diseases can be powerful tools for the discovery of specific biologic pathways relevant to human health and disease. COPA syndrome, a recently described autosomal dominant inborn error of immunity, has revealed the importance

[a] Pulmonary Division, Department of Medicine, University of California, San Francisco, 555 Mission Bay Boulevard South, CVRI 284F, Box 3118, San Francisco, CA 94158, USA; [b] Division of Rheumatology, Department of Pediatrics, Baylor College of Medicine and Center for Human Immunobiology, Texas Children's Hospital, 1102 Bates Avenue Suite 330, Houston, TX 77030, USA; [c] Cardiovascular Research Institute, University of California, San Francisco, 555 Mission Bay Boulevard South, CVRI 284F, Box 3118, San Francisco, CA 94158, USA
* Corresponding author.
E-mail address: Anthony.shum@ucsf.edu

Rheum Dis Clin N Am 49 (2023) 789–804
https://doi.org/10.1016/j.rdc.2023.06.005
rheumatic.theclinics.com
0889-857X/23/

of intracellular protein trafficking to maintaining immune homeostasis. This review will explore the clinical presentation, genetics, molecular mechanisms, organ manifestations, and treatment approaches for COPA syndrome, ending with a diagnostic framework and remaining questions.

METHODS

Published articles and conference abstracts were identified through the literature search for "COPA syndrome." No relevant results returned for "autoimmune interstitial lung joint and kidney disease" and "AILJK." Three additional abstracts were identified through searching for "COPA syndrome" plus an acronym for pulmonology, immunology, rheumatology, and primary immunodeficiency-focused conferences. Two additional articles were identified through being referenced by other studies. Every effort was made to avoid duplicate reporting of individual patients. Scrutinizing author lists and patient-level information identified the following duplicate reports: 1. patients from original publication also reported upon in 2 early follow-up studies[1–3]; 2. kindred (1 affected, 1 unaffected) with the D243N mutation[4,5]; 3. Kindred (5 affected, 3 unaffected) with the R233H mutation[5,6]; 4. kindred (1 affected, 1 unaffected) with the R233H mutation[5,7,8]; 5. patients who underwent lung transplant from kindred (4 affected) with the V242G mutation[9,10]; 6: only novel patients from an institutional registry were reported (patients 3, 4, 5, 6, and 10 per T.P.V.).[1,11–13] A P145S mutation is excluded as the referenced publication[14,15] could not be found via search or via the website of the named journal. An abstract reporting 6 individuals with one of the 3 additional C terminal tail mutations[16] was excluded due to insufficient patient information.

DETAILED DESCRIPTION

Clinical Presentation

COPA syndrome was first reported in 2015 after mutations in the *coatomer subunit alpha* (*COPA*) gene were identified in 5 kindreds in which multiple individuals had childhood onset interstitial lung disease, high titer autoantibodies, and inflammatory arthritis,[1] almost half of whom also developed renal disease. Subsequently, additional reported patients generally share these features, with most showing childhood onset of symptoms, 64% up to age 5% and 89% up to age 12 for those with reported ages. Four individuals with symptom onset in their 50s have been reported, generally showing milder disease and identified through familial sequencing after mutations were identified in young probands.[6,9,12] One individual, published as a case report, was identified through sequencing lung transplant recipients, with age available for ILD diagnosis but not arthritis onset.[17]

Presenting symptoms are typically pulmonary, ranging from tachypnea to respiratory failure, and/or musculoskeletal, ranging from arthralgias to deforming arthritis (**Table 1**). One patient presented with renal failure.[6] Several infants and toddlers presented with nonspecific lethargy, failure to thrive, and/or anemia (from insidious alveolar hemorrhage), at times years prior to developing localizing symptoms.[8] All patients have high levels of autoantibodies, including one or more of anti-nuclear antibodies (ANA), anti-neutrophil cytoplasmic antibodies (ANCA), rheumatoid factor (RF), and anti-cyclic citrullinated peptide antibodies (CCP). Antibodies to extractable nuclear antigens (ENAs) and ANCA subtype results were more variable, both between patients and within an individual over time.

Disease manifestations can evolve in individual patients over time, with the detection of additional autoantibodies and/or involvement of additional organ systems.

Table 1
Features of patients by mutation

Highest Level of Evidence		# Affected (% Male)	# Unaffected (% Male)	Cause of Death (Age)	Countries	Age (y) at Symptom Onset or Diagnosis	Presenting Symptoms	Refs
Experimentally Validated	K230N	6 (17%)	1 (100%)		USA	7	Lethargy (n = 1) abdominal pain (n = 1)	1,3
	R233H	29 (55%)	6 (67%)	Lung disease (29) Lung disease (63) Suicide (unk) Unk (unk)	USA France England	0.83, 1, 2, 2, 2, 2, 2.5, 3, 3, 5, 5, 5, 7, 7, 8, 10, 11, 16, 26, 50[a], 56[a], 59[b,c]	Pulmonary (n = 15) Joint symptoms (n = 11) Anemia (n = 3) Renal failure (n = 1) Fever (n = 1)	1,3,5,6,8,11–13,17,23,24
	E241K	9 (33%)	3 (66%)	Unk (unk)	USA Iceland	1.5, 2, 4, 11, 32[c]	Joint symptoms (n = 4) Pulmonary (n = 3)	1,3,19
	V242G	4 (75%)		Lung disease (4) Lung disease(21)	Japan	0.17, 0.33, 0.58, 53[a]	Pulmonary (n = 3) Joint symptoms (n = 1)	9,10
	D243G	5 (0%)	4 (100%)	Unk (unk) Unk (unk)	USA	0.5	Pulmonary (n = 1)	1,3
	D243N	1 (0%)	1 (0%)		England	2.5	Joint symptoms (n = 1)	5,51
Published Case Reports	H199R	3 (100%)	1 (50%)		China	0.25	Pulmonary (n = 2) Joint symptoms (n = 1)	34
	K238E	1 (100%)			China	7	Pulmonary (n = 1) Joint symptoms (n = 1)	34
	A239P	3 (100%)			USA Canada China	0.75, 2, 3	Pulmonary (n = 3) FTT (n = 2)	15,38,43
	W240L	1 (0%)			Germany	2	Pulmonary (n = 1)	40
	W240R	1 (100%)			USA	12	Pulmonary (n = 1) FTT (n = 1)	52
	W240S	1 (0%)			Germany	14	Pulmonary (n = 1) Joint symptoms (n = 1)	40
	E241A	2 (100%)			USA	0.5, 7	Pulmonary (n = 2)	39

(*continued on next page*)

Table 1
(continued)

Highest Level of Evidence		# Affected (% Male)	# Unaffected (% Male)	Cause of Death (Age)	Countries	Age (y) at Symptom Onset or Diagnosis	Presenting Symptoms	Refs
	R281W	5 (80%)	2 (0%)	Lung disease (11) Lung disease (38)	India China Germany Italy	1.5, 5, 7, 9, <12	Joint symptoms (n = 3) Pulmonary (n = 2) Anemia (n = 1)	14,20,36,40
	Q285H	1 (0%)			France	6	Joint symptoms (n = 1)	35
Mutations not Reported		3 (33%)			USA Canada Brazil	"childhood"	Pulmonary (n = 3) Joint symptoms (n = 1)	18,41,53

[a] Identified by family sequencing after mutation found in proband.
[b] Identified by the sequencing of lung transplant cohort.
[c] COPA syndrome identified after additional organ involvement, age unknown for initial symptoms.

Organ-specific manifestations also change with time, especially for pulmonary disease in which interstitial lung disease involving cysts (on imaging) and follicular bronchitis, lymphocytic interstitial pneumonia, and/or interstitial fibrosis (on biopsy) are often later findings than alveolar hemorrhage. These findings can progress despite immune suppression, even while symptoms are controlled,[3,18,19] and represent the main cause of death in COPA syndrome. Indeed, of the six patients with COPA syndrome with a reported cause of death, 5 passed away from lung disease (3 despite bilateral lung transplants),[1,9–11,14,17,18,20] while one passed away from suicide.[5] A total of eleven (14%) patients have passed away.

Genetics and Genotype-Phenotype Correlations

The first report of COPA syndrome identified four distinct disease-causing mutations with autosomal dominant inheritance and reduced penetrance. In the past 8 years, an additional 15 mutations have been described, often as case reports though 2 of these have been functionally validated experimentally and shown to statistically differ from unmutated COPA (see **Table 1**). The six validated mutations cluster tightly within exons 8 and 9 of the large COPA protein, all falling within the fifth and sixth WD repeats in the WD-40 domain that is involved in target protein recognition (**Fig. 1**). An additional mutation hotspot has been reported in exon 10 coding for part of the seventh WD repeat, with reported patients showing similar organ involvement.

One patient with a mutation in the C terminal tail, present in 172 individuals in gnomad[21] and reported in association with a different phenotype, is not included in this review of COPA syndrome. Three additional C terminal mutations have also been reported, however available clinical information was not sufficient for evaluation.[16] Indeed, there may be a spectrum of clinical phenotypes associated with an individual gene, as has been described for other immune dysregulation syndromes (ex: *TREX1* mutations causing increased susceptibility to systemic lupus erythematosus (SLE), chilblain lupus, Aicardi-Goutières syndrome, or retinal vasculopathy with cerebral leukodystrophy[22]). However, "COPA syndrome" should typically be reserved for the clinical phenotype of lung disease in the presence or absence of inflammatory arthritis and/or renal disease. Future functional validation of COPA variants outside the WD-

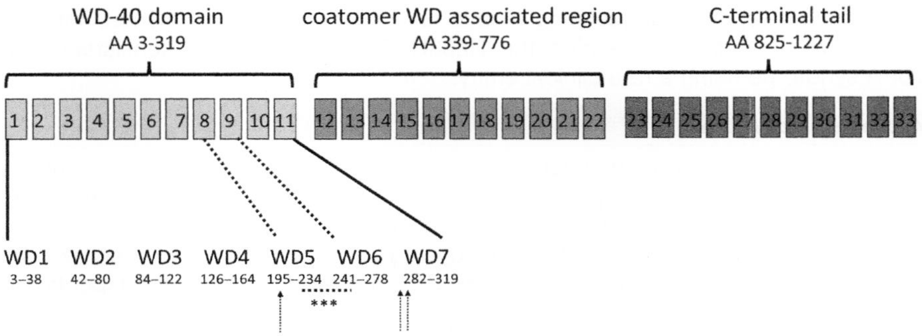

Fig. 1. Structure of COPA locus, exons are marked in boxes shaded to correspond with protein motifs. Detail of WD regions containing COPA mutations highlighted. Validated mutations (K230 N, R233H, E241 K, V242 G, D243 G, D243 N) and variants from case report tightly cluster between amino acids 230 to 243, underlined and marked with asterisks. Arrows point to additional mutations from case reports describing patients with consistent phenotypic features (see **Table 1** for full details). (*Data from Quek et. al.* in Cytogenetic and Genome Research, 1997.)

40 domain may provide support for the conclusion that additional human immune disease phenotypes are also the result of pathogenic mutations in COPA.

COPA mutations do not appear to show genotype-phenotype correlations for the common symptoms of COPA syndrome, though the strength of any conclusions is obviously limited by the small patient numbers. For example, 31 patients from 12 families (48% of all reported patients) have the R233H mutation.[1,5,6,8,11–13,17,23,24] These individuals show variable disease expressivity, with clinical presentations ranging from severe recurrent alveolar hemorrhage[7] to severe nephritis necessitating transplant in childhood.[6] Disease manifestations differ within families as well, with relatives of the patient presenting with renal failure having pulmonary but not renal involvement.[5,6] In contrast, none of 9 patients (12%) from 2 families with the E241K mutation are yet to be reported to have renal involvement, though it may subsequently develop.[1,19] Several patients have additional findings, shared by at most 2 individuals, either first degree relatives or those bearing different COPA mutations, such that these findings may or may not be part of COPA syndrome.

Epidemiology

The true frequency of COPA syndrome is hard to determine given its recent discovery, as well as the absence of experimental validation for most of the mutations reported in the literature. Nevertheless, it appears to be ultra-rare, with a total of 77 patients reported (see **Table 1**). Patients sharing core COPA syndrome features do not show a gender preference among cases (38 males and 39 females). An additional 18 unaffected carriers have been reported, males twice as commonly as females, with a resultant 15% clinical non-penetrance rate that is almost certainly an underestimate as family members were not systematically tested in many reports. The cause of non-penetrance is currently unknown, with healthy mutation carriers variably reported as indistinguishable from other family members or with minor elevations in type I interferon (IFN) signature.[1,5] Those with described racial and ethnic backgrounds are mostly Caucasian, with East Asian ancestry second most common. Cases have also been reported in individuals with South Asian, Native American, Hispanic, and African American ancestry (see **Table 1**).

Severe lung disease is a prominent feature of COPA syndrome, with the evaluation of lung transplant recipients potentially informative about disease frequency. A conference abstract reported sequencing results for 77 individuals transplanted for ILD, identifying one individual bearing the R233H COPA mutation,[17] consistent with COPA syndrome being a rare clinical entity.

Mechanisms of Disease

The International Union of Immunologic Societies (IUIS) expert committee on Inborn Errors of Immunity has grouped COPA syndrome under the “auto-inflammatory, other” category since 2015, including in the most recent update in 2022.[25] It is more accurate to describe it as a syndrome of dysregulated immunity, however, as both innate[5,26,27] (autoinflammatory) and adaptive[1,28] (autoimmune) immune aspects are aberrant.

COPA codes for the coatomer subunit alpha protein, a part of the coat protein complex I (COPI) that coats vesicles to mediate retrograde protein transport from the Golgi back to the endoplasmic reticulum (ER). How altered intracellular protein trafficking led to autoimmunity was unclear at the onset,[1] however subsequent studies unveiled a critical role for failed retrieval of stimulator of interferon genes (STING) in pathogenesis.[27] STING, a master regulator of innate immunity activated downstream of cytosolic DNA,[26,27,29,30] requires ER to Golgi transport upon activation to initiate downstream signaling, including a potent type I interferon response.[31] Termination of signaling requires transport out of the Golgi, either back to the ER, mediated by COPI, or to lysosomes for degradation.[31] Of note, COPA does not bind STING directly, instead complexing with the intermediate cargo receptor protein surfeit 4 (SURF4).[27,29]

In the presence of pathogenic COPA mutations, activated STING accumulates in the Golgi, resulting in increased type I IFN signaling, altered T cell thymic selection, T_H17 skewing, ER stress, and impaired autophagy.[1,9,23,27,28] How these processes result in immune dysregulation and clinical symptoms remains poorly understood. Nevertheless, disease clearly depends on STING as knocking it out rescued mice from the embryonic lethality of a homozygous COPA E241K mutation.[27] Data from humans further supports this link with STING as COPA syndrome shares many features with STING-associated vasculopathy with onset in infancy (SAVI), a Mendelian disorder driven by STING gain-of-function mutations.[32] Interestingly, among monogenic type I interferonopathies ILD and alveolar hemorrhage are seen only in COPA syndrome and SAVI,[33] suggesting interferon independent aspects of STING signaling may drive lung disease.

DETAILED DISEASE INVOLVEMENT BY ORGAN SYSTEM

Laboratory testing

Many patients with COPA syndrome have elevated inflammatory markers, with mild to moderately elevated erythrocyte sedimentation rate (ESR) seen in 95% of 22 reported patients, with results rarely above 90 mm/h. In contrast, C-reactive protein (CRP) was generally normal to mildly elevated, under 15 mg/L in 91% of 22 reported patients. Both ESR and CRP are reported to vary within an individual, with elevations somewhat tracking with disease activity, such as one patient with improvement but not the normalization of ESR a year after the resolution of severe arthritis.[24]

Levels of IFNα measured by ultra-sensitive digital ELISA were elevated in 100% of 6 patients, generally in the 150 to 1700 fg/mL range.[5] Several patients had elevated interleukins (IL): IL-6 in 3 patients, IL-1β in one patient, and soluble IL2 receptor α in one patient. Additional results obtained from research-based testing included 100% of 12 patients having elevated interferon signatures,[5,9,34–36] one of whom showed resolution with baricitinib treatment.[9] An additional patient was reported to have elevated IFNα2.[35]

Autoantibodies

All but one patient with COPA syndrome had elevated ANA, ANCA, and/or RF/CCP. Autoantibody results were explicitly reported for 57 patients, 74% of whom were ANA positive, somewhat higher than the 67% to 70% reported previously.[1,37] Titers, when reported, were almost universally 1:160 or higher, and often 1:640 or higher. Reported staining patterns were highly variable, including homogeneous, diffuse, and speckled appearances. ENAs were reported less frequently, though dsDNA, Smith, and RNP antibodies were each found in at least one patient. These can vary with time and disease activity, as demonstrated in an individual in which each of these antibodies was only identified once during serial testing over 14 months.[38] In contrast, ANA positivity has been reported to be durable.

ANCA or MPO/PR3 were positive in 61% of reported patients, including several patients with negative MPO and PR3 testing in whom ANCA testing was not performed. Most ANCA-positive individuals were MPO and PR3 negative (70%), potentially explaining the discrepancy from prior ANCA positivity in 64% to 71% of patients.[1,37]

MPO was identified in eleven individuals, generally at high titer, while PR3 was seen in six individuals, including at low titer and with variable positivity.[38] MPO and PR3 can fluctuate with disease activity, while ANCA remains positive.[38]

RF and/or CCP were positive in 65% of reported patients, similar to the 43% to 61% previously reported.[1,37] When reported, titers were generally markedly elevated to over 100 IU/mL for RF and over 50 U/mL for CCP, with multiple results above the limit of detection.

In conclusion, a high titer ANA is a feature of COPA syndrome, while extractable nuclear antigens are not common. When serially evaluated, ANA remained positive, while ENAs showed significant variability, with none predicting disease activity. ANCA is often positive, and can be seen in isolation or associated with MPO more commonly than PR3. RF and CCP are also common, again at high titer. A relatively unique feature of COPA syndrome is the presence of multiple autoantibodies regardless of phenotype, with many individuals reported to have high titer ANA, ANCA, and RF/CCP.

Pulmonary Disease

One of the more unique aspects of COPA syndrome is pulmonary involvement, especially among monogenic type I interferonopathies where it is only seen in COPA syndrome and SAVI. ILD, however, can be an extra-articular feature of rheumatoid arthritis (RA), while pulmonary hemorrhage can be seen in ANCA-associated vasculitis (AAV) and, less commonly, in SLE. Presentation with a combined pulmonary-renal syndrome, a hallmark of AAV, has also been reported.[3,13] Pulmonary involvement is nearly universally reported, seen in 98% of 58 individuals in which clinical descriptions are available. The sole unaffected individual was aged 9 years at the time of report, with prior publications identifying a lag of up to 20 years between the development of arthritis and ILD.[3,35]

Alveolar hemorrhage (AH) is often the earliest pulmonary manifestation, occurring as early as infancy.[9] AH recognition is often delayed as hemoptysis is infrequently seen in these children, who are often diagnosed with pulmonary infections in the setting of respiratory symptoms and patchy ground glass opacities (GGOs) on imaging.[7,39] When it occurs, hemoptysis is a major clue to AH diagnosis.[7] Interestingly AH was more common in earlier reports about COPA syndrome,[1,3] likely reflecting phenotypic expansion, something that typically follows the identification of a novel monogenic disorder, into individuals with less early or dramatic pulmonary presentations. AH may be severe, and children have presented with respiratory failure.[2] In mechanically ventilated individuals, bronchoalveolar lavage (BAL) has been demonstrated to be a sensitive tool for detecting occult AH.[3] Capillaritis was seen on biopsy in the setting of AH in 2 related and 2 unrelated individuals, with 3 additional patients demonstrating alveolar hemorrhage without capillaritis, potentially due to resolution while awaiting biopsy.[2,3,7,11]

Cough, tachypnea, shortness of breath, wheezing, and/or exercise intolerance are also common in patients with COPA syndrome, associated either with occult AH or with findings of ILD on imaging. ILD develops over time in COPA syndrome,[3] potentially from recurrent hemorrhage and inflammation and potentially from a yet unidentified direct injury to the lungs from COPA mutations. It is important to recognize that ILD may be clinically silent in young children, even when prominent on imaging.[36] Imaging features relatively unique to COPA syndrome include cystic changes, while GGOs, septal thickening, centrilobular nodules, lymphadenopathy (LAD), and fibrosis can also be seen in other clinical entities.[3,11] Crazy paving has also been reported, though it was seen in fewer than 20% of patients.[11] Imaging findings often match nonspecific interstitial pneumonia (NSIP) or lymphocytic interstitial pneumonia (LIP) patterns.[2,3,11] The usual interstitial pneumonia (UIP) pattern of fibrosis has only been reported, in a conference abstract, in one individual: an atypical case of a woman who developed lung disease diagnosed as RA-ILD in her 50s whose COPA mutation was identified through sequencing lung transplant recipients.[17]

Pulmonary function testing (PFT) results in COPA syndrome are variable, most often mixed obstruction and restriction, followed by restriction, and only occasionally isolated obstruction.[3] Results of diffusion capacity of the lung for carbon monoxide (DLCO) are infrequently reported and almost always reduced (93% of 14 patients). For individuals old enough to perform them, serial PFTs can help screen for clinically silent progressive pulmonary impairment.

Immune suppression is associated with improvement in GGOs, nodules, and LAD, but not in cystic changes or fibrosis.[3,11] This has enormous clinical implications as lung disease, the major cause of death in COPA syndrome, can have subclinical progression.[3,18,19] This progression has been documented in the context of multiple combinations of immune suppressive medications, including in patients receiving a janus kinase (JAK) inhibitor.[37]

Lung pathology, whether by surgical or transbronchial approaches, can show features of alveolar hemorrhage, as discussed above, with additional common patterns of follicular bronchiolitis (lymphoid follicles associated with bronchioles and the peribronchiolar interstitium) and airspace enlargement with cystic changes.[1,3,12,40] Fibrosis patterns were in non-usual interstitial pneumonitis pattern (histologic NSIP), other than the above-mentioned adult-onset individual that was reported in a conference abstract to have UIP on imaging and histology.[17] Histologic and radiographic patterns for individual patients are generally concordant.[3] Three individuals had additional neuroendocrine cell abnormalities on biopsy, including neuroendocrine hyperplasia and a carcinoid tumor in a 56-year-old man[12] and diffuse neuroendocrine cell hyperplasia (DIPNECH) in 2 individuals.[2]

Several patients with COPA syndrome have progressed to bilateral lung transplant (BLTx). Nine patients have been reported to undergo transplant, many with a limited duration of follow up. Patient outcomes vary from a standard post-transplant course[2,41] to death, including 3 patients who passed away within the first post-transplant year[9,18] and a fourth who passed away later in her post-transplant course.[17] Two of these early deaths were from related individuals in Japan whose detailed peri-transplant courses are published.[9,10] While there is a wide range of survival between lung transplant centers, 1- year survival in the United States is roughly 85%,[42] higher than the 67% seen in these patients with COPA syndrome. In general, sicker patients have poorer transplant outcomes, and 2 post-transplant deaths in this COPA syndrome cohort were in patients bridged to transplant on long-term mechanical ventilation and/or extracorporeal membrane oxygenation (ECMO),[9,18] one of whom further required increased immune suppression due to sensitization and presence of a positive antibody crossmatch.[18] The third early death was in a young boy with severe mycobacterial infection pre transplant.[9] Therefore, it is not clear that outcomes for patients transplanted for COPA syndrome are inferior to those transplanted for other indications. While obviously limited by sample size, outcomes in COPA syndrome are better than in SAVI, where only one of the 5 BLTx recipients survived the first post-transplant year.[10]

The question of whether COPA syndrome recurs post-transplant is important. One of the Japanese transplant patients died from overwhelming infection, without recurrence of ILD, and the other had diffuse alveolar damage, associated with pulmonary hemorrhage, and mild bronchiolitis obliterans (BO), overall consistent with chronic lung allograft dysfunction (CLAD). Follicular bronchitis and cystic changes consistent with COPA syndrome were not seen.[9,10] A third patient had CLAD on autopsy, after several documented infections and after treating cellular and antibody-mediated rejection.[18] Detailed information was not reported for the fourth patient.

Overall, there is no definitive proof of COPA syndrome recurrence post-transplant, though immune dysregulation from COPA syndrome could have contributed to accelerated CLAD and/or heightened susceptibility or severity of post-transplant infections. More information about post-transplant clinical courses is needed, including the evaluation of interferon signatures and potentially trials of JAK inhibitors (see therapy section later in discussion). Future research is also needed to determine the extent to which ILD in COPA syndrome is lung intrinsic, driven by hematopoietic cells, or both, and whether combined lung and bone marrow transplants should be considered.

Arthritis

Joint symptoms are very common in COPA syndrome, and have been reported to appear before, after, or in conjunction with pulmonary disease. Of 44 patients for whom clinical data were available, 82% had joint symptoms, ranging from arthralgias to symmetric polyarthritis to deforming arthritis, both erosive and non-erosive. Joint involvement in 3 additional patients may have resulted from steroid exposure, including avascular necrosis in 2 individuals[1,12] and a spinal compression fracture in a third.[14] If these individuals are included, 89% of patients had musculoskeletal involvement.

Affected joints in patients with arthritis are variable, including proximal interphalangeal joints, metacarpophalangeal joints, wrists, ankles, knees, hips, and spine. Non-erosive arthritis was almost always seen, 87% of 15 patients for which the type was specified, but can be severely deforming.[20] Fortunately, immune suppression of various sorts can be effective at controlling symptoms and debility from joint disease. Erosive disease which was only reported in 2 patients,[11,39] including one in whom it evolved from non-erosive arthritis while he was lost to follow up and off therapy for 8 years.[39]

Renal Disease

Renal disease as the predominant presenting symptom of COPA syndrome is atypical but has been reported, with COPA syndrome suspected due to a known familial mutation. That patient did have pulmonary involvement, albeit asymptomatic, with alveolar hemorrhage seen on BAL.[5,6] Published details on renal disease are sparser than for other main COPA syndrome manifestations, often limited to presence or absence and to biopsy results. Nephritis can, nevertheless, be severe, with the above individual and a second patient requiring renal transplantation.[1,6] It is largely unclear from the literature whether kidney biopsies were performed to further evaluate abnormal laboratory testing or to obtain a tissue diagnosis in the setting of elevated autoantibodies. Within these limitations, 40% of 43 patients have renal involvement, representing 22% of the full patient cohort. Given underreporting on renal phenotypes, a prevalence rate of 40% is likely more accurate based on prior cohort studies reporting rates of 42% (9 of 21) and 47% (9 of 19).[2,37]

All renal biopsies reported show an immune-mediated glomerulopathy, though various histopathological patterns have been seen. Three patients showed crescentic glomerulonephritis with negative immune fluorescence, while 2 showed crescentic glomerulonephritis with positive immunofluorescence (one low positive mesangial IgM, IgG, and C3, and one with "full house" IgM, IgG, IgA, C3, and C1q).[1,6,11,13] A sixth patient showed focal mesangial hypercellularity with C3 and C4 staining, a seventh showed IgA nephropathy, and an eight individual (with asymptomatic proteinuria biopsied as a potential kidney donor) had membranous glomerulonephritis.[1,2,6] One individual with normal renal function underwent a partial nephrectomy for a nodule identified on imaging, finding clear cell carcinoma in the background of normal kidney tissue,[12] a finding that may or may not relate to COPA syndrome.

Other Findings

Various additional clinical findings have been reported in 1 or 2 individuals with COPA syndrome. Neurologic involvement includes paroxysmal exertional dyskinesia,[1] neuromyelitis optica,[12,15] and disruptive behavior disorder.[40] Gastrointestinal involvement includes severe gastroesophageal reflux necessitating surgery,[24,41] hepatic cysts with cytolytic hepatitis,[5] and persistent transaminitis.[43] Cutaneous manifestations include leukocytoclastic vasculitis,[1] chilblain lupus,[15] polymorphic rash,[19] eczema,[34] and vitiligo.[5] Immune and infectious manifestations include macrophage activation syndrome,[5] thyroiditis,[1] and bacterial and viral infections.[9,12] Cardiac hypertrophy[5] has also been reported. The extent to which these represent manifestations of COPA syndrome is unclear.

THERAPIES

There is no specific therapeutic at this time for COPA syndrome, and manifestations are treated with immune suppression as extrapolated from the care of other immune disorders with overlapping features. Life-threatening alveolar hemorrhage is generally controlled with pulse dose IV steroids that are subsequently converted to an oral maintenance regimen, with doses in many patients significantly weaned.[3] Some patients have also received cyclophosphamide and/or intravenous immunoglobulin (IVIG). Various steroid-sparing agents have been reported, often as part of a 2- to 3-drug regimen using standard dosing, with variable success for any given agent or combination even among related individuals. No single regimen has emerged to be superior among standard immunosuppressives including corticosteroids, azathioprine, mycophenolate mofetil/mycophenolic acid, methotrexate, hydroxychloroquine, cyclophosphamide, cyclosporine, azithromycin, sirolimus, and IVIG. Many patients also received combination therapy with biologics, including tumor necrosis factor alpha inhibitors, IL-1 blockers, rituximab, and abatacept, again with varying success reported. It should be noted that many patients were able to achieve symptom remission with combination therapies, but without preventing ILD progression.

Jakinibs are a relatively new drug class of small molecule inhibitors of JAKs, kinases that activate intracellular signaling in response to surface receptor engagement by cytokines. Type I interferon signaling, clearly elevated in the blood of patients with COPA syndrome, is modulated by baricitinib, ruxolitinib, and upadacitinib, all of which have been used in patients with COPA syndrome.

Baricitinib was reported to require higher dosing in pediatric patients with other interferonopathies (chronic atypical neutrophilic dermatosis with lipodystrophy and elevated temperature and SAVI).[44] Following this approach, *Krtuzke and colleagues* increased baricitinib dosing from 4 to 6 mg daily in a 10-year-old girl with refractory arthritis, resulting in rapid symptom resolution while the stabilization of lung disease occurred more gradually.[24] This patient had previously failed multiple agents in combination therapy that included corticosteroids, methotrexate (continued alongside baricitinib), golimumab, etanercept, adalimumab, abatacept, tocilizumab, rituximab, leflunomide, and azithromycin. Success with baricitinib has been subsequently reported for 2 more patients, one of whom transitioned to upadacitinib for unspecified reasons.[9,36]

Ruxolitinib was described in an 11-year-old girl with recurrent steroid-refractive severe alveolar hemorrhage failing the addition of hydroxychloroquine, azathioprine, mycophenolate mofetil, and cyclophosphamide. She was transitioned to ruxolitinib 0.25 mg/kg twice daily, with steroids weaned within 3 months and exercise intolerance resolving. She was able to avoid hospitalization, in stark contrast to prior severe exacerbations requiring ECMO, though she required brief steroid courses for 2 mild exacerbations. Careful examination showed ongoing alveolar hemorrhage, with PFTs initially reported to be stable[8] but with subsequent progression of fibrosis necessitating change to baricitinib and addition of IL-1 inhibition.[37]

In summary, patients may respond to standard immune suppression regimens, especially in the setting of life-threatening alveolar hemorrhage where other regimens have not been trialed. It is important to evaluate for occult progression of lung disease even when patients achieve disease control, with the consideration of escalation or change in therapy if identified. Jakinibs hold promise for COPA syndrome, at least in the short-term outcomes currently reported, though more clinical experience is needed before these can be broadly recommended. More robust results for jakinibs have been reported in SAVI, with most patients improving lung function though some patients did not respond or worsened.[45–47] In COPA syndrome it remains to be seen whether these can durably control disease manifestations, with treatment periods longer than 1 year needed to truly evaluate ILD.

STING inhibitors, which are in late phase clinical development, may be a more promising drug class when available, targeting not only interferon-dependent but also interferon-independent functions of STING. Another potential treatment approach worth exploring is the adjunct use of antifibrotics, whether nintedanib, which is FDA approved to slow the progression of scleroderma ILD[48] and, more broadly, of progressive pulmonary fibrosis,[49] or pirfenidone, which has been shown to slow ILD progression in rheumatoid arthritis ILD.[50]

DISCUSSION AND RECOMMENDATIONS FOR TESTING

COPA syndrome is a relatively new genetic disease of immune dysregulation with common features of high autoantibody titers, pulmonary disease, and arthritis. Diagnosis is confirmed via sequencing of *COPA*. In **Table 2**, we outline a framework for when to consider testing an individual with lung disease for COPA syndrome. Familial testing of at-risk healthy individuals should be considered once a mutation is identified

Table 2
When to consider genetic testing for COPA syndrome in a patient with lung disease

Pulmonary Features	Non-Pulmonary Features
1. Clinical: Diffuse Alveolar Hemorrhage	1. Early Age of Onset (<12 y)
2. Imaging: Cysts	2. Arthritis
3. Histology: Evidence of Follicular Bronchitis	3. Positive ANA, ANCA, and/or RF/CCP
	4. Family History of Lung Disease, Inflammatory Arthritis, or Glomerulonephritis

Consider testing:
At least 1 pulmonary and 2 non-pulmonary features -or- recurrent alveolar hemorrhage in infancy
Strongly consider testing:
At least 1 pulmonary and 3 non-pulmonary features

as there is a non-penetrance rate of at least 15%. Additional research is needed to inform the causes of disease non-penetrance. The hallmark of treatment is immune suppression, with active evaluation for progressive lung disease needed even if symptoms are otherwise controlled. Further understanding of COPA syndrome would benefit from patient registries to help clarify rates of disease prevalence and penetrance, to enrich the understanding of disease manifestations, and to guide treatments.

Many of the reported *COPA* mutations have not undergone experimental validation, and it remains to be determined whether all mutations cause disease through identical disease mechanisms. Future work is needed to characterize each reported mutation, including future novel variants obtained from sequencing additional individuals with lung disease.

SUMMARY

COPA syndrome is a recently described autosomal dominant inborn error of immunity characterized by high titer autoantibodies and interstitial lung disease, with many individuals also having arthritis and nephritis. Onset is usually in early childhood, with unique disease features including alveolar hemorrhage, which can be insidious, pulmonary cyst formation, and progressive pulmonary fibrosis in nonspecific interstitial pneumonia or lymphocytic interstitial pneumonia patterns. This review explores the clinical presentation, genetics, molecular mechanisms, organ manifestations, and treatment approaches for COPA syndrome, and presents a diagnostic framework of suggested indications for patient testing.

CLINICS CARE POINTS

- COPA syndrome is a rare autosomal dominant disorder characterized by high autoantibody levels and interstitial lung disease in the presence or absence of inflammatory arthritis and renal disease.
- Prominent pulmonary manifestations of COPA syndrome include cough, tachypnea/exercise intolerance, alveolar hemorrhage (which can be insidious), respiratory failure, and interstitial lung disease characterized by cysts, centrilobular nodules, and/or pulmonary fibrosis.
- Arthritis in COPA syndrome is indistinguishable from rheumatoid arthritis or juvenile arthritis.
- Immune suppression is critical for patients with COPA syndrome.
- JAK inhibitors may be an option to slow the progression of ILD, the most common cause of death for patients with COPA syndrome and typically the most refractory aspect of the disease.

DISCLOSURE

T.P. Vogel has consulted for Novartis, Pfizer, Moderna, and SOBI and receives research support from AstraZeneca.

ACKNOWLEDGMENTS

A.K. Shum is supported by NIH, United States grants R21AI160107 and R01AI168299, and the ATD/chILD, Canada, referring to the American Thoracic Society and to the

Children's Interstitial Lung Disease Foundation N. Simchoni is supported by NIH T32AR007304.

REFERENCES

1. Genomics BHC for M, Watkin LB, Jessen B, et al. COPA mutations impair ER-Golgi transport and cause hereditary autoimmune-mediated lung disease and arthritis. Nat Genet 2015;47(6):654–60.
2. Vece TJ, Watkin LB, Nicholas SK, et al. Copa Syndrome: a Novel Autosomal Dominant Immune Dysregulatory Disease. J Clin Immunol 2016;36(4):377–87.
3. Tsui JL, Estrada OA, Deng Z, et al. Analysis of pulmonary features and treatment approaches in the COPA syndrome. Erj Open Res 2018;4(2):00017–2018.
4. Brennan M, McDougall C, Walsh J, et al. G426 A Case report: Copa mutation – a new condition to consider with polyarthritis and interstitial lung disease. Arch Dis Child 2017;102(Suppl 1):A167.
5. Lepelley A, Martin-Niclós MJ, Bihan ML, et al. Mutations in COPA lead to abnormal trafficking of STING to the Golgi and interferon signaling. J Exp Med 2020;217(11):e20200600.
6. Khalifi SBE, Viel S, Lahoche A, et al. COPA Syndrome as a Cause of Lupus Nephritis. Kidney Int Reports 2019;4(8):1187–9.
7. Nathan N, Legendre M, Amselem S, et al. COPA syndrome restricted to life-threatening alveolar hemorrhages: clinical, pathological, molecular and biological characterization. Rare Ild Dpld 2018;PA2236. https://doi.org/10.1183/13993003.congress-2018.pa2236.
8. Frémond ML, Legendre M, Fayon M, et al. Use of ruxolitinib in COPA syndrome manifesting as life-threatening alveolar haemorrhage. Thorax 2020;75(1):92.
9. Kato T, Yamamoto M, Honda Y, et al. Augmentation of Stimulator of Interferon Genes–Induced Type I Interferon Production in COPA Syndrome. Arthritis Rheumatol 2021;73(11):2105–15.
10. Matsubayashi T, Yamamoto M, Takayama S, et al. Allograft dysfunction after lung transplantation for COPA syndrome: A case report and literature review. Mod Rheumatology Case Reports 2022;6(2):rxac004.
11. Nguyen HN, Salman R, Vogel TP, et al. Imaging findings of COPA Syndrome. Pediatr Radiol 2023;1–10. https://doi.org/10.1007/s00247-023-05600-1.
12. Taveira-DaSilva AM, Markello TC, Kleiner DE, et al. Expanding the phenotype of COPA syndrome: a kindred with typical and atypical features. J Med Genet 2019; 56(11):778–82.
13. Cabrera-Pérez JS, Branch J, Reyes A, et al. A Zebra at the Rodeo: Dyspnea, Hematuria, and a Family History of Arthritis. Arthrit Care Res 2022;74(2):165–70.
14. Zeng J, Hao J, Zhou W, et al. A Novel Mutation c.841C>T in COPA Syndrome of an 11-Year-Old Boy: A Case Report and Short Literature Review. Frontiers Pediatrics 2021;9:773112.
15. Li X, Tang Y, Zhang L, et al. Case report: COPA syndrome with interstitial lung disease, skin involvement, and neuromyelitis spectrum disorder. Frontiers Pediatrics 2023;11:1118097.
16. Delafontaine S, Bigley T, Iannuzzo A, et al. C-Terminal Domain COPA Mutations in Six Children From Three Unrelated Families With Autosomal Dominant COPA Syndrome. Gothenburg, Sweden on October 2022;12:2022.
17. Beshay S, Smith J, Osuna I, et al. Copa syndrome-associated mutations in lung transplant recipients for interstitial lung disease. Chest 2021;160(4):A1265–6.

18. Riddell P, Moshkelgosha S, Levy L, et al. IL-6 receptor blockade for allograft dysfunction after lung transplantation in a patient with COPA syndrome. Clin Transl Immunol 2021;10(2):e1243.
19. Jensson BO, Hansdottir S, Arnadottir GA, et al. COPA syndrome in an Icelandic family caused by a recurrent missense mutation in COPA. BMC Med Genet 2017; 18(1):129.
20. Banday AZ, Kaur A, Jindal AK, et al. Splice-site mutation in COPA gene and familial arthritis – a new frontier. Rheumatology 2020;60(1):e7–9.
21. Chen S, Francioli LC, Goodrich JK, et al. A genome-wide mutational constraint map quantified from variation in 76,156 human genomes. bioRxiv 2022;2022: 485034.
22. Rice GI, Rodero MP, Crow YJ. Human Disease Phenotypes Associated With Mutations in TREX1. J Clin Immunol 2015;35(3):235–43.
23. Volpi S, Tsui J, Mariani M, et al. Type I interferon pathway activation in COPA syndrome. Clin Immunol 2018;187:33–6.
24. Germany D of GP Centre for Paediatric Rheumatology, Clinic Sankt Augustin, Sankt Augustin, Krutzke S, Rietschel C, Germany D for PR Clementine Kinderhospital, Horneff G, Germany D of P and A medicine University Hospital of Cologne, Cologne. Baricitinib in therapy of COPA syndrome in a 15-year-old girl. European J Rheumatology 2019;7(1):78–81.
25. Bousfiha A, Moundir A, Tangye SG, et al. The 2022 Update of IUIS Phenotypical Classification for Human Inborn Errors of Immunity. J Clin Immunol 2022;42(7): 1508–20.
26. Rivara S, Ablasser A. COPA silences STING. J Exp Med 2020;217(11): e20201517.
27. Deng Z, Chong Z, Law CS, et al. A defect in COPI-mediated transport of STING causes immune dysregulation in COPA syndrome. J Exp Med 2020;217(11): e20201045.
28. Deng Z, Law CS, Ho FO, et al. A Defect in Thymic Tolerance Causes T Cell–Mediated Autoimmunity in a Murine Model of COPA Syndrome. J Immunol 2020;204(9):2360–73.
29. Mukai K, Ogawa E, Uematsu R, et al. Homeostatic regulation of STING by retrograde membrane traffic to the ER. Nat Commun 2021;12(1):61.
30. Steiner A, Hrovat-Schaale K, Prigione I, et al. Deficiency in coatomer complex I causes aberrant activation of STING signalling. Nat Commun 2022;13(1):2321.
31. Jeltema D, Abbott K, Yan N. STING trafficking as a new dimension of immune signaling. J Exp Med 2023;220(3):e20220990.
32. Frémond ML, Crow YJ. STING-Mediated Lung Inflammation and Beyond. J Clin Immunol 2021;41(3):501–14.
33. Crow YJ, Stetson DB. The type I interferonopathies: 10 years on. Nat Rev Immunol 2022;22(8):471–83.
34. Guan Y, Liu H, Tang X, et al. Effective sirolimus treatment of 2 COPA syndrome patients. J Allergy Clin Immunol Pract 2021;9(2):999–1001.e1.
35. Bader-Meunier B, Bustaffa M, Iskounen T, et al. Rheumatoid factor positive polyarticular juvenile idiopathic arthritis associated with a novel COPA mutation. Rheumatology 2020;60(5):e171–3.
36. Basile P, Gortani G, Taddio A, et al. A toddler with an unusually severe polyarticular arthritis and a lung involvement: a case report. BMC Pediatr 2022;22(1):639.
37. Frémond ML, Nathan N. COPA syndrome, 5 years after: Where are we? Joint Bone Spine 2021;88(2):105070.

38. Psarianos P, Kwan JYY, Dell S, et al. COPA Syndrome (Ala239Pro) Presenting with Isolated Follicular Bronchiolitis in Early Childhood: Case Report. J Clin Immunol 2021;41(7):1660–3.
39. Patwardhan A, Spencer CH. An unprecedented COPA gene mutation in two patients in the same family: comparative clinical analysis of newly reported patients with other known COPA gene mutations. Pediatric Rheumatology Online J 2019; 17(1):59.
40. Prenzel F, Harfst J, Schwerk N, et al. Lymphocytic interstitial pneumonia and follicular bronchiolitis in children: A registry-based case series. Pediatr Pulmonol 2020;55(4):909–17.
41. Mallea JM, Kornafeld A, Khoor A, et al. Lung Transplantation in a Patient with COPA Syndrome. Case Reports Transplant 2020;2020:3624795.
42. Valapour M, Lehr CJ, Schladt DP, et al. OPTN/SRTR 2021 Annual Data Report: Lung. Am J Transplant 2023;23(2):S379–442.
43. Thaivalappil SS, Garrod AS, Borowitz SM, et al. Persistent Unexplained Transaminitis in COPA Syndrome. J Clin Immunol 2021;41(1):205–8.
44. Kim H, Brooks KM, Tang CC, et al. Pharmacokinetics, Pharmacodynamics, and Proposed Dosing of the Oral JAK1 and JAK2 Inhibitor Baricitinib in Pediatric and Young Adult CANDLE and SAVI Patients. Clin Pharmacol Ther 2018; 104(2):364–73.
45. Sanchez GAM, Reinhardt A, Ramsey S, et al. JAK1/2 inhibition with baricitinib in the treatment of autoinflammatory interferonopathies. J Clin Invest 2018;128(7): 3041–52.
46. Frémond ML, Hadchouel A, Berteloot L, et al. Overview of STING-Associated Vasculopathy with Onset in Infancy (SAVI) Among 21 Patients. J Allergy Clin Immunol Pract 2021;9(2):803–18.e11.
47. Gómez-Arias PJ, Gómez-García F, Hernández-Parada J, et al. Efficacy and Safety of Janus Kinase Inhibitors in Type I Interferon-Mediated Monogenic Autoinflammatory Disorders: A Scoping Review. Dermatology Ther 2021;11(3): 733–50.
48. Distler O, Highland KB, Gahlemann M, et al. Nintedanib for Systemic Sclerosis–Associated Interstitial Lung Disease. New Engl J Med 2019;380(26):2518–28.
49. Flaherty KR, Wells AU, Cottin V, et al. Nintedanib in Progressive Fibrosing Interstitial Lung Diseases. New Engl J Med 2019;381(18):1718–27.
50. Solomon JJ, Danoff SK, Woodhead FA, et al. Safety, tolerability, and efficacy of pirfenidone in patients with rheumatoid arthritis-associated interstitial lung disease: a randomised, double-blind, placebo-controlled, phase 2 study. Lancet Respir Medicine 2023;11(1):87–96.
51. Brennan M, McDougall C, Walsh J, et al. COPA syndrome - a new condition to consider when features of polyarthritis and interstitial lung disease are present. Rheumatology 2017;56(suppl_6). https://doi.org/10.1093/rheumatology/kex356.059.
52. Noorelahi R, Perez G, Otero HJ. Imaging findings of Copa syndrome in a 12-year-old boy. Pediatr Radiol 2018;48(2):279–82.
53. Oliveira FR, Sciortino ADS, Nascimento Y, et al. Copa Syndrome in a 20-Year-Old Man: A Case Report. D23 Not Usual Suspects Case Reports Rare Lung Dis 2022;A5128. https://doi.org/10.1164/ajrccm-conference.2022.205.1_meetingabstracts.a5128.

NF-κB and Related Autoimmune and Autoinflammatory Diseases

George E. Freigeh, MD, MA[a,*], Thomas F. Michniacki, MD[b]

KEYWORDS

• NF-κB • Autoinflammation • Autoimmunity • Immunodeficiency
• Inborn errors of immunity

KEY POINTS

- The NF-κB pathway is a central signaling pathway involved in countless physiologic functions.
- Disruptions in the NF-κB pathway can cause any combination of autoimmunity, autoinflammation, immunodeficiency, and malignancy.
- New disease processes involving the NF-κB pathway are being continually defined and reported.

Nuclear factor kappa-light-chain-enhancer of activated B cells (NF-κB) is a protein family of transcription factors that is involved in a diverse range of cellular functions. NF-κB was first described over 35 years ago by Ranjan Sen and David Baltimore,[1] and since then has been implicated in hundreds of cellular pathways, especially in those impacting immune function and inflammation. Dysregulation of the NF-κB system can lead to immunodeficiency, autoimmunity, autoinflammation, malignancy, and any combination of these.

In this review, we briefly describe the normal physiologic function of NF-κB. Then, we describe the genetics and clinical manifestations of defined diseases grouped by the primary purpose of the affected gene in the NF-κB pathway. Finally, we briefly discuss therapeutics in NF-κB related syndromes.

NF-κB PATHWAYS

The NF-κB protein family consists of five proteins: NFKB1 (p105, p50), NFKB2 (p100, p52), RelA (p65), RelB, and c-Rel.[2] These proteins associate into 15 possible dimers,

[a] Division of Allergy and Clinical Immunology, Department of Internal Medicine, University of Michigan, Lobby H Suite 2100, 24 Frank Lloyd Wright Drive, Ann Arbor, MI 48105, USA; [b] Division of Hematology and Oncology, Department of Pediatrics, University of Michigan, 1522 Simpson Road East, Ann Arbor, MI 48109, USA
* Corresponding author.
E-mail address: gfreigeh@med.umich.edu

Rheum Dis Clin N Am 49 (2023) 805–823
https://doi.org/10.1016/j.rdc.2023.06.008 rheumatic.theclinics.com
0889-857X/23/

although only 13 are described.[3] The protein complex is ready-formed in the cytoplasm in an inactive state. This allows a rapid response to cellular damage and pathogen invasion without a need to be transcribed on demand. NF-κB signaling occurs through two primary pathways, classical and alternative. The classical pathway responds rapidly to a large number of cellular stimuli and is critical for inflammatory response and cell proliferation.[4] The main protein complex that directly regulates NF-κB in the classical pathway is IκB kinase, which consists of three proteins: IKKα, IKKβ, and nuclear factor-kappa B essential modulator (NEMO).[2] On activation, IκB kinase phosphorylates inhibitory proteins on the NF-κB complex, leading to their degradation and thus freeing NF-κB to enter the nucleus to begin cellular transcription.[4] Several NF-κB inhibitors are target genes of NF-κB transcription, allowing for tight regulatory feedback control of the pathway. In contrast, the alternative pathway is characteristically slower, and responds only to a handful of specific stimuli. The alternative pathway is typically associated with immune cell formation and lymphoid development.[4] NF-κB-inducing kinase (NIK) serves as the central regulator in the alternative pathway and is responsible for the phosphorylation of the NF-κB complex to allow nuclear entry.[4]

Several signaling pathways converge and/or intersect with NF-κB, including the tumor necrosis factor (TNF) family, toll-like receptor 4 (TLR4), and IL-1 receptor type I.[4] The primary end targets of NF-κB are genes that prevent apoptosis and promote cell survival and are involved in immune responses in both the innate and adaptive immune systems. Interference in any of these phases in the NF-κB pathway produce variable phenotypes dependent on where the disruption occurs. However, the complexity of the pathways and the functions of NF-κB are so diverse that gene mutations produce sometimes unexpected and paradoxic results. A focused overview of the NF-κB pathway can be found in **Fig. 1**.

NF-κB-RELATED AUTOIMMUNE AND AUTOINFLAMMATORY DISEASES

NF-κB Protein Complex

NFKB1

Heterozygous mutations in *NFKB1* are well described and are a leading monogenic cause of common variable immunodeficiency (CVID) and hypogammaglobulinemia in patients with European ancestry.[5] The mechanism is thought to be due to both an absolute reduction in B cells as well as impaired memory B cell generation.[5] Interestingly, there is variable penetrance of *NFKB1* variants. As with all CVID, the degree of immune compromise is variable, even in patients with the same mutation. Patients with CVID due to *NFKB1* are more likely to have extra immune manifestations of CVID and concomitant autoimmune disease, including immune-mediated cytopenias, autoimmune enteropathy, inflammatory bowel disease, and autoimmune thyroiditis.[6]

Recently defined mutations have demonstrated an increasing association with additional autoinflammatory diseases. These are associated with a variable level of immune compromise and infection burden. These autoinflammatory conditions include a Bechet's-like disease with aphthous ulcers, recurrent fever, and small vessel vasculitis; familial non-infectious necrotizing cellulitis; and non-specific systemic inflammation with recurrent fevers, vasculitis, and persistently elevated inflammatory markers.[7]

NFKB2

Autosomal dominant mutations in *NFKB2* also lead to CVID. Along with the known immunodeficiency manifestations of CVID, these patients have an increased risk of alopecia areata, nail dystrophy, and central adrenal insufficiency. The mechanism of adrenal insufficiency in particular is unknown.[8]

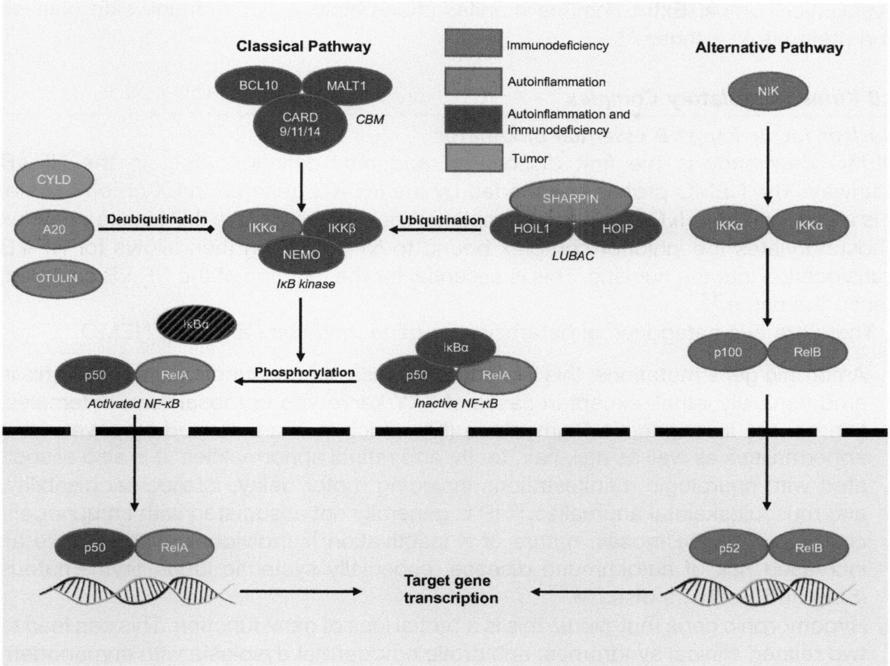

Fig. 1. Focused representation of the NF-κB pathway. Proteins are color coded by the primary type of disorder caused by defined gene mutations. In the classical pathway, the IκB kinase regulatory complex (NEMO, IKKα, IKKβ) phosphorylates the NF-κB protein complex (RelA, p50/NFKB1), causing dissociation and degradation of IκBα. This allows the NF-κB protein complex to enter the nucleus and promote target gene transcription. The LUBAC complex (SHARPIN, HOIL-1, HOIP) activates IκB activity via ubiquitination. The deubiquitinases (A20, OTULIN, CYLD) serve as downregulators of LUBAC and IκB kinase activity. The CBM complex (CARD protein, BCL10, MALT1) also serve as NF-κB activators. In the alternative pathway, NIK stimulates IKKα and activation of the NF-κB protein complex (RelB, p52/p100/NFKB2) allowing for nuclear translocation and target gene transcription. The classical pathway responds rapidly to cellular stimuli, whereas the alternative pathway is characteristically slower.

Of note, NFKB2 is a downstream target of B-cell activating factor (BAFF), which is as one of the key signaling molecules in the alternative pathway. NFKB2, along with c-Rel and RelB, serve as crucial mediators of BAFF-dependent B cell maturation.[9,10]

RelA

RELA mutations have been recently described in the literature and cause an autoinflammatory disorder termed RelA-associated autoinflammatory disease (RAID). Clinical manifestations of this disorder include oral and genital ulcers, rash, recurrent fever, colitis, and conjunctivitis.[11] A case series studying multiple members of the same family also demonstrated neuromyelitis optica.[12]

RelB

RELB mutations are extremely rare and have been described in the literature in only three individuals all from the same family.[13] Affected individuals have a primarily immunodeficiency phenotype with severe combined immunodeficiency (SCID) and dysplastic thymus. Extra immune manifestations include autoimmune skin disease and rheumatoid arthritis.[13]

IκB Kinase Regulatory Complex

Nuclear factor-kappa B essential modulator

NEMO deficiency is the first discovered and best-defined defect in the NF-κB pathway. The NEMO protein is encoded by the *IKBKG* gene on the X chromosome. It is a subunit of the IκB regulatory complex. When activated, the IkB kinase complex phosphorylates the inhibitor complex bound to NF-κB which then allows for NF-κB translocation into the nucleus. This is essential for the function of the NF-κB complex, hence the name.[14]

There are two categories of heterozygous gene mutations affecting NEMO.

1. Amorphic gene mutations: this is a complete loss of gene function. In males, this is embryonically lethal, except in cases of XXY karyotype or mosaicism. In females, this causes Incontinentia Pigmentosa (IP), which is characterized by severe skin abnormalities as well as nail, hair, teeth, and retinal abnormalities. It is also associated with neurologic manifestations including motor delay, intellectual disability, and musculoskeletal anomalies.[15] IP is generally not associated with immunodeficiency due to the mosaic nature of X inactivation.[16] Individuals with IP have an increased risk of autoimmune disease, especially systemic lupus erythematous (SLE) and Bechet's disease.[17]
2. Hypomorphic gene mutations: this is a partial loss of gene function. This can lead to two related clinical syndromes: anhidrotic ectodermal dysplasia with immunodeficiency (EDA-ID) or immunodeficiency without EDA. The location of the gene mutation typically determines which phenotype the patient presents with.[18] EDA-ID almost exclusively affects males, since a female with a heterozygous gene mutation typically has enough NEMO function from the wild type and hypomorphic alleles for appropriate NF-κB activity, although female carriers can sometimes have autoinflammatory manifestations such as oral ulcers due to skewed X inactivation.[19] A particularly well-described autoinflammatory association in EDA-ID is inflammatory colitis, sometimes referred to as "NEMO colitis." This is due to both dysfunctional gut immune cell activation and loss of NF-κB activity necessary for intrinsic epithelial function.[20] Interestingly, while hematopoietic stem cell transplant (HSCT) can be curative for the immunodeficiency seen in EDA-ID, colitis is unchanged or even worsened after transplant.[20]

EDA-ID is characterized by abnormalities in the ectodermal structures, including skin, nail, hair, and exocrine glands. Patients also have distinctive facies including frontal bossing, low nasal bridge, and sunken cheeks.[15] Extraimmune manifestations typically occur in more severe disease and include osteoporosis.[18,21]

Immune dysfunction effects both the innate and acquired immune systems, and patients are at increased risk of severe viral, bacterial, and mycobacterial infections. Patients with EDA-ID have impaired cellular responses to multiple immune mediators, including IL-1β, IL-18, TNF-α, and lipopolysaccharides. Interestingly, hypogammaglobulinemia occurs in only approximately half of patients, although they have impaired specific antibody responses.[18]

IKKα

IKKα is one of the 2 enzymatic subunits of the IκB regulatory complex. Previously described IKKα mutations have all been linked to fetal encasement syndrome which is embryonically lethal.[22] However, a more recent article[23] reported a consanguineous patient with a homozygous IKKα mutation leading to SCID, absent secondary lymphoid structures, and skeletal abnormalities.

IKKβ

IKKβ is the other enzymatic subunit of the IκB regulatory complex. Homozygous IKKβ deficiency leads to aSCID phenotype, with normal T and B cell development but impaired activation of mature cells. Patients with homozygous IKKβ mutations lack the extraimmune manifestations present in NEMO deficiency, implying that IKKα can compensate for some, but not all, of the functions of IKKβ.[22] Interestingly, there also exists patients with heterozygous gain of function mutations in IKKβ. Their clinical phenotype involves ectodermal dysplasia, severe combined immunodeficiency, premature cataracts, and progressive cystic lung changes and bronchiectasis.[24,25]

There is a recent report of a patient with a heterozygous gain of function variant in IKKβ associated mainly with autoimmunity and autoinflammation.[26] The patient presented with recurrent autoimmune hemolytic anemia, fevers, and inflammatory rash. Functional studies demonstrated increased levels of chemokines associated with monocyte and macrophage recruitment and activation. The patient's symptoms spontaneously resolved after age 3.

Linear Ubiquitin Chain Assembly Complex (LUBAC)

LUBAC is composed of three proteins: heme-oxidized IRP2 ubiquitin ligase-1 (HOIL-1), HOIL-1-interacting protein (HOIP), and Shank-associated RH domain-interacting protein (SHARPIN). This complex is responsible for the ubiquitination and thus the activation of NEMO and downstream NF-κB activity.[27]

HOIL-1

Autosomal recessive disease has been identified in 3 individuals from 2 different families.[28] These patients suffered from severe pyogenic bacterial infections. They also developed an autoinflammatory syndrome characterized by periodic fevers, hepatosplenomegaly, colitis, and concomitant increase in serum inflammatory markers (elevated CRP, thrombocytosis, and neutrophilia).[28] Interestingly, these patients also had muscular amylopectinosis, consisting of glycogen deposition in developed muscle with resultant cardiomyopathy and myopathy. This was the first instance of amylopectinosis associated with any inborn error of immunity.

Functional studies in patients with *HOIL-1* demonstrated reduced NF-κB activity and NF-κB-specific response to TNF and IL-1. However, hematopoietic cells showed hyperresponsiveness to IL-1 in these patients *ex vivo*, serving as a potential explanation for severe autoinflammation in the setting of immunodeficiency.[28]

HOIP

Two unrelated cases of *HOIP* deficiency are described in the literature. The first patient had a homozygous missense mutation and a similar phenotype as patients with *HOIL-1*. The second patient had a compound heterozygous mutation and the same immune phenotype without amylopectinosis.[29]

SHARPIN

SHARPIN deficient mice have been designated *chronic proliferative dermatitis in mice* (*cpdm*), characterized by severe inflammatory skin lesions, splenomegaly, absence of secondary lymphoid tissue, and hypogammaglobulinemia.[27] *SHARPIN* variants in humans have not previously been reported. However, an article in preprint[30] identifies the first reported human mutation in *SHARPIN*. The patient demonstrated an autoinflammatory phenotype similar to HOIL-1 and HOIP deficiency with less severe immunodeficiency and without the dermatologic manifestations seen in mouse models.

Deubiquitinases (DUBs)

There are several DUBs that provide negative feedback to downregulate NF-κB. The most clinically relevant of these include A20, Otulin, and CYLD. These proteins target M1 and K63 polyubiquitin chains on multiple NF-κB intermediates, including NEMO, LUBAC, and TNF receptor cytoplasmic constituents.[31] Thus, mutations affecting these genes lead to increased inflammatory processes and cellular proliferation. While the DUBs have largely overlapping substrates, defects lead to specific and variable phenotypes.

A20

A comprehensive case series of patients with A20 deficiency was published in 2018.[32] All patients experienced some combination of autoimmune and/or autoinflammatory symptoms and prior to the discovery of their A20 variants, they held diagnoses of juvenile idiopathic arthritis, Bechet's disease, SLE, and rheumatoid arthritis. All family members with haploinsufficiency that were sequenced were symptomatic, though the clinical presentation was heterogenous, even amongst family members with the same mutations. All patients experienced recurrent, painful, oral, genital, and/or gastrointestinal ulcers. Other common symptoms included colitis, polyarthritis, rash, and recurrent fever. Less common presentations included uveitis and pericardial effusion.

OTULIN

Homozygous mutations in *OTULIN* result in OTULIN-related autoinflammatory syndrome (ORAS) with a phenotype characterized by fever, panniculitis, and diarrhea. Patients can also have rashes, lipodystrophy, joint inflammation, and weight loss, as well as leukocytosis and neutrophilia.[33] As in A20 deficiency, these patients have elevated inflammatory markers and a similar cytokine profile with elevated TNF-a, IL-6, GCSF, and CXCL1.[33,34]

A recent case series published last year[35] demonstrated impaired immunity to *staphylococcus* alpha toxin in OTULIN haploinsufficient patients. This is thought to be due to the disruption of OTULIN and NF-κB function in skin fibroblasts.

CYLD

Interestingly, though OTULIN and A20 share many similar functions with CYLD as a DUB, *CYLD* mutations lead to tumor syndromes as opposed to autoinflammation. The mechanism for this divergence is not known.

CYLD mutations cause cylindromas, spiradenomas, and/or trichoepitheliomas involving the head, neck, face, and salivary glands. Though previously known by various names (Brooke-Spiegler syndrome, familial cylindromatosis, and multiple familial trichoepithelioma), the clinical spectrum of disease is now known as CYLD cutaneous syndrome. These tumors are typically benign, although malignant transformation has been reported in a minority of patients.[36]

CBM Complex

This is a protein complex consisting of a CARD protein, BCL10, and MALT1. The primary purpose of this complex is NF-κB activation. Gain of function mutations thus lead to constitutive NF-κB activation and malignancy, while loss of function mutations are associated with autoinflammatory syndromes and immunodeficiency.

BCL10 and MALT1

Loss of function mutations in BCL10 and MALT1 lead to combined immunodeficiency and autoimmune enteropathy.[20,37] MALT1 has also been associated with an IPEX-like syndrome combining immunodeficiency with severe eczema, enteropathy, and extremely elevated levels of immunoglobulin E.[20]

CARD9

CARD9 loss of function mutations result in invasive fungal disease. The mutation was first identified in a family with invasive candida infections involving the central nervous system, though more recent data indicate overall susceptibility to various fungal species.[38]

Interestingly, *CARD9* loss of function mutations do not seem to promote autoimmune and autoinflammatory diseases in mouse models. Conversely, certain polymorphisms that increase CARD9 activity have been associated with Crohn's disease.[38]

CARD11

CARD11 is the typical CARD protein associated with CBM.[4] *CARD11* mutations are associated with a wide spectrum of clinical disease dependent on the individual gene mutation and subsequent protein expression and activity.

1. Homozygous loss of function mutations lead to SCID.[39,40]
2. Hypomorphic dominant negative mutations with subsequent diminished, but not absent, protein expression lead to immunodeficiency, severe atopy, and are a recognized cause of Hyper IgE syndrome.[41]
3. *CARD11* gain of function mutations cause B cell expansion with NF-κB and T cell anergy (BENTA). These patients experience polyclonal B cell lymphocytosis, splenomegaly, and an increased risk of lymphoma.[39]

CARD14

Autosomal dominant *CARD14* mutations are associated with psoriasis and familial pityriasis ruba pilaris. Gene variants in *CARD14* are also associated with an increased risk of pustular psoriasis and psoriasis with arthritis.[42,43]

NF-κB Inhibitors

IκBα

The IκBα protein binds to the NF-κB protein complex resulting in cytoplasmic retention and thus inhibiting its function. Phosphorylation and ubiquitination of IκBα lead to its degradation and the propagation of the NF-κB pathway.[44]

Heterozygous dominant negative mutations have been described in humans causing phosphorylation resistant IκBα and lead to EDA-ID similar to NEMO deficiency.[45] As it is an autosomal mutation, this should especially be considered in females who present with EDA-ID.

Upstream Signaling Pathways

There are several upstream signaling pathways that do not directly act on the NF-κB protein complex, but rather upregulate or downregulate mediators that eventually converge on NF-κB and modulate its activity.

IL-36 receptor

IL-36 is an upstream activator of NF-κB, and the IL-36 receptor antagonist downregulates its function. Thus, deficiency in this antagonist leads to the inappropriate activation of the NF-κB pathway.[46]

Deficiency of interleukin-36 receptor antagonist (DITRA) is characterized by recurrent generalized pustular psoriasis (GPP) and fever. There have been approximately 200 reported cases of DITRA, mostly in Asia.[47] GPP in DITRA patients differs from non-monogenic causes of GPP in that DITRA patients usually have an earlier age of onset and high degree of systemic inflammation.[47]

Nucleotide-binding leucine-rich repeat-containing receptor 12 (NLRP12)

NLRP12 serves as a regulator of immune responses to pathogen invasion and cellular damage. Autosomal dominant loss of function mutations lead to decreased functional activity of NLRP12 and thus decreases the inhibition of NF-κB with increased levels of IL-1β and IL-18.[48]

The condition falls within the autoinflammatory category of disorders known as inflammasomopathies, with the mutation causing a clinical disease called familial cold autoinflammatory syndrome 2 (FCAS2) characterized by recurrent fever induced by cold temperatures. Patients have signs/symptoms of polyarthralgia/arthritis, abdominal pain and diarrhea, lymphadenopathy, splenomegaly, headache, neurosensory deafness, aphthous stomatitis, and rash.[48]

ALPK1

Retinal dystrophy, optic nerve edema, splenomegaly, anhidrosis, and headache (ROSAH) syndrome is a more recently described condition resulting from autosomal dominant mutations in the *ALPK1* gene. This gene encodes a protein that identifies bacterial sugars and leads to the downstream activation of NF-κB.[49]

ROSAH syndrome was originally identified as a form of familial blindness. Almost all patients experience some form of ophthalmologic dysfunction, including optic nerve elevation, uveitis, retinal vasculitis, and retinal degeneration.[49] However, recent cohort studies show that patients typically exhibit multiple autoinflammatory and autoimmune features, including episodic fevers, xerostomia with associated dental caries, arthritis, and episodic abdominal pain. These patients have an inflammatory signature demonstrating elevated CRP, IL-6, TNF-α, CXCL10, and CXCL1.[49]

NOD2

NOD2 belongs to the nucleotide-binding oligomerization domain (NOD)-like receptors (NLRs) family of proteins. NOD2 is an intracellular receptor that is activated in response to bacterial invasion. Among other functions, it serves as an activator of NF-κB.[50]

Certain *NOD2* polymorphisms have been strongly associated with inflammatory bowel disease, namely *R702 W*, *G908 R*, and *L1007PfsX2*.[51] Gain of function mutations are also associated with systemic inflammatory syndromes, including Blau syndrome and sarcoidosis. Blau syndrome (sometimes referred to as early onset sarcoidosis) is characterized by early onset of disease, typically before age 5. The classic triad of Blau syndrome includes granulomatous arthritis, uveitis, and rash.[52] There are over 30 known mutations in *NOD2* that lead to Blau syndrome, most commonly *R334 W* and *R334Q*.[52]

UBA1

Vacuoles, E1 enzyme, X-linked, autoinflammatory, somatic (VEXAS) is a newly defined disease process resulting from a heterozygous, loss of function mutation in the *UBA1* gene which encodes the UBA1 protein, an E1 ubiquitination protein necessary for the initial step in protein ubiquitination. In this disorder, aberrant ubiquitination leads to the unfolded protein response and ultimately an increased production of proinflammatory cytokines IL-6, TNF-α, IFN-γ. This in turn results in overstimulation of the NF-κB pathway.[53,54]

Table 1
Summary of NF-κB related conditions

Gene	Protein	Inheritance	Condition	Autoimmune/ Autoinflammatory Manifestations	Other Clinical Manifestations	Treatments	References
NFKB1	NFKB1	AD (LOF)	CVID, Bechet's-like disease, familial non-infectious necrotizing cellulitis	Immune-mediated cytopenias, autoimmune enteropathy, IBD, autoimmune thyroiditis, Bechet-like disease (aphthous ulcers, fevers, vasculitis), familial non-infectious necrotizing cellulitis	Immunodeficiency	Immunoglobulin replacement; corticosteroids	Tuijnenburg P et al,[5] 2018; Lorenzini T et al,[6] 2020; Kaustio M et al,[7] 2017
NFKB2	NFKB2	AD (LOF)	CVID	Alopecia areata, nail dystrophy, central adrenal insufficiency	Immunodeficiency	Immunoglobulin replacement	Shi C et al,[8] 2016
RELA	RelA	AD (LOF)	RAID (RelA-associated autoinflammatory disease)	Oral and genital ulcers, fever, rash, colitis, conjunctivitis	NMO	Corticosteroids; colchicine; etanercept; rituximab (NMO)	An JW et al,[11] 2023; Adeeb F et al,[12] 2021
RELB	RelB	AR	SCID	Autoimmune skin disease, rheumatoid arthritis	Immunodeficiency, FTT	Immunoglobulin replacement; HSCT	Sharfe N et al,[13] 2015

(continued on next page)

Table 1
(*continued*)

Gene	Protein	Inheritance	Condition	Autoimmune/ Autoinflammatory Manifestations	Other Clinical Manifestations	Treatments	References
IKBKG	NEMO	XL (amorphic)	Incontinentia Pigmentosa	Increased risk of SLE, Bechet's disease. Single case reports of macrophage activation syndrome, myasthenia gravis	Characteristic inflammatory skin changes, ophthalmologic abnormalities (retinal detachments, retinal vascular anomalies), neurologic abnormalities (seizures, intellectual disability, motor delay), malignancy (Wilm's tumor, retinoblastoma, squamous cell carcinoma)	Supportive	Maubach G et al,[14] 2017; Pescatore et al,[15] 2022; Ohnishi et al,[16] 2017; Gibson et al,[17] 2020
IKBKG	NEMO	XL (hypomorphic)	EDA-ID, Immunodeficiency without EDA	Autoinflammatory colitis (NEMO colitis)	Anhidrosis, immunodeficiency, ectodermal anomalies (skin, nail, hair) and distinctive facies (frontal bossing, low nasal bridge, sunken cheeks), osteoporosis	Immunoglobulin replacement; HSCT	Maubach G et al,[14] 2017; Pescatore et al,[15] 2022; Kawai T et al,[18] 2012; Surucu et al,[21] 2022; Miot C et al,[57] 2017
CHUK	IKKα	AR	SCID with congenital anomalies	Possibly associated with autoimmune enteropathy	Immunodeficiency, skeletal anomalies (fusion abnormalities, incomplete ossification), liver failure	Immunoglobulin replacement	Bainter W et al,[23] 2021

IKBKB	IKKβ	AR	SCID	N/A	Immunodeficiency	Immunoglobulin replacement; HSCT	Pannicke U et al,[22] 2013
IKBKB	IKKβ	AD (GOF)	Ectodermal dysplasia with immunodeficiency	Uveitis, infiltrative lung disease, inflammatory skin changes, autoimmune cytopenias	Immunodeficiency, ectodermal anomalies	Immunoglobulin replacement	Abbott J et al,[24] 2021; Cardinez C et al,[25] 2018; Sacco K et al,[26] 2023
HOIL1	HOIL-1	AR	Immunodeficiency with autoinflammation and amylopectinosis	Periodic fevers, inflammatory colitis	Immunodeficiency, amylopectinosis, FTT, hepatosplenomegaly	Immunoglobulin replacement; corticosteroids; TNF inhibitors (ineffective)	Boisson B et al,[28] 2012
HOIP	HOIP	AR; compound heterozygous	Immunodeficiency with autoinflammation with and without amylopectinosis	Periodic fevers, inflammatory colitis, inflammatory arthritis,	Immunodeficiency, amylopectinosis, severe eczema, lymphangiectasia,	Immunoglobulin replacement; corticosteroids; etanercept	Oda H et al,[29] 2019
SHARPIN	SHARPIN	AR	Sharpenia	Periodic fevers, inflammatory colitis, inflammatory arthritis, parotitis	Hypoplastic secondary lymphoid structures	Methotrexate (ineffective); etanercept; adalimumab	Oda H et al,[30] 2022
TNFAIP3	A20	AD (LOF)	Haploinsufficiency of A20	Oral, genital, and/or gastrointestinal ulcers, inflammatory colitis, inflammatory arthritis, recurrent rash, periodic fever, uveitis	Pericardial effusion, gynecologic abnormalities (irregular menses, possibly premature ovarian failure)	Corticosteroids; methotrexate; colchicine; infliximab; anakinra	Aeschlimann FA et al,[32] 2018
OTULIN	OTULIN	AR	ORAS (OTULIN-related autoinflammatory syndrome)	Periodic fever, panniculitis, inflammatory rash, inflammatory arthritis	FTT	Etanercept; infliximab; anakinra (ineffective); HSCT	Verboom L et al,[33] 2021; Damgaard RB et al,34 2016.
CYLD	CYLD	AD (GOF)	CYLD cutaneous syndrome	N/A	Cutaneous tumors (cylindromas, spiradenomas, trichoepitheliomas) appearing in the second/third decade of life	Supportive	Dubois A et al,[36] 2020

(*continued on next page*)

Table 1
(*continued*)

Gene	Protein	Inheritance	Condition	Autoimmune/ Autoinflammatory Manifestations	Other Clinical Manifestations	Treatments	References
BCL10	BCL10	AR	SCID	Autoimmune enteropathy	Immunodeficiency, FTT, secondary diffuse leukoencephalopathy	Immunoglobulin replacement	Torres JM et al,[37] 2014
MALT1	MALT1	AR	SCID, IPEX-like syndrome	Autoimmune enteropathy	Immunodeficiency, severe eczema, FTT, facial dysmorphia	Immunoglobulin replacement; HSCT	Charbit-Henrion F et al,[20] 2017
CARD9	CARD9	AR	Susceptibility to invasive fungal disease	N/A	Chronic mucocutaneous candidiasis, candida meningoencephalitis, deep dermatophytosis	Directed antifungal therapy	Liu X et al,[38] 2022
CARD11	CARD11	AR	SCID	N/A	FTT	Immunoglobulin replacement; HSCT	Béziat V et al. 2019; Greil et al. 2013
CARD11	CARD11	AD (LOF)	Combined immunodeficiency with atopy	Alopecia areata, bullous pemphigoid, autoimmune thrombocytopenic purpura, oral ulcers	Immunodeficiency, atopic propensity (eczema, food allergy, asthma), neutropenia (possibly autoimmune)	Various	Béziat V et al. 2019; Dorjbal B et al. 2019
CARD11	CARD11	AD (GOF)	BENTA (B-cell expansion with NF-κB and T cell Anergy)	N/A	Polyclonal lymphocytosis, splenomegaly, and increased risk of lymphoma	Various	Béziat V et al,[39] 2019
CARD14	CARD14	AD	Familial pityriasis ruba pilaris, psoriasis	Psoriasis and psoriasis associated with arthritis	N/A	Ustekinumab; methotrexate (varied response); etanercept (not effective)	Mellett M et al,[42] 2020; Craiglow BG et al,[43] 2018

NFKBIA	IκBα	AD	EDA-ID	Autoinflammatory colitis	Anhidrosis, immunodeficiency, ectodermal anomalies (skin, nail, hair) and distinctive facies (frontal bossing, low nasal bridge, sunken cheeks)	Immunoglobulin replacement; HSCT	Schimke LF et al,[44] 2013; Moriya K et al,[45] 2018
IL36RN	IL-36RA	AR	DITRA (deficiency of interleukin-36 receptor antagonist)	Recurrent generalized pustular psoriasis, recurrent fever	N/A	Various biologics targeting TNF-α, IL-17, IL-12/23, IL-1	Marrakchi S et al,[46] 2011; Hospach T et al,[47] 2019
NLRP12	NLRP12	AD	FCAS2 (familial cold autoinflammatory syndrome 2)	Recurrent fever induced by cold temperatures, arthritis, aphthous stomatitis, inflammatory rash	Splenomegaly, headache, neurosensory deafness, lymphadenopathy	Corticosteroids; colchicine (varied response); anakinra; canakinumab	Wang HF et al,[48] 2022
ALPK1	ALPK1	AD (GOF)	ROSAH (retinal dystrophy, optic nerve edema, splenomegaly, anhidrosis, and headache)	Recurrent fever, uveitis, retinal vasculitis, xerostomia and associated dental caries, inflammatory arthritis	Ocular disease (optic nerve elevation, retinal degeneration), recurrent abdominal pain, headaches, splenomegaly, premature cerebral mineralization, anhidrosis, agalactorrhea	Anakinra; adalimumab; tocilizumab (particularly for ocular manifestations)	Kozycki CT et al,[49] 2022
NOD2	NOD2	AD (GOF)	Blau syndrome	Uveitis, arthritis, and non-granulomatous skin rash, recurrent fever, vasculitis	Coarse facies, hepatosplenomegaly, hypertension	Corticosteroids; TNF inhibitors (infliximab, adalimumab); IL-1 and IL-6 inhibitors (varied response)	Kaufman KP et al,[52] 2021
UBA1	UBA1	Somatic (X chromosome)	VEXAS (vacuoles, E1 enzyme, X-linked,	Recurrent fever, cutaneous vasculitis,	Macrocytic anemia, thrombocytopenia,	Corticosteroids; ruxolitinib; HSCT;	Beck DB et al,[53] 2020;

(*continued on next page*)

Table 1
(continued)

Gene	Protein	Inheritance	Condition	Autoimmune/ Autoinflammatory Manifestations	Other Clinical Manifestations	Treatments	References
			autoinflammatory, somatic)	neutrophilic dermatosis, ear and nose chondritis, pulmonary involvement (interstitial pneumonia, bronchiolitis obliterans), arthritis	increased risk of hematologic malignancy especially myelodysplastic syndrome, sensorineural hearing loss	IL-1 inhibitors avoided due to paradoxic cutaneous reactions	Koster MJ et al,[55] 2022; Koster MJ et al,[56] 2021;

Abbreviations: AD, autosomal dominant; AR, autosomal recessive; CVID, combined variable immunodeficiency; EDA-ID, anhidrotic ectodermal dysplasia with immunodeficiency; FTT, failure to thrive; GOF, gain of function; HSCT, hematopoietic stem cell transplant; IBD, inflammatory bowel disease; LOF, loss of function; NMO, neuromyelitis optica; SCID, severe combined immunodeficiency; XL, X-linked.

This syndrome is unique in this review as it arises exclusively from somatic mutations. It generally affects patients over the age of 50. The *UBA1* gene is on the X chromosome, and so it almost entirely affects males.[54]

The clinical syndrome is characterized by severe autoinflammation, including recurrent fever, cutaneous involvement (cutaneous vasculitis, neutrophilic dermatosis), ear and nose chondritis, pulmonary involvement (interstitial pneumonia, bronchiolitis obliterans, cryptogenic organizing pneumonia, bronchial vessel vasculitis), sensorineural hearing loss, and arthritis.[55] It is important to note that many patients with VEXAS meet diagnostic criteria for other rheumatologic diseases, especially relapsing polychondritis.[55]

Patients with VEXAS also develop hematologic disease, typically macrocytic anemia and thrombocytopenia with an increased risk of hematologic malignancy. Many patients go on to develop myelodysplastic syndrome.[55,56] VEXAS is an aggressive condition with high mortality.[56] It is an emerging disease, having first been defined in 2020, though there have been hundreds of patients diagnosed since.

THERAPEUTICS

Treatment of NF-κB related syndromes is understandably complicated given the centrality of the pathway to countless cellular functions. In general, the clinical manifestations of NF-κB syndromes are treated similarly to other rheumatologic and immunologic disease through usage of immunosuppressive and immunomodulatory therapies. Accordingly, immunodeficiencies such as in NEMO deficiency or NFKB1-associated CVID are treated with supplemental immunoglobulins with or without prophylactic antibiotics.[3] Severe NEMO deficiency in particular is currently being treated increasingly with HSCT.[57] Autoimmunity and autoinflammation in NF-κB syndromes typically respond partially/temporarily to corticosteroid therapy.[58] As monoclonal antibody therapies are becoming more widespread in use, these have also been applied to the treatment of NF-κB syndromes. Further details of specific therapies reported in the literature for each disease can be found in **Table 1**.

SUMMARY

NF-κB is at the intersection of a number of diverse cellular pathways integral to innumerable physiologic functions. Beyond its involvement in immune regulation, there is data implicating its connection to a myriad of processes including obesity,[59] preeclampsia,[60] depression,[61] and addiction.[62] New diseases involving NF-κB continue to be discovered and elucidate further the intersection of immunodeficiency, autoimmunity, and autoinflammation.

CLINICS CARE POINTS

- NF-κB is implicated in a growing body of disorders encompassing autoimmunity, autoinflammation, and immunodeficiency. Often, pathway defects lead to presentations that cross disease categories.
- The first subspecialist a patient with an NF-κB pathway defect may come to is a rheumatologist, and the practicing clinician should be familiar with the common presentations of defined NF-κB diseases.
- Evaluation of these patients is often multidisciplinary, given the broad range of symptomatology. Patients presenting with features of autoimmunity and autoinflammation should undergo evaluation for NF-κB disorders.

DISCLOSURE

There are no commercial or financial conflicts of interest to disclose. No funding sources were utilized in the creation of this article.

REFERENCES

1. Sen R, Baltimore D. Inducibility of kappa immunoglobulin enhancer-binding protein Nf-kappa B by a posttranslational mechanism. Cell 1986;47(6):921–8.
2. Li Q, Verma IM. NF-kappaB regulation in the immune system. Nat Rev Immunol 2002;2(10):725–34.
3. Zhang Q, Lenardo MJ, Baltimore D. 30 years of NF-κB: a blossoming of relevance to human pathobiology. Cell 2017;168(1–2):37–57.
4. Yu H, Lin L, Zhang Z, et al. Targeting NF-κB pathway for the therapy of diseases: mechanism and clinical study. Signal Transduct Target Ther 2020;5(1):1–23.
5. Tuijnenburg P, Lango Allen H, Burns SO, et al. Loss-of-function nuclear factor κB subunit 1 (NFKB1) variants are the most common monogenic cause of common variable immunodeficiency in Europeans. J Allergy Clin Immunol 2018;142(4): 1285–96.
6. Lorenzini T, Fliegauf M, Klammer N, et al. Characterization of the clinical and immunologic phenotype and management of 157 individuals with 56 distinct heterozygous NFKB1 mutations. J Allergy Clin Immunol 2020;146(4):901–11.
7. Kaustio M, Haapaniemi E, Göös H, et al. Damaging heterozygous mutations in NFKB1 lead to diverse immunologic phenotypes. J Allergy Clin Immunol 2017; 140(3):782–96.
8. Shi C, Wang F, Tong A, et al. NFKB2 mutation in common variable immunodeficiency and isolated adrenocorticotropic hormone deficiency. Medicine (Baltim) 2016;95(40):e5081.
9. De Silva NS, Anderson MM, Carette A, et al. Transcription factors of the alternative NF-κB pathway are required for germinal center B-cell development. Proc Natl Acad Sci 2016;113(32):9063–8.
10. Almaden JV, Liu YC, Yang E, et al. B-cell survival and development controlled by the coordination of NF-κB family members RelB and cRel. Blood 2016;127(10): 1276–86.
11. An JW, Pimpale-Chavan P, Stone DL, et al. Case report: Novel variants in RELA associated with familial Behcet's-like disease. Front Immunol 2023;14:1127085.
12. Adeeb F, Dorris ER, Morgan NE, et al. A Novel RELA Truncating Mutation in a Familial Behçet's Disease–like Mucocutaneous Ulcerative Condition. Arthritis Rheumatol 2021;73(3):490–7.
13. Sharfe N, Merico D, Karanxha A, et al. The effects of RelB deficiency on lymphocyte development and function. J Autoimmun 2015;65:90–100.
14. Maubach G, Schmädicke AC, Naumann M. NEMO Links Nuclear Factor-κB to Human Diseases. Trends Mol Med 2017;23(12):1138–55.
15. Pescatore A, Spinosa E, Casale C, et al. Human Genetic Diseases Linked to the Absence of NEMO: An Obligatory Somatic Mosaic Disorder in Male. Int J Mol Sci 2022;23(3):1179.
16. Ohnishi H, Kishimoto Y, Taguchi T, et al. Immunodeficiency in Two Female Patients with Incontinentia Pigmenti with Heterozygous NEMO Mutation Diagnosed by LPS Unresponsiveness. J Clin Immunol 2017;37(6):529–38.
17. Gibson DC, Couser NL, King KB. Co-occurrence of incontinentia pigmenti and down syndrome: examining patients' potential susceptibility to autoimmune

disease, autoinflammatory disease, cancer, and significant ocular disease. Ophthalmic Genet 2021;42(1):92–5.

18. Kawai T, Nishikomori R, Heike T. Diagnosis and treatment in anhidrotic ectodermal dysplasia with immunodeficiency. Allergol Int Off J Jpn Soc Allergol 2012;61(2):207–17.
19. Kohn LL, Braun M, Cordoro KM, et al. Skin and Mucosal Manifestations in NEMO Syndrome: A Case Series and Literature Review. Pediatr Dermatol 2022;39(1): 84–90.
20. Charbit-Henrion F, Jeverica AK, Bègue B, et al. Deficiency in Mucosa-associated Lymphoid Tissue Lymphoma Translocation 1: A Novel Cause of IPEX-Like Syndrome. J Pediatr Gastroenterol Nutr 2017;64(3):378–84.
21. Surucu Yilmaz N, Bilgic Eltan S, Kayaoglu B, et al. Low Density Granulocytes and Dysregulated Neutrophils Driving Autoinflammatory Manifestations in NEMO Deficiency. J Clin Immunol 2022;42(3):582–96.
22. Pannicke U, Baumann B, Fuchs S, et al. Deficiency of innate and acquired immunity caused by an IKBKB mutation. N Engl J Med 2013;369(26):2504–14.
23. Bainter W, Lougaris V, Wallace JG, et al. Combined immunodeficiency with autoimmunity caused by a homozygous missense mutation in inhibitor of nuclear factor κB kinase alpha (IKKα). Sci Immunol 2021;6(63):eabf6723.
24. Abbott J, Ehler AC, Jayaraman D, et al. Heterozygous IKKβ activation loop mutation results in a complex immunodeficiency syndrome. J Allergy Clin Immunol 2021;147(2):737–40.e6.
25. Cardinez C, Miraghazadeh B, Tanita K, et al. Gain-of-function IKBKB mutation causes human combined immune deficiency. J Exp Med 2018;215(11):2715–24.
26. Sacco K, Kuehn HS, Kawai T, et al. A Heterozygous Gain-of-Function Variant in IKBKB Associated with Autoimmunity and Autoinflammation. J Clin Immunol 2023;43(2):512–20.
27. Tokunaga F. Linear ubiquitination-mediated NF-κB regulation and its related disorders. J Biochem (Tokyo) 2013;154(4):313–23.
28. Boisson B, Laplantine E, Prando C, et al. Immunodeficiency, autoinflammation and amylopectinosis in humans with inherited HOIL-1 and LUBAC deficiency. Nat Immunol 2012;13(12):1178–86.
29. Oda H, Beck DB, Kuehn HS, et al. Second Case of HOIP Deficiency Expands Clinical Features and Defines Inflammatory Transcriptome Regulated by LUBAC. Front Immunol 2019;10:479.
30. Oda H, Manthiram K, Chavan PP, et al. Human LUBAC deficiency leads to autoinflammation and immunodeficiency by dysregulation in TNF-mediated cell death. Published online November 14, 2022:2022. doi:10.1101/2022.11.09.22281431.
31. Lork M, Verhelst K, Beyaert RCYLD. A20 and OTULIN deubiquitinases in NF-κB signaling and cell death: so similar, yet so different. Cell Death Differ 2017;24(7): 1172–83.
32. Aeschlimann FA, Batu ED, Canna SW, et al. A20 haploinsufficiency (HA20): clinical phenotypes and disease course of patients with a newly recognised NF-kB-mediated autoinflammatory disease. Ann Rheum Dis 2018;77(5):728–35.
33. Verboom L, Hoste E, van Loo G. OTULIN in NF-κB signaling, cell death, and disease. Trends Immunol 2021;42(7):590–603.
34. Damgaard RB, Walker JA, Marco-Casanova P, et al. The Deubiquitinase OTULIN Is an Essential Negative Regulator of Inflammation and Autoimmunity. Cell 2016; 166(5):1215–30.e20.

35. Spaan AN, Neehus AL, Laplantine E, et al. Human OTULIN haploinsufficiency impairs cell-intrinsic immunity to staphylococcal α-toxin. Science 2022;376(6599): eabm6380.
36. Dubois A, Rajan N. CYLD cutaneous syndrome. In: Adam MP, Mirzaa GM, Pagon RA, et al, editors. GeneReviews®. Seattle: University of Washington; 2020. 1993-2023. http://www.ncbi.nlm.nih.gov/books/NBK555820/. 1993-2023.
37. Torres JM, Martinez-Barricarte R, García-Gómez S, et al. Inherited BCL10 deficiency impairs hematopoietic and nonhematopoietic immunity. J Clin Invest 2014;124(12):5239–48.
38. Liu X, Jiang B, Hao H, et al. CARD9 Signaling, Inflammation, and Diseases. Front Immunol 2022;13:880879.
39. Béziat V, Jouanguy E, Puel A. Dominant negative CARD11 mutations: Beyond atopy. J Allergy Clin Immunol 2019;143(4):1345–7.
40. Greil J, Rausch T, Giese T, et al. Whole-exome sequencing links caspase recruitment domain 11 (CARD11) inactivation to severe combined immunodeficiency. J Allergy Clin Immunol 2013;131(5):1376–83.e3.
41. Dorjbal B, Stinson JR, Ma CA, et al. Hypomorphic caspase activation and recruitment domain 11 (CARD11) mutations associated with diverse immunologic phenotypes with or without atopic disease. J Allergy Clin Immunol 2019;143(4): 1482–95.
42. Mellett M. Regulation and dysregulation of CARD14 signalling and its physiological consequences in inflammatory skin disease. Cell Immunol 2020;354:104147.
43. Craiglow BG, Boyden LM, Hu R, et al. CARD14-associated papulosquamous eruption: A spectrum including features of psoriasis and pityriasis rubra pilaris. J Am Acad Dermatol 2018;79(3):487–94.
44. Schimke LF, Rieber N, Rylaarsdam S, et al. A novel gain-of-function IKBA mutation underlies ectodermal dysplasia with immunodeficiency and polyendocrinopathy. J Clin Immunol 2013;33(6):1088–99.
45. Moriya K, Sasahara Y, Ohnishi H, et al. IKBA S32 Mutations Underlie Ectodermal Dysplasia with Immunodeficiency and Severe Noninfectious Systemic Inflammation. J Clin Immunol 2018;38(5):543–5.
46. Marrakchi S, Guigue P, Renshaw BR, et al. Interleukin-36–Receptor Antagonist Deficiency and Generalized Pustular Psoriasis. N Engl J Med 2011;365(7):620–8.
47. Hospach T, Glowatzki F, Blankenburg F, et al. Scoping review of biological treatment of deficiency of interleukin-36 receptor antagonist (DITRA) in children and adolescents. Pediatr Rheumatol Online J 2019;17:37.
48. Wang HF. NLRP12-associated systemic autoinflammatory diseases in children. Pediatr Rheumatol Online J 2022;20(1):9.
49. Kozycki CT, Kodati S, Huryn L, et al. Gain-of-function mutations in ALPK1 cause an NF-κB-mediated autoinflammatory disease: functional assessment, clinical phenotyping and disease course of patients with ROSAH syndrome. Ann Rheum Dis 2022;81(10):1453–64.
50. Hugot JP, Chamaillard M, Zouali H, et al. Association of NOD2 leucine-rich repeat variants with susceptibility to Crohn's disease. Nature 2001;411(6837):599–603.
51. Girardelli M, Loganes C, Pin A, et al. Novel NOD2 Mutation in Early-Onset Inflammatory Bowel Phenotype. Inflamm Bowel Dis 2018;24(6):1204–12.
52. Kaufman KP, Becker ML. Distinguishing Blau Syndrome from Systemic Sarcoidosis. Curr Allergy Asthma Rep 2021;21(2):10.
53. Beck DB, Ferrada MA, Sikora KA, et al. Somatic Mutations in UBA1 and Severe Adult-Onset Autoinflammatory Disease. N Engl J Med 2020;383(27):2628–38.

54. Rodolfi S, Nasone I, Folci M, et al. Autoinflammatory manifestations in adult patients. Clin Exp Immunol 2022;210(3):295–308.
55. Koster MJ, Samec MJ, Warrington KJ. VEXAS Syndrome—A Review of Pathophysiology, Presentation, and Prognosis. JCR J Clin Rheumatol 2022. https://doi.org/10.1097/RHU.0000000000001905.
56. Koster MJ, Warrington KJ. VEXAS within the spectrum of rheumatologic disease. Semin Hematol 2021;58(4):218–25.
57. Miot C, Imai K, Imai C, et al. Hematopoietic stem cell transplantation in 29 patients hemizygous for hypomorphic IKBKG/NEMO mutations. Blood 2017;130(12):1456–67.
58. Gupta SC, Sundaram C, Reuter S, et al. Inhibiting NF-κB activation by small molecules as a therapeutic strategy. Biochim Biophys Acta 2010;1799(10–12):775–87.
59. Nisr RB, Shah DS, Ganley IG, et al. Proinflammatory NFkB signalling promotes mitochondrial dysfunction in skeletal muscle in response to cellular fuel overloading. Cell Mol Life Sci CMLS 2019;76(24):4887–904.
60. Sakowicz A, Hejduk P, Pietrucha T, et al. Finding NEMO in preeclampsia. Am J Obstet Gynecol 2016;214(4):538.e1–7.
61. Caviedes A, Lafourcade C, Soto C, et al. BDNF/NF-κB Signaling in the Neurobiology of Depression. Curr Pharm Des 2017;23(21):3154–63.
62. Nennig SE, Schank JR. The Role of NFkB in Drug Addiction: Beyond Inflammation. Alcohol Alcohol Oxf Oxfs 2017;52(2):172–9.

Expanding IPEX: Inborn Errors of Regulatory T Cells

Holly Wobma, MD, PhD[a], Erin Janssen, MD, PhD[b,*]

KEYWORDS

- Regulatory T cells • Tregopathy • Autoimmune disease
- Primary immune regulatory disorder • Inborn error of immunity • IPEX
- Stem cell transplantation • Gene therapy

KEY POINTS

- Tregopathies often present with early-onset polyautoimmunity, increased infections, and atopic disease. There may be a positive family history of related, but not identical symptoms.
- Genetic testing should be pursued in patients with suspicion for Tregopathies or those with polyautoimmunity and poor responses to established treatments.
- Hematopoietic cell transplantation is the only curative treatment for patients with a Tregopathy, although gene therapies are in development.
- Agents that enhance Treg activity, such as rapamycin, or partially "substitute" for a Treg deficiency, such as CTLA4-Ig, may be effective for certain autoimmune manifestations.

INTRODUCTION

Regulatory T cells (Tregs) play a crucial role in enforcing immune tolerance in the periphery, preventing the activation of autoreactive cells, production of autoantibodies, and development of autoimmune and allergic diseases. Through both cell contact-dependent and independent mechanisms, Tregs downmodulate responses of autoreactive T and B cells, shift antigen presenting cells (APCs) from being immune stimulatory to tolerogenic, and achieve their agenda of maintaining immune tolerance.[1] It is thus not surprising that disorders of Tregs, or "Tregopathies," lead to widespread immune dysfunction. In this review, we focus on monogenic inborn errors of immunity (IEIs) leading to impaired Treg development, stability, and function with subsequent immune dysregulation. These conditions may present throughout life with autoimmune, atopic, and infectious manifestations.

[a] Division of Immunology, Boston Children's Hospital, 300 Longwood Avenue, Boston, MA 02115, USA; [b] Department of Pediatrics, Division of Pediatric Rheumatology, Michigan Medicine, C.S. Mott Children's Hospital, 1500 East Medical Center Drive, SPC 5718, Ann Arbor, MI 48109, USA
* Corresponding author.
E-mail address: ejanssen@med.umich.edu

Rheum Dis Clin N Am 49 (2023) 825–840
https://doi.org/10.1016/j.rdc.2023.06.009
rheumatic.theclinics.com

IPEX SYNDROME, THE "CLASSIC" TREGOPATHY

The first well-described Tregopathy, Immunodysregulation, polyendocrinopathy, enteropathy, X-linked (IPEX) syndrome, is caused by hemizygous mutations in *FOXP3,* the lineage defining transcriptional regulator in Tregs.[2] FOXP3 expression leads to the upregulation of the high affinity Interleukin-2 (IL-2) receptor containing CD25 (IL-2Rα) as well as CTLA-4, and it suppresses expression of certain cell cycle and cytokine genes (including the *IL2* gene).[3–5] This expression profile is important for the differentiation and suppressive function of Tregs.[4,6,7]

IPEX syndrome was first described by Powell and colleagues in 1982.[8] In an extended family, numerous boys died in infancy with profound secretory diarrhea as well as type I diabetes (T1D), anemia, atopic dermatitis, and recurrent infections. Based on the family pedigree, an X-linked inheritance pattern was suggested.[8] In 2000, pathogenic variants in the *FOXP3* gene were found to be associated with IPEX.[9–11]

Most patients with IPEX syndrome present in infancy with a combination of autoimmune and atopic manifestations, with autoimmune enteropathy, T1D, and atopic dermatitis being the classic triad.[12] Other manifestations may include autoimmune cytopenias, thyroid disease, adrenal insufficiency, hepatitis, arthritis, alopecia, and food allergies. Neurologic and renal abnormalities have also been reported[12,13] (**Table 1**). Serious infections are common, especially staphylococcal, viral, and fungal infections. This may be, in part, due to a breakdown of the barrier of the gastrointestinal tract and skin.[13]

The myriad of allergic and autoimmune manifestations in patients with IPEX syndrome dramatically illustrates the importance of Tregs in controlling the immune system. Since the identification of *FOXP3* variants associated with the development of IPEX syndrome, several IEIs reviewed here have been identified that affect Treg development, stability, and function.

IPEX syndrome has also served a model for the treatment of Tregopathies, with experience reported on the use of small molecules, biologic agents, hematopoietic cell transplantation (HCT), and now one of the first gene therapy trials for a Tregopathy.[14]

ADDITIONAL DISORDERS OF TRANSCRIPTION FACTORS LEADING TO TREGOPATHIES

In addition to FOXP3, other transcription factors have been identified that are important for Treg differentiation and/or function, and deficiencies of these transcription factors are associated with autoimmune disease (**Fig. 1**A).

BACH2 Deficiency

BACH2 is a transcription factor that is important for T cell differentiation[15] and B cell class switching and somatic hypermutation.[16] BACH2 expression stabilizes Tregs, promoting their survival and high expression of FOXP3.[17] BACH2 can also downmodulate signals through the IL-2R, coordinating the myriad of signals important for Treg homeostasis.[18]

Haploinsufficiency of BACH2 results in BACH2-related immunodeficiency and autoimmunity (BRIDA). Patients from 2 families with BRIDA and *Bach2*$^{-/+}$ mice have hypogammaglobulinemia with impaired responses to immunization and reduced percentages of memory B cells. Consistent with a pattern of poor B cell differentiation, increased infections have been reported in patients with BRIDA. In addition, the reported patients developed colitis. They also have a significant reduction in the percentage of FOXP3^{+} Tregs compared with healthy individuals.[16]

Table 1
Features associated with reported Tregopathies

	Year Described	Gene	Inheritance	Infection	Allergy	Autoimmunity	Lympho-Proliferation	Malignancy	Other/Notable	Targeted Therapy
Disorders of Treg Transcriptional Programs										
IPEX Syndrome	1982	FOXP3	XL	Bacterial, viral, fungal	Atopic dermatitis, asthma, food allergy	Cytopenias, alopecia, T1D, hypoparathyroidism, ILD, neurologic, kidney	Yes		Often presents by 2 mo of age	Gene therapy (clinical trial)
BRIDA	2017	BACH2	AD	Recurrent sinopulmonary infection	Not reported	Colitis	Yes			
Ikaros Gain-of-Function (GOF)	2021	Ikaros	AD, incomplete penetrance	Sinopulmonary infections; otitis media	Asthma, allergic rhinitis, eosinophilic esophagitis, dermatitis, food allergy	Cytopenias, alopecia, vitiligo, T1D, thyroid disease, hepatitis, celiac disease, colitis	Yes			IL-2 (Future?)
Disorders of IL-2 Signaling										
IL2Ra (CD25) Deficiency	1997	IL2RA	AR	Sinopulmonary infections; chronic CMV	Atopic dermatitis, asthma	Cytopenias, alopecia, psoriasiform dermatitis, thyroid disease, T1D, enteropathy	Yes		No CD25+ cells on flow cytometry	IL-2 (Future?)
IL2Rb (CD122) Deficiency	2019	IL2RB	AR	Otitis media, sinopulmonary, GI, and urinary infections, CMV, EBV	Dermatitis, food allergy	Cytopenias, ANCA vasculitis, thyroid disease, enteropathy	Yes		IUGR in some; high IgG	IL-2 (Future?)
STAT5b Deficiency	2006	STAT5B	AR	Recurrent respiratory infection, varicella/zoster, PJP	Atopic dermatitis	Cytopenias, thyroid disease, enteropathy, arthritis, ILD			Severe short stature, delayed puberty, severe pulmonary disease	

(*continued on next page*)

Table 1
(continued)

	Year Described	Gene	Inheritance	Infection	Allergy	Autoimmunity	Lympho-Proliferation	Malignancy	Other/Notable	Targeted Therapy
Disorders of CTLA-4 Surface Expression										
CTLA4 Haploinsufficiency	2014	CTLA4	AD, incomplete penetrance	CVID, sinopulmonary infection, EBV, CMV	Atopic dermatitis	Cytopenias, alopecia, thyroid disease, T1D, enteropathy, ILD, arthritis, psoriasis, vasculitis, neurologic, kidney	Yes	Lymphoma and gastric cancer (small subset)		CTLA4-Ig
LRBA Deficiency	2012	LRBA	AR	CVID, viral, bacterial, and fungal infections	Atopic dermatitis	Cytopenias, alopecia, thyroid disease, T1D, enteropathy, ILD, arthritis, psoriasis, vitiligo, vasculitis, uveitis, neurologic	Yes	Gastric cancer, melanoma, astrocytic tumor, CNS lymphoma described (small subset)		CTLA4-Ig
DEF6 Deficiency	2019	DEF6	AR	Bacterial, viral	Not reported	Cytopenias, enteropathy	Not reported			CTLA4-Ig
Disorders of the Cytoskeleton										
WAS	1937	WASP	XL	Bacterial, viral	Atopic dermatitis	Cytopenias, arthritis, vasculitis, IgA nephropathy, dermatomyositis, uveitis	Possible	Viral driven malignancy	Thrombocytopenia with small platelets	Gene therapy
DOCK8 Deficiency	2009	DOCK8	AR	Severe cutaneous and visceral viral infections, staphylococcal skin infections, opportunistic bacterial and fungal infections	Atopic dermatitis, asthma, eosinophilic esophagitis, food allergy	Cytopenias, thyroid disease, enteropathy, uveitis, vasculitis, SLE	Possible	Viral-driven malignancy	High IgE with eosinophilia, severe infections	
DOCK11 Deficiency	2023	DOCK11	XL	Not reported	Not reported	Cytopenias, SLE, RF + arthritis, colitis, panniculitis, oral ulcers	Not reported	Not reported		

Abbreviations: AD, autosomal dominant; AR, autosomal recessive; ILD, interstitial lung disease; IUGR, intrauterine growth restriction; RF, rheumatoid factor; SLE, systemic lupus erythematosus; XL, X-linked.

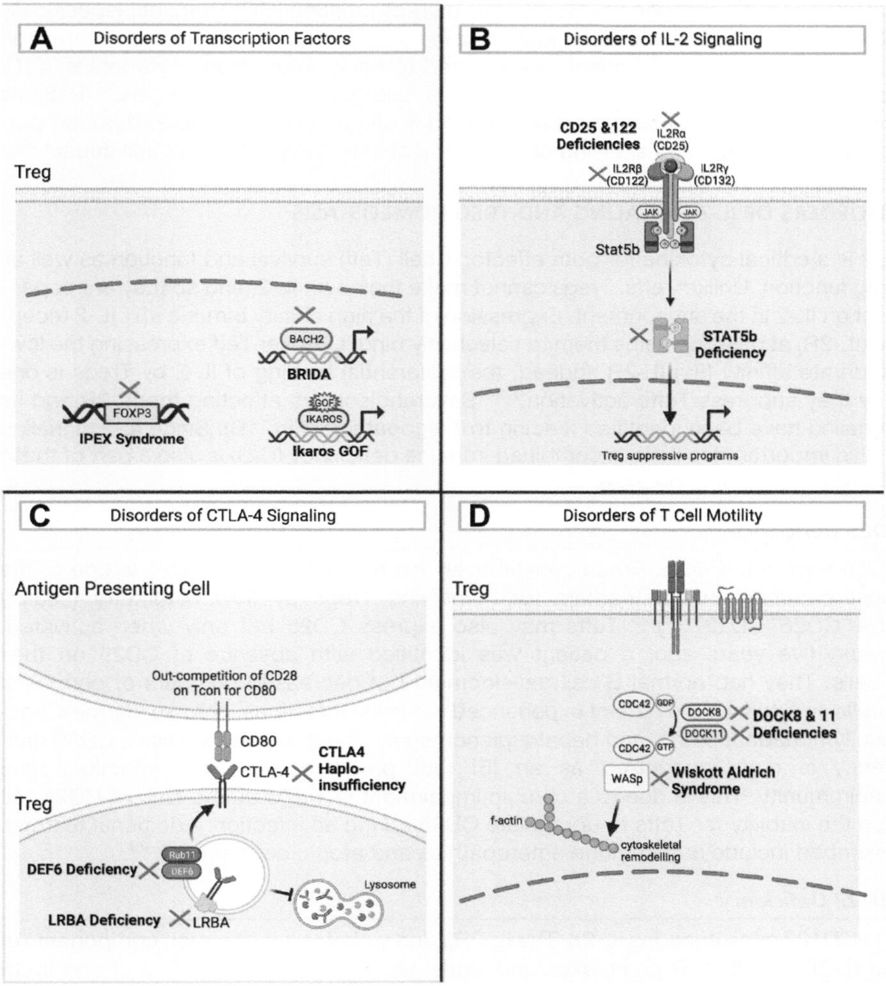

Fig. 1. Schematic of different categories of Tregopathy based on general mechanism. Red X's indicate deficiency of the related protein. Disorders of transcription factors (*A*), IL-2 signaling (*B*), CTLA-4 regulation (*C*), and T cell motility (*D*) that affect Treg function are shown. (Created with BioRender.com.)

Polymorphisms in the *BACH2* region have been associated with an increased risk in developing autoimmune diseases such as autoimmune endocrinopathies,[19] vitiligo, systemic lupus erythematosus (SLE), and multiple sclerosis.[20,21] This suggests that, in addition to monogenic immune dysregulation, variants in *BACH2* may confer genetic risk for autoimmunity.

IKAROS Gain-of-Function

IKAROS is a transcription factor important for lymphocyte development encoded by *IKZF1*. While haploinsufficiency of IKAROS and dominant-negative mutations in *IKZF1* have been associated with humoral and combined immunodeficiencies

(CID),[22] recently described heterozygous gain-of-function (GOF) variants (specifically (R183C/H)) in *IKZF1* have been identified in patients from 4 families with atopy and autoimmune disease.[23] Patients were noted to have autoimmune cytopenias, T1D, colitis, autoimmune and atopic skin disease, asthma, and food allergies.[23] Patients with *IKAROS* GOF mutations have impaired T cell production of IL-2, reduced percentages of Tregs, and skewing of T helper (Th) cells toward the Th2 cell subset.[23]

DISORDERS OF IL-2 SIGNALING AND TREG HOMEOSTASIS

IL-2 is a critical cytokine for both effector T cell (Teff) survival and function as well as Treg function. Unlike Teffs, Tregs cannot make their own IL-2, and so they are dependent on IL-2 in the environment. Expression of the high affinity trimeric $\alpha\beta\gamma$ IL-2 receptor (IL-2R) at baseline helps them to selectively bind IL-2 over Teff expressing the low-moderate affinity ($\beta\gamma$) IL-2R. Indeed, the preferential binding of IL-2 by Tregs is one way they suppress Teffs activation.[7,24] Several disorders affecting the IL-2R and its signaling have been identified leading to Tregopathies (**Fig. 1**B). Since IL-2 signaling is also important for Teffs, a combined immune deficiency (CID) is also a part of these disorders to varying degrees.

CD25 Deficiency

CD25 encodes IL-2Rα. Tregs constitutively express CD25, and CD25 is one of the most commonly used markers for identifying Tregs by flow cytometry (usually $CD4^+CD25^+CD127^{low}$).[25] Teffs may also express CD25 but only when activated. Twenty-five years ago, a patient was identified with absence of CD25 on their T cells. They had normal B cell development but decreased numbers of peripheral T cells. In addition, the patient experienced recurrent infections, chronic diarrhea, anemia, lymphadenopathy, and hepatosplenomegaly.[26] Autosomal recessive CD25 deficiency is now recognized as an IEI that presents with both infections and autoimmunity. This is due to a chronic impairment in Tregs due to lack of CD25 but also the inability for Teffs to upregulate CD25 during an infection. Additional features described include autoimmune enteropathies and atopic dermatitis.[26–29]

CD122 Deficiency

The *CD122* gene encodes IL-2β. The IL-2Rβ and γ chains are common components of the IL-2R and IL-15R complexes and signal via JAK3 and STAT5.[30] IL-2 and IL-15 signaling are important for T and natural killer (NK) cell development, and IL-2Rγ and JAK3 deficiencies both result in severe combined immunodeficiency (SCID) with absent T and NK cells.[31] Two groups have identified individuals from unrelated families with homozygous *CD122* mutations. These children had recurrent pulmonary infections as well as cytomegalovirus (CMV) and Epstein-Barr virus (EBV) infections. They also developed hypergammaglobulinemia and autoantibodies along with autoimmune disease (predominantly enteropathy and hemolytic anemia) and atopic features (atopic dermatitis and food allergies).[32,33] Patient T cells were shown to have reduced phosphorylation of STAT5 after stimulation with IL-2, and the percentage of $CD4^+FOXP3^+CD25^+$ Tregs were severely reduced compared with healthy controls.[32,33] This is consistent with the significant role of IL-2 signaling in Treg cell maintenance.

STAT5B Deficiency

STAT5 is activated by signaling through receptors for various cytokines including IL-2, hematopoietic growth factors, as well as growth hormone.[34] There are 2 highly homologous *STAT5* genes, *STAT5A* and *STAT5B*, with overlapping but not identical functions. Absence of STAT5B, compared with STAT5A, was found to have a more profound effect on immune cell proliferation in response to IL-2.[35] STAT5B is also an important regulator of FOXP3 expression.[36] STAT5B deficiency was first described in a young girl with extreme short stature who had recurrent infections and chronic pulmonary disease.[37] Subsequent reports have identified patients with autosomal recessive inactivating mutations as well as heterozygous, dominant negative mutations in *STAT5B*, with growth hormone insensitivity, lymphopenia and infections, interstitial lung disease, autoimmune disease (thyroid disease, immune thrombocytopenia (ITP), and arthritis), and atopic dermatitis. STAT5B-deficient Tregs have impaired IL-2R signaling as well low expression of FOXP3 and impaired *in vitro* suppressive abilities leading to impaired peripheral immune tolerance.[38]

DISORDERS OF CTLA-4 SIGNALING

CTLA-4 is a co-inhibitory molecule expressed on activated Teffs and Tregs. CTLA-4 competes with the positive co-stimulatory molecule, CD28, for binding to CD80 and CD86 on APCs. This is one mechanism by which Tregs suppress immune responses[39] (**Fig. 1**C).

CTLA-4 Haploinsufficiency

CTLA-4 haploinsufficiency is an autosomal dominant condition with variable expressivity and incomplete penetrance. The initial cases were described in 2014 in several families with affected members having lymphoproliferation, increased infections, malignancy, and polyautoimmunity. Individuals with heterozygous mutations in *CTLA4* were found to have Tregs with decreased CTLA-4 expression and impaired *in vitro* suppressive function. In addition, affected patients had decreased circulating B cells, a reduced memory B cell percentage, and hypogammaglobulinemia.[40,41]

Manifestations of CTLA-4 haploinsufficiency present throughout childhood and adulthood. The penetrance rate was suggested to be at least 67% in one study of 133 individuals from 54 unrelated families.[42] Many patients are initially diagnosed with common variable immunodeficiency (CVID). Over time, they develop infections (eg, CMV, EBV) and acquire autoimmune manifestations (eg, autoimmune enteropathies, cytopenias, skin disease, interstitial lung disease, and neurologic manifestations) with an increased risk for malignancy.[42,43]

LRBA Deficiency

A related disease illustrates the importance of CTLA-4 in the down-modulation of immune responses. LPS-responsive beige-like anchor (LRBA) is a trafficking protein that is critical for CTLA-4 recycling to the cell surface.[44] Patients with biallelic *LRBA* mutations may present initially with infections and/or autoimmunity. While having similar clinical phenotypes, life threatening infections, faltering growth, and autoimmune enteropathy are more common in LRBA deficiency, whereas malignancies, atopy, and skin and neurologic disorders are more common in CTLA-4 haploinsufficiency.[45]

DEF6 Deficiency

DEF6 is a guanine nucleotide exchange factor that activates Rho/Ras family members downstream of the T cell receptor. DEF6 also interacts with the GTPase RAB11, which co-localizes with CTLA-4 containing vesicles and is crucial for CTLA-4 containing vesicle recycling to the cell surface.[44,46] Patients from 3 families have been reported with DEF6 deficiency and severe EBV infections, recurrent infections, and autoimmunity (autoimmune hemolytic anemia, arthritis, and colitis).[46,47]

DISORDERS OF REGULATION OF THE ACTIN CYTOSKELETON

The actin cytoskeleton is a critical support needed for cells to maintain their proper shape and motility, and it is crucial for phagocytosis and the development of cell-cell interactions.[48] While not classic Tregopathies, deficiencies of actin-regulatory proteins lead to CIDs and have been associated with Treg dysfunction and the development of autoimmunity (**Fig. 1**D).

Wiskott–Aldrich Syndrome

Wiskott–Aldrich syndrome protein (WASP) is exclusively expressed in hematopoietic cells and is a key regulator of the actin cytoskeleton. It activates the Actin Related Protein 2/3 complex, which is essential for actin filament nucleation and branching. In the absence of WASP, cells have impaired homing to sites of infection.[49] WASP-deficient T cells have decreased IL-2 production,[50] and WASP-deficient Tregs have impaired stability and suppressive activity.[51] In addition, WASP-deficient mice have decreased Treg and regulatory B cells and exacerbated disease in an arthritis model.[52]

Patients with hemizygous variants in *WASP* lie on a clinical spectrum depending on the variant. Hypomorphic variants, with some WASP expression, may present solely with thrombocytopenia (X-linked thrombocytopenia), whereas significantly depressed/absent WASP results in WAS with severe and recurrent infections, high IgE, atopic dermatitis, and autoimmune disease.[53]

Approximately 40% of patients with WAS develop autoimmunity, including over half of those having polyautoimmunity. The most common autoimmune manifestations are autoimmune hemolytic anemia, arthritis, vasculitis, renal disease, and IgA nephropathy.[54,55]

DOCK8 Deficiency

DOCK8 is a guanine nucleotide exchange factor that forms a complex with WASP and its stabilizing factor WIP. DOCK8 activates the GTPase, CDC42, facilitating CDC42 mediated WASP activation.[56]

Patients with DOCK8 deficiency have biallelic pathologic variants and deletions in DOCK8 leading to autosomal recessive hyper-IgE syndrome.[57,58] Patients present with recurrent infections, skin disease, food allergies, and highly elevated serum IgE levels. Over time, patients may develop autoantibodies as well as autoimmune disease (most commonly cytopenias, autoimmune thyroiditis, uveitis, vasculitis).[59,60]

Like patients with WAS, DOCK8-deficient patient Tregs are present at reduced percentages in the blood and have impaired *in vitro* suppressive abilities.[59] In a mouse model of DOCK8 deficiency, Tregs were found to form unstable immune synapses and have impaired transendocytosis of co-stimulatory molecules from APCs. In addition, DOCK8-deficient Tregs had impaired phosphorylation and nuclear localization of STAT5 after IL-2 stimulation.[61]

DOCK11 Deficiency

Another DOCK-family member, DOCK11, was recently linked to autoimmunity.[62] Like DOCK8, DOCK11 is also primarily expressed in immune cells and activates CDC42.[63]

Eight boys from 7 unrelated families were identified who had early-onset autoimmunity (cytopenias, arthritis, SLE, and lymphoproliferation) along with skin disease. They were all found to have hemizygous missense variants in *DOCK11*. Unlike patients with WASP or DOCK8 deficiency, patients with DOCK11 deficiency did not have increased infections or atopic disease. Activated T and B cells from patients with DOCK11 deficiency had abnormal protrusions and impaired actin polymerization. Their Tregs had reduced FOXP3 expression along with impaired STAT5 phosphorylation after IL-2 stimulation.[62]

CHARACTERISTICS AND LABORATORY FINDINGS SUGGESTIVE OF TREGOPATHIES

Atopic Features

Tregs are not only important for curbing the development of autoimmune conditions but also atopic disorders (ie, atopic dermatitis, allergy, asthma). Patients with the Treg dysfunction often present with a combination of these conditions and may also have laboratory features such as high IgE.[64]

Immune Deficiency

Since many Tregopathies are due to genetic variants that affect other immune cells, another clue may be the presence of a comorbid immune deficiency, as evidenced by recurrent and/or severe infections. When B cell maturation is disturbed, patients may also have decreased immunoglobulin levels, poor antibody responses to vaccines, a reduced percentage of memory B cells, and meet criteria for CVID.

Treatment Resistance

A poor response to conventional immunosuppressive agents may suggest the involvement of pathways outside those targeted with the usual disease modifying agents and point the clinician toward further investigation of Treg cell numbers, function, as well as genetic studies.

Polyautoimmunity

While there are classic autoimmune associations (eg, juvenile arthritis and uveitis) that are rarely due to an IEI, if a patient develops multiple autoimmune diseases that are less commonly associated or more numerous than expected, this may raise suspicion for Tregopathy. Enteropathy is a common feature to most described Treg disorders, and one of the first involved organs may be the GI tract leading to faltering growth.

Family History

An X-linked inheritance pattern, as seen with IPEX, and autosomal recessive patterns are most commonly seen. However, certain conditions, such as CTLA-4 haploinsufficiency, show an autosomal dominance inheritance pattern. While this may be helpful if there are affected family members, due to incomplete penetrance, the inheritance pattern may not always be clear.

Laboratory Testing

Laboratory findings vary widely between different Tregopathies and even within a given condition. In healthy individuals, ~5 to 7% of $CD4^+$ T cells in the blood express the surface markers ($CD4^+CD25^+CD127^{low}$) found on Tregs.[65] For instance, in patients with IPEX syndrome, the percentage of $CD4^+CD25^+CD127^{low}$ cells out of $CD4^+$ cells in the blood can vary widely from almost zero to a higher-than-expected percentage.[12] FOXP3 expression assessed by flow cytometry also varies widely in patients with IPEX syndrome. Depending on the pathogenic variant, FOXP3 protein may be absent, or it may be present at normal levels in patients with expressed but dysfunctional FOXP3.[13] Patients with *CD25* variants tend to have expected percentages of $CD4^+FOXP3^+$ Tregs, while $CD4^+CD25^+$ T cells are absent,[13] suggesting that Tregs are present but with impaired function. Thus, lymphocyte subset data, especially Treg percentages, must be interpreted with caution.

Demethylation of the *FOXP3* locus has also been found to be important for persistent FOXP3 expression and Treg stability,[66] and analyzing this demethylation may be useful in the future for determining the ratios of Tregs to Teffs and better characterizing Tregopathies.[67] *In vitro* Treg function testing may also be helpful in identifying Treg dysfunction but is currently only available on a research basis. Circulating T follicular helper cells have also been found to be elevated in patients with autoimmune disorders[68] and Tregopathies.[69]

TREATMENT FOR TREGOPATHIES

Hematopoietic Cell Transplantation

Except for a limited number of gene therapies available on a clinical trial basis (discussed later), the only cure for monogenic Tregopathies is allogeneic HCT. HCT will not cure established T1D or manifestations due to defects in non-hematopoietic cells.[42] Given that most Tregopathies have only been described in the last decade, large published cohorts include patients for whom genetic diagnoses were made after HCT.[13,70] These patients tended to have extensive autoimmunity and/or opportunistic infections prompting transplant, and outcomes were likely worse based on their higher disease severity prior to transplantation. With greater recognition of Tregopathies and earlier genetic diagnoses, outcomes may be improving. For example, in a cohort of 24 patients with LRBA deficiency who underwent HCT between 2005 and 2019, the transplant related mortality was 42.9% prior to 2015 (6/14) and 10% (1/10) between 2015 and 2019.[70]

While this is encouraging, the decision to pursue HCT even with a known genetic diagnosis can be challenging. Many IEIs affecting Tregs have variable expressivity, and specific genetic variants are poor predictors of future disease severity.[42,70,71] Thus, pursuing HCT early, prior to significant disease burden, comes with the risks of allogeneic HCT without a guarantee that a patient is avoiding a severe disease course. HCT may also feel less urgent if targeted therapies are available. In general, while HCT tends to have higher up-front mortality, with most deaths occurring in the first few months, there is greater long-term disease-free survival. In a cohort of 96 patients with IPEX syndrome, the 5-year disease-free survival after HCT was 71.6% versus 65.1% in the immune-suppression only arm, and pre-transplant organ involvement score was the only predictor of survival.[12]

Gene Therapy

The principle behind gene therapy is to gene-correct harvested autologous stem cells and then provide them back to a patient, thus avoiding potential toxicities intrinsic to allogeneic HCT, such as the potential need for myeloablative conditioning, the risk of graft-versus-host disease (GVHD), and the risk of infection while giving prophylaxis or treatment for GVHD. After decades of progress, current gene therapies are based on lentiviral vectors and have strong safety data relative to first-generation gene therapies that were hampered by developments of leukemia. Gene therapies currently exist for several causes of SCID (Artemis, IL-2Rγ, and Adenosine Deaminase deficiencies), X-linked chronic granulomatous disease, and WAS.[72]

Regarding the treatment of WAS, long-term follow up (median 7.6 years) of 9 patients who received gene therapy was recently published. Treatment led to a reduction in atopic dermatitis and the incidence of severe infections. While platelet counts did not fully normalize, there was a reduction in significant bleeding. Features of autoimmunity also improved, although one patient had persistent (albeit improved) lower extremity vasculitis, and another patient developed new nephrotic syndrome.

Overall, the study showed promising long-term outcomes using gene therapy for WAS.[73]

Thus far, gene therapies appear safe and can ameliorate the most severe features of an underlying disorder, with better outcomes associated with a higher fraction of corrected cells. Currently, they are best suited for gene replacement in the setting of a "loss-of-function" scenario based on lentiviral strategies to provide a highly expressed gene replacement. Treatment of Tregopathies due to missense GOF (eg,IKAROS GOF) variants will depend on further development of tools for gene correction by means of techniques such as homology-directed repair (HDR).[74,75]

Small Molecules and Biologics

Historically, both calcineurin and mTOR inhibitors were used for the medical management of Tregopathies. The mTOR inhibitor sirolimus (a.k.a. rapamycin) is attractive due to its "Treg-sparing" effects thought to be related to differential effects on cell survival and metabolism in Tregs versus Teffs.[76] Indeed, current *ex-vivo* expansion protocols for Treg cell products use rapamycin to help keep the products "pure."[77,78]

Given the favorable effect of sirolimus on Tregs, it may seem unclear if it would be beneficial in scenarios in which there are intrinsic defects in Tregs. However, this appears to still be true. In IPEX syndrome, sirolimus was shown to enhance Treg function independent of FOXP3 expression.[79] In a large CTLA-4 haploinsufficiency cohort, improvement primarily in lymphoproliferation and enteropathy were seen in 8 out of 13 patients treated with sirolimus.[42] Similarly, in a cohort of 76 patients with LRBA deficiency, 26 patients received sirolimus with the most consistent benefit shown for enteropathy and neurologic manifestations.[70]

While CTLA-4 and LRBA deficiencies have shown partial response to sirolimus, a targeted treatment is available in the form of CTLA-4 Ig, either abatacept or belatacept. Abatacept is available in a subcutaneous form and is currently FDA approved for rheumatoid arthritis and GVHD prophylaxis in children.[80] When used off-label for CTLA-4 haploinsufficiency, 11/14 patients receiving CTLA-4 Ig showed a clinical response.[42] As with sirolimus, the most improvement was in the enteropathy and lymphoproliferation; however, there was also improvement in granulomatous lymphocytic interstitial lung disease in 2 patients. Six patients had to stop therapy – 3 to go to HCT and another 3 due to infections. Meanwhile, in a cohort of 22 LRBA-deficient patients, 18/22 were treated with abatacept with the best responses seen for features of chronic diarrhea and lymphoproliferation with a more moderate response for other autoimmune features.[81] Complete responses were more commonly seen when abatacept was given on a weekly regimen. Given its theoretic role as a targeted therapy, a Phase IIa, prospective, non-randomized ABACHAI trial in Germany (DRKS00017736) will further investigate the use of abatacept in these disorders.[82]

Other biologic agents used to treat Tregopathies include rituximab, which is particularly useful for managing features of lymphoproliferation. In the future, low dose IL-2 (aldesleukin) may be attempted for Tregopathies that specifically have impaired IL-2 signaling such as IKAROS GOF and CD25 deficiency. While FDA approved at high doses for the treatment of renal cell carcinoma and melanoma, at low doses, aldesleukin has shown promise to selectively expand Tregs in the setting of chronic GVHD, with particularly impressive results demonstrated in children.[83,84] At present, it is still difficult to obtain insurance approval, and there are logistic hurdles to its preparation. However, longer acting versions of "low-dose" IL-2 are currently in development and may be available in the next 2 decades.

SUMMARY

Since the description of IPEX syndrome in the 1980s, there is an ever-expanding number of disorders that are related to Treg dysfunction with varying degrees of polyautoimmunity, atopy, and infection. The combination of these features, along with positive family history and/or treatment refractory disease may suggest a strong underlying genetic driver of immune dysregulation. With earlier recognition and genetic diagnosis, patients may be started on a targeted therapy or considered for HCT.

CLINICS CARE POINTS

- It is important for rheumatologists to take a detailed family history, as well as a history of atopy and infection for patients presenting with autoimmune features.
- Laboratory studies are often insufficient to make a definitive diagnosis, so when a Tregopathy is suspected, genetic testing should be pursued.
- Early involvement of stem cell transplant physicians may help assess the risk-benefit profile for this curative approach for a given patient.

DISCLOSURE

The authors have declared no conflict of interest.

REFERENCES

1. Cheru N, Hafler DA, Sumida TS. Regulatory T cells in peripheral tissue tolerance and diseases. Front Immunol 2023;14:1154575.
2. Gavin MA, Rasmussen JP, Fontenot JD, et al. Foxp3-dependent programme of regulatory T-cell differentiation. Nature 2007;445(7129):771–5.
3. Camperio C, Caristi S, Fanelli G, et al. Forkhead transcription factor FOXP3 upregulates CD25 expression through cooperation with RelA/NF-kappaB. PLoS One 2012;7(10):e48303.
4. Tang AL, Teijaro JR, Njau MN, et al. CTLA4 expression is an indicator and regulator of steady-state CD4+ FoxP3+ T cell homeostasis. J Immunol 2008;181(3):1806–13.
5. Hench VK, Su L. Regulation of IL-2 gene expression by Siva and FOXP3 in human T cells. BMC Immunol 2011;12:54.
6. Wing K, Onishi Y, Prieto-Martin P, et al. CTLA-4 control over Foxp3+ regulatory T cell function. Science 2008;322(5899):271–5.
7. Furtado GC, Curotto de Lafaille MA, Kutchukhidze N, et al. Interleukin 2 signaling is required for CD4(+) regulatory T cell function. J Exp Med 2002;196(6):851–7.
8. Powell BR, Buist NR, Stenzel P. An X-linked syndrome of diarrhea, polyendocrinopathy, and fatal infection in infancy. J Pediatr 1982;100(5):731–7.
9. Chatila TA, Blaeser F, Ho N, et al. JM2, encoding a fork head-related protein, is mutated in X-linked autoimmunity-allergic disregulation syndrome. J Clin Invest 2000;106(12):R75–81.
10. Bennett CL, Christie J, Ramsdell F, et al. The immune dysregulation, polyendocrinopathy, enteropathy, X-linked syndrome (IPEX) is caused by mutations of FOXP3. Nat Genet 2001;27(1):20–1.
11. Wildin RS, Ramsdell F, Peake J, et al. X-linked neonatal diabetes mellitus, enteropathy and endocrinopathy syndrome is the human equivalent of mouse scurfy. Nat Genet 2001;27(1):18–20.

12. Barzaghi F, Amaya Hernandez LC, Neven B, et al. Long-term follow-up of IPEX syndrome patients after different therapeutic strategies: An international multicenter retrospective study. J Allergy Clin Immunol 2018;141(3):1036–1049 e5.
13. Gambineri E, Ciullini Mannurita S, Hagin D, et al. Clinical, Immunological, and Molecular Heterogeneity of 173 Patients With the Phenotype of Immune Dysregulation, Polyendocrinopathy, Enteropathy, X-Linked (IPEX) Syndrome. Front Immunol 2018;9:2411.
14. Goodwin M, Lee E, Lakshmanan U, et al. CRISPR-based gene editing enables FOXP3 gene repair in IPEX patient cells. Sci Adv 2020;6(19). https://doi.org/10.1126/sciadv.aaz0571. eaaz0571.
15. Tsukumo S, Unno M, Muto A, et al. Bach2 maintains T cells in a naive state by suppressing effector memory-related genes. Proc Natl Acad Sci U S A 2013;110(26):10735–40.
16. Afzali B, Gronholm J, Vandrovcova J, et al. BACH2 immunodeficiency illustrates an association between super-enhancers and haploinsufficiency. Nat Immunol 2017;18(7):813–23.
17. Kim EH, Gasper DJ, Lee SH, et al. Bach2 regulates homeostasis of Foxp3+ regulatory T cells and protects against fatal lung disease in mice. J Immunol 2014;192(3):985–95.
18. Li Y, Rao X, Tang P, et al. Bach2 Deficiency Promotes Intestinal Epithelial Regeneration by Accelerating DNA Repair in Intestinal Stem Cells. Stem Cell Rep 2021;16(1):120–33.
19. Fichna M, Zurawek M, Slominski B, et al. Polymorphism in BACH2 gene is a marker of polyglandular autoimmunity. Endocrine 2021;74(1):72–9.
20. Zhang H, Hu Q, Zhang M, et al. Bach2 Deficiency Leads to Spontaneous Expansion of IL-4-Producing T Follicular Helper Cells and Autoimmunity. Front Immunol 2019;10:2050.
21. Consiglio A, Nuzziello N, Liguori M. Dysregulation of Gene Expressions in Multiple Sclerosis: TNFSF13B and Other Candidate Genes. J Integr Neurosci 2022;22(1):4.
22. Yamashita M, Morio T. Inborn errors of IKAROS and AIOLOS. Curr Opin Immunol 2021;72:239–48.
23. Hoshino A, Boutboul D, Zhang Y, et al. Gain-of-function IKZF1 variants in humans cause immune dysregulation associated with abnormal T/B cell late differentiation. Sci Immunol 2022;7(69):eabi7160.
24. Hofer T, Krichevsky O, Altan-Bonnet G. Competition for IL-2 between Regulatory and Effector T Cells to Chisel Immune Responses. Front Immunol 2012;3:268.
25. Santegoets SJ, Dijkgraaf EM, Battaglia A, et al. Monitoring regulatory T cells in clinical samples: consensus on an essential marker set and gating strategy for regulatory T cell analysis by flow cytometry. Cancer Immunol Immunother 2015;64(10):1271–86.
26. Sharfe N, Dadi HK, Shahar M, et al. Human immune disorder arising from mutation of the alpha chain of the interleukin-2 receptor. Proc Natl Acad Sci U S A 1997;94(7):3168–71.
27. Goudy K, Aydin D, Barzaghi F, et al. Human IL2RA null mutation mediates immunodeficiency with lymphoproliferation and autoimmunity. Clin Immunol 2013;146(3):248–61.
28. Caudy AA, Reddy ST, Chatila T, et al. CD25 deficiency causes an immune dysregulation, polyendocrinopathy, enteropathy, X-linked-like syndrome, and defective IL-10 expression from CD4 lymphocytes. J Allergy Clin Immunol 2007;119(2):482–7.

29. Bezrodnik L, Caldirola MS, Seminario AG, et al. Follicular bronchiolitis as phenotype associated with CD25 deficiency. Clin Exp Immunol 2014;175(2):227–34.
30. Lin JX, Leonard WJ. The role of Stat5a and Stat5b in signaling by IL-2 family cytokines. Oncogene 2000;19(21):2566–76.
31. Buckley RH. Molecular defects in human severe combined immunodeficiency and approaches to immune reconstitution. Annu Rev Immunol 2004;22:625–55.
32. Fernandez IZ, Baxter RM, Garcia-Perez JE, et al. A novel human IL2RB mutation results in T and NK cell-driven immune dysregulation. J Exp Med 2019;216(6): 1255–67.
33. Zhang Z, Gothe F, Pennamen P, et al. Human interleukin-2 receptor beta mutations associated with defects in immunity and peripheral tolerance. J Exp Med 2019;216(6):1311–27.
34. Able AA, Burrell JA, Stephens JM. STAT5-Interacting Proteins: A Synopsis of Proteins that Regulate STAT5 Activity. Biology 2017;6(1). https://doi.org/10.3390/biology6010020.
35. Imada K, Bloom ET, Nakajima H, et al. Stat5b is essential for natural killer cell-mediated proliferation and cytolytic activity. J Exp Med 1998;188(11):2067–74.
36. Yao Z, Kanno Y, Kerenyi M, et al. Nonredundant roles for Stat5a/b in directly regulating Foxp3. Blood 2007;109(10):4368–75.
37. Kofoed EM, Hwa V, Little B, et al. Growth hormone insensitivity associated with a STAT5b mutation. N Engl J Med 2003;349(12):1139–47.
38. Cohen AC, Nadeau KC, Tu W, et al. Cutting edge: Decreased accumulation and regulatory function of CD4+ CD25(high) T cells in human STAT5b deficiency. J Immunol 2006;177(5):2770–4.
39. Gamez-Diaz L, Grimbacher B. Immune checkpoint deficiencies and autoimmune lymphoproliferative syndromes. Biomed J 2021;44(4):400–11.
40. Kuehn HS, Ouyang W, Lo B, et al. Immune dysregulation in human subjects with heterozygous germline mutations in CTLA4. Science 2014;345(6204):1623–7.
41. Schubert D, Bode C, Kenefeck R, et al. Autosomal dominant immune dysregulation syndrome in humans with CTLA4 mutations. Nat Med 2014;20(12):1410–6.
42. Schwab C, Gabrysch A, Olbrich P, et al. Phenotype, penetrance, and treatment of 133 cytotoxic T-lymphocyte antigen 4-insufficient subjects. J Allergy Clin Immunol 2018;142(6):1932–46.
43. Wobma H, Perkins R, Bartnikas L, et al. Genetic diagnosis of immune dysregulation can lead to targeted therapy for interstitial lung disease: A case series and single center approach. Pediatr Pulmonol 2022;57(7):1577–87.
44. Janman D, Hinze C, Kennedy A, et al. Regulation of CTLA-4 recycling by LRBA and Rab11. Immunology 2021;164(1):106–19.
45. Jamee M, Hosseinzadeh S, Sharifinejad N, et al. Comprehensive comparison between 222 CTLA-4 haploinsufficiency and 212 LRBA deficiency patients: a systematic review. Clin Exp Immunol 2021;205(1):28–43.
46. Serwas NK, Hoeger B, Ardy RC, et al. Human DEF6 deficiency underlies an immunodeficiency syndrome with systemic autoimmunity and aberrant CTLA-4 homeostasis. Nat Commun 2019;10(1):3106.
47. Fournier B, Tusseau M, Villard M, et al. DEF6 deficiency, a mendelian susceptibility to EBV infection, lymphoma, and autoimmunity. J Allergy Clin Immunol 2021; 147(2):740–743 e9.
48. Pollard TD, Goldman RD. Overview of the Cytoskeleton from an Evolutionary Perspective. Cold Spring Harb Perspect Biol 2018;10(7). https://doi.org/10.1101/cshperspect.a030288.

49. Janssen E, Geha RS. Primary immunodeficiencies caused by mutations in actin regulatory proteins. Immunol Rev 2019;287(1):121–34.
50. Azuma H, Oshima M, Ito K, et al. Impaired interleukin-2 production in T-cells from a patient with Wiskott-Aldrich syndrome: basis of clinical effect of interleukin-2 replacement therapy. Eur J Pediatr 2000;159(8):633–4.
51. Humblet-Baron S, Sather B, Anover S, et al. Wiskott-Aldrich syndrome protein is required for regulatory T cell homeostasis. J Clin Invest 2007;117(2):407–18.
52. Bouma G, Carter NA, Recher M, et al. Exacerbated experimental arthritis in Wiskott-Aldrich syndrome protein deficiency: modulatory role of regulatory B cells. Eur J Immunol 2014;44(9):2692–702.
53. Liu DW, Zhang ZY, Zhao Q, et al. Wiskott-Aldrich syndrome/X-linked thrombocytopenia in China: Clinical characteristic and genotype-phenotype correlation. Pediatr Blood Cancer 2015;62(9):1601–8.
54. Schurman SH, Candotti F. Autoimmunity in Wiskott-Aldrich syndrome. Curr Opin Rheumatol 2003;15(4):446–53.
55. Sullivan KE, Mullen CA, Blaese RM, et al. A multiinstitutional survey of the Wiskott-Aldrich syndrome. J Pediatr 1994;125(6 Pt 1):876–85.
56. Janssen E, Tohme M, Hedayat M, et al. A DOCK8-WIP-WASp complex links T cell receptors to the actin cytoskeleton. J Clin Invest 2016;126(10):3837–51.
57. Engelhardt KR, McGhee S, Winkler S, et al. Large deletions and point mutations involving the dedicator of cytokinesis 8 (DOCK8) in the autosomal-recessive form of hyper-IgE syndrome. J Allergy Clin Immunol 2009;124(6):1289–12302 e4.
58. Zhang Q, Davis JC, Lamborn IT, et al. Combined immunodeficiency associated with DOCK8 mutations. N Engl J Med 2009;361(21):2046–55.
59. Janssen E, Morbach H, Ullas S, et al. Dedicator of cytokinesis 8-deficient patients have a breakdown in peripheral B-cell tolerance and defective regulatory T cells. J Allergy Clin Immunol 2014;134(6):1365–74.
60. Biggs CM, Keles S, Chatila TA. DOCK8 deficiency: Insights into pathophysiology, clinical features and management. Clin Immunol 2017;181:75–82.
61. Janssen E, Kumari S, Tohme M, et al. DOCK8 enforces immunological tolerance by promoting IL-2 signaling and immune synapse formation in Tregs. JCI Insight 2017;2(19). https://doi.org/10.1172/jci.insight.94298.
62. Boussard C, Delage L, Gajardo T, et al. DOCK11 deficiency in patients with X-linked actinopathy and autoimmunity. Blood 2023. https://doi.org/10.1182/blood.2022018486.
63. Lin Q, Yang W, Baird D, et al. Identification of a DOCK180-related guanine nucleotide exchange factor that is capable of mediating a positive feedback activation of Cdc42. J Biol Chem 2006;281(46):35253–62.
64. Castagnoli R, Lougaris V, Giardino G, et al. Inborn errors of immunity with atopic phenotypes: A practical guide for allergists. World Allergy Organ J 2021;14(2):100513.
65. Seddiki N, Santner-Nanan B, Martinson J, et al. Expression of interleukin (IL)-2 and IL-7 receptors discriminates between human regulatory and activated T cells. J Exp Med 2006;203(7):1693–700.
66. Floess S, Freyer J, Siewert C, et al. Epigenetic control of the foxp3 locus in regulatory T cells. PLoS Biol 2007;5(2):e38.
67. Narula M, Lakshmanan U, Borna S, et al. Epigenetic and immunological indicators of IPEX disease in subjects with FOXP3 gene mutation. J Allergy Clin Immunol 2023;151(1):233–246 e10.
68. Gensous N, Charrier M, Duluc D, et al. T Follicular Helper Cells in Autoimmune Disorders. Front Immunol 2018;9:1637.

69. Alroqi FJ, Charbonnier LM, Baris S, et al. Exaggerated follicular helper T-cell responses in patients with LRBA deficiency caused by failure of CTLA4-mediated regulation. J Allergy Clin Immunol 2018;141(3):1050–1059 e10.
70. Tesch VK, Abolhassani H, Shadur B, et al. Long-term outcome of LRBA deficiency in 76 patients after various treatment modalities as evaluated by the immune deficiency and dysregulation activity (IDDA) score. J Allergy Clin Immunol 2020;145(5):1452–63.
71. Leiding JW, Vogel TP, Santarlas VGJ, et al. Monogenic early-onset lymphoproliferation and autoimmunity: Natural history of STAT3 gain-of-function syndrome. J Allergy Clin Immunol 2023;151(4):1081–95.
72. Kohn LA, Kohn DB. Gene Therapies for Primary Immune Deficiencies. Front Immunol 2021;12:648951.
73. Magnani A, Semeraro M, Adam F, et al. Long-term safety and efficacy of lentiviral hematopoietic stem/progenitor cell gene therapy for Wiskott-Aldrich syndrome. Nat Med 2022;28(1):71–80.
74. Allen D, Kalter N, Rosenberg M, et al. Homology-Directed-Repair-Based Genome Editing in HSPCs for the Treatment of Inborn Errors of Immunity and Blood Disorders. Pharmaceutics 2023;15(5). https://doi.org/10.3390/pharmaceutics15051329.
75. De Ravin SS, Brault J, Meis RJ, et al. Enhanced homology-directed repair for highly efficient gene editing in hematopoietic stem/progenitor cells. Blood 2021;137(19):2598–608.
76. Stallone G, Infante B, Di Lorenzo A, et al. mTOR inhibitors effects on regulatory T cells and on dendritic cells. J Transl Med 2016;14(1):152.
77. Fraser H, Safinia N, Grageda N, et al. A Rapamycin-Based GMP-Compatible Process for the Isolation and Expansion of Regulatory T Cells for Clinical Trials. Mol Ther Methods Clin Dev 2018;8:198–209.
78. Singh K, Stempora L, Harvey RD, et al. Superiority of rapamycin over tacrolimus in preserving nonhuman primate Treg half-life and phenotype after adoptive transfer. Am J Transplant 2014;14(12):2691–703.
79. Passerini L, Barzaghi F, Curto R, et al. Treatment with rapamycin can restore regulatory T-cell function in IPEX patients. J Allergy Clin Immunol 2020;145(4):1262–1271 e13.
80. Watkins B, Qayed M, McCracken C, et al. Phase II Trial of Costimulation Blockade With Abatacept for Prevention of Acute GVHD. J Clin Oncol 2021;39(17):1865–77.
81. Kiykim A, Ogulur I, Dursun E, et al. Abatacept as a Long-Term Targeted Therapy for LRBA Deficiency. J Allergy Clin Immunol Pract 2019;7(8):2790–2800 e15.
82. Krausz M, Uhlmann A, Rump IC, et al. The ABACHAI clinical trial protocol: Safety and efficacy of abatacept (s.c.) in patients with CTLA-4 insufficiency or LRBA deficiency: A non controlled phase 2 clinical trial. Contemp Clin Trials Commun 2022;30:101008.
83. Wobma HM, Kapadia M, Kim HT, et al. Real-world experience with low-dose IL-2 for children and young adults with refractory chronic graft-versus-host disease. Blood Adv 2023. https://doi.org/10.1182/bloodadvances.2023009729.
84. Whangbo JS, Kim HT, Mirkovic N, et al. Dose-escalated interleukin-2 therapy for refractory chronic graft-versus-host disease in adults and children. Blood Adv 2019;3(17):2550–61.

Understanding the Spectrum of Immune Dysregulation Manifestations in Autoimmune Lymphoproliferative Syndrome and Autoimmune Lymphoproliferative Syndrome-like Disorders

Christopher Failing, MD[a,b,*], Jennifer R. Blase, MD, PhD[c], Kelly Walkovich, MD[c]

KEYWORDS

• ALPS • ALPS-like • Double-negative T cells • Autoimmune cytopenias
• Chronic lymphoproliferation • Immune dysregulation

INTRODUCTION

As early as 1967, patients with the clinical hallmarks of autoimmune lymphoproliferative syndrome (ALPS), i.e., non-infectious, non-malignant chronic lymphoproliferation associated with immune cytopenias and propensity for lymphoma, were recognized as a unique clinical entity, initially dubbed Canale-Smith syndrome.[1] However, clues to the driving pathophysiology were not uncovered until 1992 when the profound expansion of double-negative alpha-beta T cells (DNTs), i.e., $CD3^+$ $TCR\alpha\beta^+$ $CD4^-$ $CD8^-$ T cells, were detected in the peripheral blood of patients with the Canale-Smith phenotype, and the parallels to the murine lymphoproliferative (*lpr*)/generalized-lymphoproliferative-disease (*gld*) models associated with defects in first apoptosis signal receptor (Fas)-mediated apoptosis were appreciated.[2]

The association of defects in Fas-mediated apoptosis with lymphoproliferative disease in humans was validated in further studies in 1995 and 1996 that demonstrated evidence of impaired apoptosis of activated T cells incubated with anti-Fas antibody, decreased FAS protein expression and identification of novel heterozygous pathogenic variants in *FAS*.[3,4] Subsequently, the term ALPS was used to describe the subset of patients with the Canale-Smith phenotype that demonstrated defective lymphocyte apoptosis secondary to defects in the Fas-Fas ligand cell death pathway.

[a] Sanford Health, Fargo, ND, USA; [b] University of North Dakota School of Medicine and Health Sciences, Grand Folks, ND, USA; [c] University of Michigan, 1500 East Medical Center Drive, D4202 Medical Professional Building, Ann Arbor, MI 48109, USA
* Corresponding author. 3955 56th Street South, Suite D, Fargo, ND 58104.
E-mail address: Christopher.Failing@sanfordhealth.org

Rheum Dis Clin N Am 49 (2023) 841–860
https://doi.org/10.1016/j.rdc.2023.07.001 rheumatic.theclinics.com

To better define the cohort, diagnostic criteria were proposed in 1999 and then revised in 2009.[5] The 2009 revised criteria rely on two required criteria of 1) nonmalignant, non-infectious lymphoproliferation with 2) elevated $CD3^+$ $TCR\alpha\beta^+$ $CD4^-$ $CD8^-$ double-negative T cells, as well as primary and secondary accessory criteria to assign a definitive or probable ALPS diagnosis (**Table 1**). Additional commentary in 2019 regarding the diagnostic criteria from the European Society of Immunodeficiencies (ESID) registry working group emphasizes a combination of clinical and laboratory supportive features to achieve an ALPS diagnosis.[6]

While the initial patients with ALPS were found to have pathogenic variants in *FAS*, germline pathogenic variants in other components of the extrinsic apoptosis pathway, i.e. Fas ligand (*FASL*) and caspase-10 (*CASP10*), were confirmed shortly thereafter.[7,8] Furthermore, in 2004, somatic heterozygous pathogenic variants in *FAS* within polyclonal double-negative T cell populations were identified.[9] Thus, the use of gene-based nomenclature is recommended when describing patients with ALPS. Despite advances in genetically defining patients with ALPS, roughly 30% of patients with an ALPS phenotype remain without an underlying genetic etiology and are termed ALPS-U. Additionally, an increasing repertoire of ALPS-like disorders are appreciated.

Table 1
Diagnostic criteria for ALPS, per 2009 NIH international workshop

	Accessory Criteria	
Required Criteria	**Primary**	**Secondary**
1. CHRONIC (>6 MONTHS), NONMALIGNANT, NONINFECTIOUS LYMPHADENOPATHY, SPLENOMEGALY, OR BOTH	1. Defective lymphocyte apoptosis (in 2 separate assays)	1. Elevated plasma sFASL levels (>200 pg/mL) OR elevated plasma interleukin-10 levels (>20 pg/mL) OR elevated serum or plasma vitamin B12 levels (>1500 ng/L) OR elevated plasma interleukin-18 levels (>500 pg/mL)
2. ELEVATED $CD3^+TCRAB^+CD4^-CD8^-$ DNT CELLS (≥1.5% OF TOTAL LYMPHOCYTES OR 2.5% OF $CD3^+$ LYMPHOCYTES) IN THE SETTING OF NORMAL OR ELEVATED LYMPHOCYTE COUNTS	2. Somatic or germline pathogenic mutation in *FAS*, *FASLG*, or *CASP10*	2. Typical immunohistological findings as review by an experienced hematopathologist
		3. Autoimmune cytopenias (hemolytic anemia, thrombocytopenia, or neutropenia) AND elevated immunoglobulin G levels (polyclonal hypergammaglobulinemia)
		4. Family history of a nonmalignant/ noninfectious lymphoproliferation with or without autoimmunity

A *definitive* diagnosis is based on the presence of both required criteria plus one primary accessory criterion.
A *probable* diagnosis is based on the presence of both required criteria plus one secondary accessory criterion.

Abbreviations: DNT, double negative; L, liter; mL, milliliter; ng, nanogram; pg, picogram; T cells.

This article aims to review the clinical and laboratory features associated with ALPS and highlight ALPS-like disorders for the practicing rheumatologist, while also providing insights to approach to diagnosis and management.

AUTOIMMUNE LYMPHOPROLIFERATIVE SYNDROME CLINICAL FEATURES

While the clinical features of ALPS can be variable and overlap with other disorders complicating or delaying diagnosis, the most common manifestations are chronic non-malignant lymphoproliferation and autoimmunity, most notably immune cytopenias. Patients often present in the first few years of life with lymphoproliferation followed by immune cytopenias, although cases with overt symptoms as young as 36 weeks gestation or in the neonatal period are reported.[10] Patients with ALPS-FAS are also at substantially increased risk of lymphoma, particularly beyond the second decade of life, warranting close monitoring for malignant transformation. While most patients come to clinical attention in childhood, more adults are being diagnosed with ALPS with increased disease awareness, especially the association of immune cytopenias with underlying inborn errors of (IEI).[11,12]

Lymphoproliferation

Non-malignant, non-infectious lymphoproliferation lasting more than 6 months is the most common clinical manifestation of patients with ALPS-FAS. Splenomegaly is documented in 94-95% and generalized lymphadenopathy in 85-97% of patients from the NIH and French ALPS-FAS cohorts.[13,14] The lymphoproliferation, which is attributed to expansion and persistence of lymphocyte populations not eliminated through apoptosis, is frequently an early manifestation of the disease presenting at a median age of 2.7-3 years, with splenomegaly often occurring prior to lymphadenopathy.[13,14]

On exam, the lymphoproliferation is non-tender and diffuse. The burden of lymphoproliferation can wax and wane by 20-30%, sometimes improving with age.[13] The adenopathy is defined via grades 1-4 with grade 1 indicating a few shotty nodes, grade 2 with multiple 1-2 cm nodes, grade 3 with multiple nodes with some more than 2 cm and grade 4 with extensive visible adenopathy.[15] In some cases, peripheral blood lymphocytosis or $CD4^+$ T cell lymphopenia can accompany the lymphadenopathy.[16,17] The splenomegaly can be massive, but splenic fracture is rare.[14]

Treatment of benign lymphoproliferation is generally not warranted, and splenectomy is highly discouraged. Of note, prior to the utilization of steroid-sparing immunosuppressive therapies, many patients with ALPS-FAS underwent splenectomy to manage cytopenias. However, patients with post-splenectomy ALPS-FAS suffer a high risk of sepsis and thrombosis.[13] To help mitigate the risk for sepsis, asplenic individuals should receive ongoing prophylaxis for encapsulated organisms, e.g. penicillin VK, as well as regular immunization against encapsulated organisms.

Autoimmune Cytopenias

Patients with ALPS may present with symptoms of hemolytic anemia (AIHA) (ie, fatigue, pallor, scleral icterus), immune thrombocytopenia (ITP) (ie, ecchymoses, purpura) or neutropenia (AIN) (ie, oral ulcers, bacterial infections). Immune cytopenias are typically multilineage in patients with ALPS, although the cytopenias may present dyssynchronously. The clinical entity of Evans syndrome, defined as the presence of a least two immune-mediated cytopenias, most commonly warm autoimmune hemolytic anemia and immune thrombocytopenia, overlaps with ALPS. In fact, in a multi-institutional study, 47% (21/45) of children who presented with Evans syndrome were diagnosed with ALPS via the measurement of peripheral blood DNTs and Fas-mediated apoptosis, with markedly elevated DNTs being the strongest predictor of ALPS.[18] Based on this study, it is recommended to screen all children with Evans syndrome for ALPS. In a large cohort of 150 patients with ALPS, 69% had at least 1 grade 3-4 cytopenia, with median age of onset of 5.6 years.[13] Grade 4 thrombocytopenia (platelet count less than 25,000/mm^3) was present in 39%, neutropenia (absolute neutrophil count less than 500/mm^3) in 37%, and anemia (hemoglobin less than 6.5 g/dL) in 36% of patients with ALPS.[13] Cytopenia frequency declines with age in patients with ALPS.

Initial treatment of either ITP or AIHA in patients with ALPS is similar to that of other autoimmune cytopenias and includes corticosteroids with or without IVIG.[19,20] However, while effective in the short-term, most patients with ALPS do not have long-term responses to corticosteroids alone. For ALPS-related cytopenias, second-line treatment typically involves immunosuppression with either mycophenolate mofetil (MMF) or sirolimus.[19] Second-line treatment for other ALPS-like disorders should be tailored to the specific pathway impacted in the IEI, leveraging targeted therapeutics when available.[20]

MMF inhibits purine synthesis in proliferating T and B lymphocytes. Several case reports of children with ALPS and refractory cytopenias demonstrate successful treatment with MMF.[21,22] Additionally, in a prospective study with 13 pediatric patients with ALPS (age 9 months – 17 years, median 10.9 years) with at least 1 immune cytopenia (9 with AIHA, 9 with ITP, 3 with AIN), MMF led to a sustained clinical response in 12 patients (92%), with a median response duration of 49 weeks.[23] Sirolimus is an mTOR inhibitor that works by blocking lymphocyte proliferation through apoptosis induction. In a study of 6 children with refractory ALPS treated with sirolimus (4 of whom had severe chronic autoimmune cytopenias), all had rapid complete or near complete response.[24] In addition to improvement in their cytopenias, 5 of the 6 patients in this study also had significant lymphoproliferation prior to the initiation of sirolimus, and 4 of those 5 (80%) had compete or near-complete response with dramatic reduction in lymphoproliferation. In the selection of a second-line agent for patients with ALPS, shared decision making between patient and provider is recommended, with the consideration of the tolerability of known side effects, the patient's ability to access routine drug level monitoring (ie, therapeutic sirolimus levels) and familiarity of the provider with each agent. Patients on MMF should be monitored for hepatotoxicity and iatrogenic immunodeficiency-associated lymphoproliferation, while patients on sirolimus should be monitored for thrombocytopenia, hyperlipidemia and the development of oral ulcers. Concurrent clinical symptoms (such as lymphadenopathy and/or splenomegaly) may help guide the selection of therapeutic agent, as sirolimus has also shown improvement in lymphoproliferation.

Other treatments for refractory cytopenias have been used in patients with ALPS, including anti-CD20$^+$ antibody therapy (eg, rituximab). In a case series of 12 patients with ALPS with refractory cytopenias treated with rituximab, 7 of the 12 responded.[25] Interestingly, 7 of the 9 patients with ITP responded, but none of the 3 patients with AIHA responded, suggesting that rituximab works better for ALPS-associated thrombocytopenia than anemia. Rituximab also resulted in prolonged hypogammaglobulinemia requiring IVIG supplementation in 3 of the 12 patients.[25] Splenectomy has historically been used for ALPS-related cytopenias, however, as noted above, incurs a substantial risk for sepsis and thrombosis. Furthermore, many patients with ALPS who undergo splenectomy suffer the relapse of their immune cytopenias. In a large cohort of patients, 56% (37/66) of patients with ALPS had cytopenia relapse following splenectomy and 41% (27/66) experienced at least one episode of sepsis.[13]

Therefore, splenectomy should be reserved for patients with severe splenic sequestration leading to cytopenias who have failed all other medical interventions.[19]

Malignancy

Patients with ALPS-FAS are noted to have a significantly increased risk of developing Hodgkin and non-Hodgkin lymphoma, although other non-hematopoietic tumors are rarely reported. In an NIH cohort of 150 patients with ALPS-FAS, 18 (12%) patients developed lymphoma at a median age of 18 years (range 5–60 years).[13] As compared to general population rates of lymphoma, the standardized incidence values for Hodgkin and non-Hodgkin lymphoma were 149 and 61, respectively.[13] Similarly, the cumulative risk of lymphoma in 90 patients with ALPS-FAS from a French cohort was 15 percent with a median age of diagnosis of 24.5 years (range 14–51 years).[14] Lymphoma is reported more frequently in males, is predominantly of B cell origin, infrequently related to Epstein-Barr virus (EBV) infection and more likely to occur in patients with pathogenic variants impacting the death domain of Fas. Importantly, family members with confirmed pathogenic variants in *FAS,* who were otherwise healthy, have been reported to develop lymphoma.[13]

Distinguishing lymphoma from background chronic lymphoproliferation in ALPS can be challenging. Routine symptom screening for classic "B symptoms" of fever, weight loss, and night sweats, along with the histological evaluation of lymph nodes with aggressive, focal or otherwise unusual growth characteristics is recommended. PET scans can be useful in identifying the extent of lymphoproliferation burden and identifying the most metabolically active node for excisional biopsy; however, routine use of PET scans for surveillance is not recommended.[26] Following the diagnosis of lymphoma, patients with ALPS-FAS can generally be treated per standard protocols as the defect in Fas-mediated apoptosis is not felt to impact the efficacy of chemotherapy nor radiation.

The risk for lymphoma in patients with ALPS-sFAS, ALPS-FASL, and ALPS-CASP10 is uncertain. Further study is needed to delineate the malignancy risk in these ALPS populations. Many of the ALPS-like conditions also have high rates of lymphoma.

Other Inflammatory Features

Although less common than lymphadenopathy and splenomegaly, lymphoproliferation in patients with ALPS may infiltrate other organs, leading to uveitis, hepatitis/hepatomegaly, glomerulonephritis, arthritis, and pulmonary lesions, among others.[24,27–32] In a case series of 29 patients with ALPS referred for ophthalmologic examination due to vision or ocular symptoms, 10 had abnormal findings, with uveitis being the most common finding.[27] In a large review of 234 patients with ALPS with available chest CT imaging, 8% (18/234) of patients had lung abnormalities present on CT, most commonly findings of bronchiectasis, ground glass opacities, consolidations and nodules.[32] Notably, most of these patients (16/18) with CT findings had no clinical symptoms of dyspnea or signs of oxygen desaturations on room air.[32] Overall, infiltrative lymphoproliferation is rare in patients with ALPS but is often a more prominent feature in the ALPS-like disorders.

AUTOIMMUNE LYMPHOPROLIFERATIVE SYNDROME LABORATORY FEATURES

Double-Negative T Cells

The accumulation and activation of T cell lymphocytes play an important role in the pathogenesis of autoimmune disorders. A majority of T cells are TCR alpha beta ($\alpha\beta$) positive, and among these cells, $CD4^+$ helper or $CD8^+$ cytotoxic T cells are the most prevalent subsets.[33] Double-negative T cells (DNTs), which represent around 3-5% of T lymphocytes in the peripheral blood, are CD3 positive, do not express the CD4 or CD8 co-receptors and can express either TCR alpha beta ($\alpha\beta$) or TCR gamma delta ($\gamma\delta$).[34,35] Although the precise function of DNTs in immune systems is still not fully understood, they are believed to be crucial for maintaining immunological homeostasis; additionally, there is growing interest in their role in the development of autoimmune disease, malignancy, and inflammation.

DNTs are a sensitive marker of ALPS but are not specific. Numerous autoimmune disorders in adults and children have demonstrated expanded DNT populations, including systemic lupus erythematosus (SLE), Sjogren's syndrome, mixed connective tissue disease (MCTD), Behcet's syndrome, juvenile idiopathic arthritis and juvenile dermatomyositis (JDM).[36–39] Expanded DNTs can be a clinical characteristic of other immunodeficiency illnesses, such as signal transducer and activator of transcription 3 gain of function (STAT3 GOF) and lipopolysaccharide responsive beige-like anchor protein (LRBA) deficiency, which both present with lymphoproliferation.[40,41]

The role DNTs play in the pathogenesis of these disorders remains unknown, but these cells infiltrate various organs in autoimmune disease, including, but not limited to, the skin, kidney and liver and may play a direct role in tissue damage.[35,42] Inflamed salivary glands of patients with Sjogren's syndrome have shown the infiltration of IL-17 producing DNTs, with the expansion of DNTs associated with disease activity.[43] Increased tissue damage and inflammation is noted in SLE with DNT expansion.[44] DNTs that produce IL-17 have also been found to infiltrate the kidney in those with lupus nephritis and in the skin of patients with psoriatic inflammation.[45,46] DNTs can also activate the production of pro-inflammatory cytokines, such as IL-17A, which can drive the production of pathogenic autoantibodies in various autoimmune disorders, such as SLE.[47,48]

Peripheral blood biomarkers

Besides defective *in vitro* Fas-mediated apoptosis, elevated levels of IL-18, vitamin B12 and soluble FASL (sFASL) were found to constitute a novel biomarker signature for ALPS in a large cohort of patients followed over a 20-year period; however, these biomarkers can also be elevated in other conditions, as described later in discussion.[13]

Vitamin B12

Vitamin B12 (cobalamin) is a microscopic nutrient linked to both transcobalamin and haptocorrin (HC), with HC binding the vast majority of endogenous plasma vitamin B12.[49] This ALPS biomarker has been found in extremely high concentrations (>2000 pg/mL) in individuals with ALPS-FAS, ALPS-sFAS, and ALPS-U.[49] Although the exact mechanisms are still unclear, lymphocytes in patients with ALPS produce more HC, which is believed to bind vitamin B12 that has been released from different tissues.[49]

Mild to modest elevations in vitamin B12 levels have also been reported in hypereosinophlic syndromes, myeloproliferative disorders, hepatic disease, and other disorders that can have ALPS-like phenotypes, such as STAT3 GOF and deficiency of adenine deaminase 2 (DADA2).[50–52]

Vitamin B12 remains a valuable screening tool for ALPS as it is inexpensive and easily accessible to most clinicians, in contrast with other ALPS biomarkers, which are not universally available to most clinicians and can be difficult to perform (eg, Fas-mediated apoptosis assay).

Interleukin-18

IL-18 is a pro-inflammatory cytokine produced by both hematopoietic and non-hematopoietic cells, including dendritic cells and macrophages, and is a member of the IL-1 family of cytokines. It plays a crucial role in host defense against infections and stimulates innate and acquired immune responses.[53,54] Given its diverse biological functions, it is believed to have a potential pathogenic role in several inflammatory, lymphoproliferative, and autoinflammatory disorders.

High circulating levels of IL-18 (>500 pg/mL) are a characteristic biomarker of ALPS, including patients with germline or somatic FAS mutations. Elevated IL-18 levels are not specific to ALPS as IL-18 is also elevated in other autoimmune disorders including, but not limited to, systemic lupus erythematosus, psoriasis, inflammatory bowel disease and rheumatoid arthritis.[54–58]

Extremely elevated concentrations of circulating IL-18 (sometimes >100,000 pg/mL) are found in a number of autoinflammatory disorders, such as systemic juvenile idiopathic arthritis, adult-onset Still's disease, and several conditions linked to recurrent/severe hemophagocytic lymphohistiocytosis (HLH)/macrophage activation syndrome (MAS), such as X-linked inhibitor of apoptosis (XIAP) and NLR Family CARD Domain Containing 4 (NLRC4) gain-of-function mutations.[59–63] New IL-18 targeted treatments, such as exogenous IL-18 binding protein (IL-18BP), are under investigation for the treatment of inflammatory conditions in which IL-18 is thought to play a vital role in disease pathogenesis.[64,65]

Fas apoptosis

The Fas-mediated assay is performed on isolated lymphocytes and measures the ability of activated T cells to experience cell death by apoptosis following the ligation of cell surface Fas. However, a normal assay does not rule out all variants of ALPS because those with somatic *FAS* variant or germline *FASLG* variant have intact lymphocyte apoptotic function.[9,66] Due to this assay's limited availability and potential technical difficulty, it is a less useful screening tool for most clinicians.

Impact of immunosuppressive therapy on testing

Immunosuppressive treatments can normalize the DNT compartment, ALPS biomarkers, and/or interfere with Fas-mediated apoptosis assays, making it prudent to exercise caution when interpreting ALPS testing results in patients on immunosuppressive drugs.[67] When compared to other immunosuppressive drugs (such TNF inhibitors), drugs routinely used to treat ALPS, including MMF or sirolimus, are more likely to have an effect on ALPS tests. Repeat testing off-immunosuppression, when feasible, should be obtained. Genetic testing is recommended upfront for suspected ALPS/ALPS-like patients on chronic immunosuppression.

Genetic Testing

The most common genetic variants in patients with ALPS are in the *FAS* gene (also known as TNFRSF6/APO1/CD95), occurring in 85% of patients with ALPS.[68] These variants are typically heterozygous and may be germline (86%) or somatic (14%). Additionally, pathogenic variants in the genes encoding FAS ligand (*FASL*) and caspase 10 (*CASP10*) cause ALPS, and account for 2.5% and 2.8% of patients with ALPS, respectively.[68] FADD and caspase 8 are also involved in the Fas-mediated apoptosis pathway, and defects in genes encoding these proteins cause an ALPS-like phenotype but are not considered classic ALPS. There are at least 173 unique variants in *FAS* that have been reported in ALPS.[68] In two different cohorts of patients with ALPS with *FAS* variants, 61-73% had variants that affected the intracellular portion of the FAS receptor, 21-

35% had variants that affected the extracellular portion, and 4-6% had variants affecting the transmembrane domain.[13,68] Patients with defects in the intracellular portion, including the death domain, are more likely to have an earlier age of disease onset.[68]

Genetic testing for ALPS is accomplished via sequencing of ALPS-related genes (*FAS, FASL, CASP10*), often in the context of a broader next-generation sequencing panel. However, if no germline variant is detected in a patient with clinical ALPS phenotype, Sanger sequencing of the *FAS* gene should be performed in isolated double-negative T cells.[69] Somatic variants, when present, are most common in exons 7, 8, and 9. While classically detectable in double-negative T cells, somatic *FAS* variants may also be detected in a minority of $CD4^+$ or $CD8^+$ T cells.[70] Since the discovery of somatic *FAS* variants in patients with ALPS, other inborn errors of immunity associated with somatic variants, such as TLR8 gain-of-function variants, have been described.[71]

Finally, ALPS has incomplete penetrance (estimated at less than 60%), as demonstrated by the presence of healthy mutation-positive relatives.[13] These healthy relatives typically have apoptosis defects and modest elevations in ALPS serum biomarkers, but without clinical symptoms of ALPS. Further investigation is needed in order to understand the other factors that lead to clinical disease in patients with pathogenic *FAS* variants.

AUTOIMMUNE LYMPHOPROLIFERATIVE SYNDROME-LIKE DISORDERS

Advances in genetic testing have rapidly expanded the repertoire of conditions outside of the Fas-FasL pathway that mimic the key clinical and laboratory features of ALPS, i.e. the ALPS-like disorders. While overlapping with ALPS, the broader phenotype of ALPS-like disorders are heterogenous and inclusive of characteristics not typical of ALPS, including increased risk of infection secondary to immunodeficiency, organ specific autoimmunity, extensive lymphocyte infiltration of non-lymphoid organs, and autoinflammation.

To date, at least 24 genetic disorders with an ALPS-like phenotype are known.[72] Of these ALPS-like disorders, CTLA4 haploinsufficiency and LRBA deficiency comprise 50% of cases, with XIAP deficiency, STAT3 GOF, RAS-associated autoimmune leukoproliferative disease (RALD), ADA2 deficiency, X-linked lymphoproliferative disease 1 (XLP-1) and activated phosphoinositide 3-kinase δ syndrome (APDS) also regularly identified in patients with an ALPS-like presentation.[72] Other disorders, e.g. caspase 8 deficiency and common variable immunodeficiency (CVID) can present with features suggestive of ALPS. As the identification of an ALPS-like disorder can have significant therapeutic and prognostic ramifications, it is crucial to consider these disorders in the differential diagnosis of ALPS. Many of the conditions highlighted later in discussion have autoimmune and other inflammatory complications that can also be manifestations of rheumatologic disorders, making them highly relevant to the practicing rheumatologist. Key clinical and laboratory features of these ALPS-like disorders are summarized in **Table 2**.

Cytotoxic T Cell Antigen Haploinsufficiency

Cytotoxic T cell antigen (CTLA-4) haploinsufficiency is an autosomal dominant immune dysregulation syndrome due to a heterozygous germline pathogenic variant in *CTLA4* that encodes the inhibitory receptor CTLA-4 found predominantly on regulatory T lymphocytes. CTLA-4 and CD28 compete in binding two common ligands on antigen-presenting cells, CD80 and CD86, and have opposing effects on T cell

Table 2
Clinical and laboratory features of ALPS and ALPS-like disorders

	Clinical Features				Laboratory Parameters				
Disorder	LP	AIC	Inflammatory Symptoms	Other Features	DNT	Vit B12	IL-18	Igs	Functional Assays
ALPS	++	++	Rare uveitis, hepatitis, GN, bronchiectasis	Lymphoma	↑↑	↑	↑	↑/nl	↑ sFASL, defective Fas-mediated apoptosis
CTLA-4 HAPLOINSUFFICIENCY	++	++	Enteropathy, GLILD, endocrinopathy, psoriasis/eczema	Lymphoma, gastric cancer	↑/nl	nl	nl	↓	↓ CTLA-4 protein by flow cytometry
LRBA DEFICIENCY	++	++	Enteropathy, endocrinopathy	Respiratory infections, FTT	↑/nl	nl	nl	↓	↓ LRBA protein by flow cytometry
XIAP DEFICIENCY	+	+	HLH, enteropathy	Skin lesions, severe EBV	nl	nl	↑↑	↓/nl	↓ XIAP protein by flow cytometry
STAT3 GOF	+	++	Hepatitis, enteropathy, arthritis, vasculitis, ILD, psoriasis, vitiligo	Lymphoma, respiratory infections, FTT	↑/nl	↑/nl	nl	↓/nl	↑ sCD25, ↑ STAT3 phosphorylation
RALD	+	+	Pericarditis, arthritis, enteropathy	Lymphoma, skin lesions	↑/nl	nl	nl	↑/nl	
DADA2	+	+	Vasculitis (polyarteritis nodosa, livedo racemosa)	Early onset stroke	↑/nl	↑	nl	↓/nl	↓ ADA2 enzyme activity
XLP-1	+	+	HLH, vasculitis, gastritis	Lymphoma, severe EBV	nl	nl	↑/nl	↓/nl	↓ SAP protein by flow cytometry
APDS 1/2	++	+	Bronchiectasis, arthritis, enteropathy, GN	Herpesvirus, respiratory infections, lymphoma, DD	nl	nl	nl	↓/nl	(*research level only*)
CASPASE 8 DEFICIENCY	+	+	Asthma, eczema	Herpesvirus, respiratory infections, FTT	ND	ND	ND	↓	Defective Fas-mediated apoptosis
CVID	+	+	Enteropathy, GLILD, arthritis, SLE, Sjogren's	Lymphoma	nl	nl	nl	↓↓	

Abbreviations: AIC, autoimmune cytopenias; ALPS, autoimmune lymphoproliferative syndrome; APDS, activated phosphoinositide 3-kinase δ syndrome; CTLA-4, cytotoxic T cell antigen-4; CVID, common variable immunodeficiency; DADA2, deficiency of adenosine deaminase 2; DD, developmental delay; DNT, double-negative T cells; EBV, Epstein-Barr virus; FTT, failure to thrive; GLILD, granulomatous lymphocytic interstitial lung disease; GN, glomerulonephritis; HLH, hemophagocytic lymphohistiocytosis; Igs, immunoglobulins; ILD, interstitial lung disease; LP, lymphoproliferation; LRBA, lipopolysaccharide-responsive beige-like anchor; ND, not determined (*due to small cohort*); nl, normal; RALD, RAS-associated autoimmune leukoproliferative disease; SAP, SLAM-associated protein; sFASL, soluble Fas ligand; SLE, systemic lupus erythematosus; STAT3 GOF, signal transducer and activator of transcription 3 gain-of-function; Vit B12, vitamin B12; XIAP, X-linked inhibitor of apoptosis; XLP-1, X-linked lymphoproliferative disease 1.

lymphocyte function. In contrast to CD28, which sends signals that promote T-cell activation and proliferation, CTLA-4 downregulates immune activation.[73,74] Those with CTLA-4 haploinsufficiency have hyperactivation of effector T cells and dysregulation of $FOXP3^+$ regulatory T cells (Tregs).[75]

Lymphoproliferation and autoimmune cytopenias are the most common clinical features of CTLA-4 haploinsufficiency. Abnormal T cell infiltration of non-lymphoid organs can also occur, leading to autoimmune enteropathies, endocrinopathies, and inflammatory arthritis.[76–84] Laboratory features include normal to expanded DNTs, normal vitamin B12 level, normal soluble Fas-Ligand. Immunologic features include recurrent infections, hypogammaglobulinemia, hyperactivation of effector T cells, decreased absolute NK cell counts, decreased switched memory B cells and progressive loss of circulating B cells.[75,82] Diagnosis is made via *CTLA4* gene sequencing. Treatment includes immunosuppressive therapy (most commonly abatacept or sirolimus) and supportive care (eg, intravenous immunoglobulin). Hematopoietic stem cell transplantation (HSCT) has been used in refractory cases.[85]

Lipopolysaccharide-responsive beige-like anchor deficiency

Lipopolysaccharide-responsive beige-like anchor (LRBA) deficiency is an autosomal recessive IEI with phenotypic overlap with CTLA-4 haploinsufficiency, with patients presenting with lymphoproliferation, autoimmune enteropathy, and recurrent respiratory infections. The LRBA protein binds to the cytoplasmic portion of CTLA-4 and prevents the lysosomal degradation of CTLA-4; therefore, LRBA deficiency leads to CTLA-4 loss.[86] This, in turn, leads to T cell dysregulation (increased follicular T helper cells, reduced T regulatory cells), progressive loss of B cells, and hypogammaglobulinemia.[87,88] Compared to CTLA-4 haploinsufficiency, the symptoms of autoimmunity, infectious complications, and lymphoproliferation all developed earlier in patients with LRBA deficiency.[88] Additionally, enteropathy and failure to thrive are more common in LRBA deficiency compared to CTLA-4 deficiency.[88] Treatment includes targeted immunosuppressive therapy, most commonly with abatacept.[88] HSCT has been used for definitive treatment.

X-linked inhibitor of apoptosis deficiency

X-linked inhibitor of apoptosis (XIAP) deficiency, also known as X-linked lymphoproliferative disease 2 (XLP-2), is caused by pathogenic variants in the *XIAP/BIRC4* gene. XIAP has anti-apoptotic functions through the inhibition of caspases 3, 7, and 9; therefore, T cells (specifically invariant natural killer T cells and mucosal-associated invariant T cells) from patients with XIAP deficiency have increased sensitivity to activation-induced cell death.[89–91] XIAP also plays a role in innate immunity through NOD2-mediated NF-κB activation and regulation of the NLR family pyrin domain containing 3 (NLRP3) inflammasome.[92,93] XIAP deficiency is characterized by chronic hyperinflammation, leading to hemophagocytic lymphohistiocytosis (HLH) and inflammatory bowel disease (IBD), as well as increased susceptibility to infections and hypogammaglobulinemia.[90,94] Key laboratory features include markedly elevated IL-18 levels, and diagnosis is confirmed via flow cytometric analysis of XIAP expression and *XIAP/BIRC4* gene sequencing.[63,94] Treatment involves immunosuppression (ie, with corticosteroids, anti-$CD20^+$ antibody therapy, azathioprine), with the only curative treatment being allogeneic HSCT, typically reserved for those with severe HLH and IBD.[90] Recently, inflammasome inhibition, i.e. quercetin, has shown promise at controlling inflammation in XIAP deficiency in animal models.[95]

Signal Transducer and Activator of Transcription 3 Gain of Function

Signal transducer and activator of transciption 3 (STAT3) belongs to a 7-member family of transcription factors essential for the regulation of numerous crucial and diverse cellular processes, such as cellular differentiation (including B-cell differentiation into plasma cells), survival, and proliferation.[96–98] Various cytokines, including IL-6 and IL-10, activate Janus kinase (JAK), which then leads to STAT3 phosphorylation and DNA binding.[99] Lymphoproliferation is the most common clinical manifestation in patients with STAT3 GOF, with 76% of patients in a large international cohort study having diffuse lymphadenopathy and 72% having splenomegaly.[40]

Post-natal growth failure is usually very profound in STAT3 GOF; in a large international cohort, over 50% had a concurrent endocrinopathy or enteropathy.[40] Autoimmune cytopenia is the most common autoimmune manifestation. Others include autoimmune hepatitis, endocrinopathies, enteropathies, inflammatory arthritis mimicking juvenile idiopathic arthritis, psoriasis, vitiligo, uveitis, and myasthenia gravis. Interstitial lung disease is the most common non-infectious pulmonary manifestation in STAT3 GOF.[51,100,101] A wide range of vasculopathy and central nervous system manifestations have been reported as well, including CNS and systemic vasculitis, stroke, optic neuritis, MoyaMoya syndrome and isolated white matter lesions.[40]

Patients are at increased risk for infections, with a majority have recurrent respiratory tract infections.[40,102,103] Immunologic laboratory features, while variable, include hypogammaglobulinemia, reduced memory B cells, moderate T, B, and/or NK cell lymphopenia, reduced T cell lymphoproliferative responses and elevated DNTs, without Fas apoptosis defects.[40,102,104]

RAS-associated autoimmune leukoproliferative disease

RAS-associated autoimmune leukoproliferative disease (RALD) is caused by gain-of-function somatic variants in either *NRAS* or *KRAS*.[5] Activating somatic *NRAS* variants have been described in 3 patients since 2007 with lymphadenopathy and normal to mildly elevated DNTs.[5,105] While germline *KRAS* variants are associated with Noonan syndrome, somatic activating *KRAS* variants present in mononuclear cells were first described in 2011 in 2 patients with ALPS-like phenotypes.[106] These patients had splenomegaly and autoimmune cytopenias, but no elevation of DNTs nor defect in the Fas-mediated apoptosis.[106]

Deficiency of adenosine deaminase 2

Deficiency of adenosine deaminase 2 (DADA2) is caused by biallelic loss-of-function variants in the *ADA2* gene, which encodes the adenosine deaminase 2 (ADA2) protein, produced by activated myeloid cells. The most common clinical manifestation is small- to medium-vessel vasculitis, classically polyarteritis nodosa, early onset stroke, livedo racemosa, and fever.[107] Other clinical findings include hypogammaglobulinemia, pure red cell aplasia, cytopenias, and lymphadenopathy. Treatment consists of immunosuppression, mainly with TNF inhibitors, and HSCT has also been performed as curative therapy.[108]

X-linked Lymphoproliferative Disease 1

X-linked lymphoproliferative disease 1 (XLP-1, SAP deficiency) is charactered by SLAM-associated protein (SAP) deficiency due to pathogenic variants in the *SH2D1A* gene. SAP is highly expressed in T and NK cells and binds to the SLAM family of receptors on B cells and other hematopoietic cells.[109–111] Absence of SAP leads to defective killing of EBV-infected B cells.[110,112] Clinical manifestations of XLP-1 include EBV-triggered lymphoproliferation, HLH, lymphoma, aplastic anemia, vasculitis, chronic gastritis, and skin lesions.[111] Laboratory features include generalized hypogammaglobulinemia or impaired antibody response to immunizations, decreased memory B cells, and impaired CD8^{+} cytotoxic T cell and NK cell activity. Diagnosis is made via flow cytometric analysis of SAP expression and *SH2D1A* gene sequencing. The only curative treatment for XLP-1 is allogeneic hematopoietic stem cell transplant.[113]

Activated phosphoinositide 3-kinase δ syndrome 1 and 2

Activated phosphoinositide 3-kinase δ syndrome (APDS) 1 and 2 are caused by autosomal dominant GOF variants in *PIK3CD* and *PIK3R1*, respectively. *PIK3CD* encodes the p110δ catalytic subunit of phosphoinositide 3-kinase δ (PI3Kδ), while *PIK3R1* encodes the regulatory subunits (p85α, p55α, and p50α) of class IA phosphoinositide 3 kinases (PI3Ks). The p110δ catalytic subunit is restricted to leukocytes, and p85α is the predominant regulatory subunit in lymphocytes.[114] Defects in either subunit, through GOF variants in *PIK3CD* or *PIK3R1*, lead to hyperactivated PI3Kδ signaling in T and B lymphocytes.

Both APDS 1 and 2 are characterized clinically by chronic lymphadenopathy and recurrent respiratory tract infections. Additionally, they have increased rates of bronchiectasis, persistent or severe herpesvirus infections, autoimmune cytopenias, infiltrative inflammatory disease (eg, glomerulonephritis, colitis, arthritis) and lymphoma.[114–116] Neurologic features, e.g., global developmental delay, have also been observed in patients with APDS.[114,115] While many clinical features are shared with ALPS, patients with APDS do not have increased DNTs or defective Fas-mediated apoptosis. However, similar to ALPS, sirolimus may be used to treat both lymphoproliferation and autoimmune cytopenias in APDS.[116] Leniolisib, a potent oral inhibitor of the p110δ subunit of PI3Kδ, is also now approved for the treatment of APDS.[117]

Caspase 8 deficiency

Caspase 8 deficiency was first described in 2002 in two siblings with ALPS-like phenotypes, characterized by lymphadenopathy, splenomegaly, and defective Fas-induced apoptosis.[118] Additionally, these patients had recurrent sinopulmonary and herpes simplex virus infections and defective immunization responses. They were found to have homozygous germline variants in *CASP8*, with asymptomatic heterozygous relatives. The associated immunodeficiency in these patients distinguishes them clinically from patients with ALPS. Patients with caspase 8 deficiency have decreased lymphocyte proliferation to mitogens and antigens and variable degrees of hypogammaglobulinemia.[118]

Common Variable Immunodeficiency

Common variable immunodeficiency (CVID) is one of the most prevalent primary immunodeficiency disorders, and despite adequate levels of B cells, those with CVID have decreased serum levels of immunoglobulin G (IgG) and IgA or IgM and poor/absent responses to vaccinations.[119] Defective B cell function is thought to lead to impaired immunoglobulin production.[120] CVID presents with heterogenous clinical manifestations including lymphoproliferation and granulomatous lymphocytic interstitial lung disease (GLILD). Autoimmune cytopenias are the most common autoimmune manifestation of CVID, but others include systemic lupus erythematosus, inflammatory arthritis, autoimmune thyroiditis, enteropathy, vitiligo, and Sjogren's syndrome.[121] While many clinical features of CVID are shared with ALPS, patients with CVID do not have increased DNTs or defective Fas-mediated apoptosis. The mainstay of CVID treatment is immunoglobulin replacement, and patients with rheumatologic disease receive the same care as those who are not immunocompromised.[122]

SUMMARY

When rheumatologists encounter patients presenting with chronic lymphoproliferation and autoimmunity who have an unrevealing rheumatologic evaluation, it is prudent to approach these patients with a very broad differential diagnosis and to consider ALPS and the other ALPS-like disorders. If feasible, careful testing for these disorders is needed prior to starting immunosuppressive therapies, as they can potentially interfere with ALPS and/or immunologic testing. As the ALPS-like conditions have significant overlap with ALPS, the rheumatologist should have a low threshold to pursue genetic testing to rapidly identify a disorder which could have potential therapeutic and prognostic implications.

CLINICS CARE POINTS

- ALPS and the ALPS-like conditions should be considered in any patient who presents with chronic lymphoproliferation and/or autoimmune cytopenias.
- Double-negative T cells (DNTs) are a sensitive marker of ALPS but are not necessarily specific, as numerous autoimmune disorders in adults and children have demonstrated expanded DNT populations, including many rheumatologic disorders (eg, systemic lupus erythematosus)
- Rigorous testing is imperative prior to starting immunosuppressive therapy, as the medications can potentially interfere with ALPS and/or other immunologic testing.
- The rheumatologist should have a low threshold to pursue genetic testing to make a timely, accurate diagnosis, which may have potential therapeutic and prognostic implications.

DISCLOSURE

K. Walkovich discloses the following potential conflicts of interest: Local principal investigator for the mavorixafor trial (sponsored by X4 Pharmaceuticals); Member of the steering committee for Sobi; and Advisory board for Sobi, Pharming, AstraZeneca, Horizon, and X4 Pharmaceuticals.

REFERENCES

1. Canale VC, Smith CH. Chronic lymphadenopathy simulating malignant lymphoma. J Pediatr 1967;70(6):891–9.
2. Sneller MC, Straus SE, Jaffe ES, et al. A novel lymphoproliferative/autoimmune syndrome resembling murine lpr/gld disease. J Clin Invest 1992;90(2): 334–41.
3. Rieux-Laucat F, Le Deist F, Hivroz C, et al. Mutations in Fas associated with human lymphoproliferative syndrome and autoimmunity. Science 1995;268(5215): 1347–9.
4. Drappa J, Vaishnaw AK, Sullivan KE, et al. Fas gene mutations in the Canale-Smith syndrome, an inherited lymphoproliferative disorder associated with autoimmunity. N Engl J Med 1996;335(22):1643–9.

5. Oliveira JB, Bleesing JJ, Dianzani U, et al. Revised diagnostic criteria and classification for the autoimmune lymphoproliferative syndrome (ALPS): report from the 2009 NIH International Workshop. Blood 2010;116(14):e35–40.
6. Consonni F, Gambineri E, Favre C. ALPS, FAS, and beyond: from inborn errors of immunity to acquired immunodeficiencies. Ann Hematol 2022;101(3):469–84.
7. Del-Rey M, Ruiz-Contreras J, Bosque A, et al. A homozygous Fas ligand gene mutation in a patient causes a new type of autoimmune lymphoproliferative syndrome. Blood 2006;108(4):1306–12.
8. Wang J, Zheng L, Lobito A, et al. Inherited human Caspase 10 mutations underlie defective lymphocyte and dendritic cell apoptosis in autoimmune lymphoproliferative syndrome type II. Cell 1999;98(1):47–58.
9. Holzelova E, Vonarbourg C, Stolzenberg MC, et al. Autoimmune lymphoproliferative syndrome with somatic Fas mutations. N Engl J Med 2004;351(14):1409–18.
10. Hansford JR, Pal M, Poplawski N, et al. In utero and early postnatal presentation of autoimmune lymphoproliferative syndrome in a family with a novel FAS mutation. Haematologica 2013;98(4):e38–9.
11. Deutsch M, Tsopanou E, Dourakis SP. The autoimmune lymphoproliferative syndrome (Canale-Smith) in adulthood. Clin Rheumatol 2004;23(1):43–4.
12. Seidel MG. Autoimmune and other cytopenias in primary immunodeficiencies: pathomechanisms, novel differential diagnoses, and treatment. Blood 2014;124(15):2337–44.
13. Price S, Shaw PA, Seitz A, et al. Natural history of autoimmune lymphoproliferative syndrome associated with FAS gene mutations. Blood 2014;123(13):1989–99.
14. Neven B, Magerus-Chatinet A, Florkin B, et al. A survey of 90 patients with autoimmune lymphoproliferative syndrome related to TNFRSF6 mutation. Blood 2011;118(18):4798–807.
15. Rao VK, Dowdell KC, Dale JK, et al. Pyrimethamine treatment does not ameliorate lymphoproliferation or autoimmune disease in MRL/lpr-/- mice or in patients with autoimmune lymphoproliferative syndrome. Am J Hematol 2007;82(12):1049–55.
16. Volkl S, Rensing-Ehl A, Allgauer A, et al. Hyperactive mTOR pathway promotes lymphoproliferation and abnormal differentiation in autoimmune lymphoproliferative syndrome. Blood 2016;128(2):227–38.
17. Lisco A, Wong CS, Price S, et al. Corrigendum: paradoxical CD4 lymphopenia in autoimmune lymphoproliferative syndrome (ALPS). Front Immunol 2019;10:1552.
18. Seif AE, Manno CS, Sheen C, et al. Identifying autoimmune lymphoproliferative syndrome in children with Evans syndrome: a multi-institutional study. Blood 2010;115(11):2142–5.
19. Rao VK, Oliveira JB. How I treat autoimmune lymphoproliferative syndrome. Blood 2011;118(22):5741–51.
20. Seidel MG. Treatment of immune-mediated cytopenias in patients with primary immunodeficiencies and immune regulatory disorders (PIRDs). Hematology Am Soc Hematol Educ Program 2020;2020(1):673–9.
21. Kossiva L, Theodoridou M, Mostrou G, et al. Mycophenolate mofetil as an alternate immunosuppressor for autoimmune lymphoproliferative syndrome. J Pediatr Hematol Oncol 2006;28(12):824–6.

22. Arora S, Singh N, Chaudhary GK, et al. Autoimmune lymphoproliferative syndrome: response to mycophenolate mofetil and pyrimethamine/sulfadoxine in a 5-year-old child. Indian J Hematol Blood Transfus 2011;27(2):101–3.
23. Rao VK, Dugan F, Dale JK, et al. Use of mycophenolate mofetil for chronic, refractory immune cytopenias in children with autoimmune lymphoproliferative syndrome. Br J Haematol 2005;129(4):534–8.
24. Teachey DT, Greiner R, Seif A, et al. Treatment with sirolimus results in complete responses in patients with autoimmune lymphoproliferative syndrome. Br J Haematol 2009;145(1):101–6.
25. Rao VK, Price S, Perkins K, et al. Use of rituximab for refractory cytopenias associated with autoimmune lymphoproliferative syndrome (ALPS). Pediatr Blood Cancer 2009;52(7):847–52.
26. Carrasquillo JA, Chen CC, Price S, et al. 18F-FDG PET imaging features of patients with autoimmune lymphoproliferative syndrome. Clin Nucl Med 2019; 44(12):949–55.
27. Ucar D, Kim JS, Bishop RJ, et al. Ocular inflammatory disorders in autoimmune lymphoproliferative syndrome (ALPS). Ocul Immunol Inflamm 2017;25(5):703–9.
28. Chandramati J, Sidharthan N, Ponthenkandath S. Neonatal autoimmune lymphoproliferative syndrome: a case report and a brief review. J Pediatr Hematol Oncol 2021;43(2):e227–9.
29. Kianifar HR, Khalesi M, Farid R, et al. Autoimmune lymphoproliferative syndrome (ALPS) in a boy with massive lymphadenopathy. Iran J Allergy, Asthma Immunol 2010;9(3). 181-63.
30. Naveed M, Khamis Butt UB, Mannan J. Autoimmune lymphoproliferative syndrome with neonatal onset. J Coll Physicians Surg Pak 2014;24(Suppl 2): S124–6.
31. Kanegane H, Vilela MM, Wang Y, et al. Autoimmune lymphoproliferative syndrome presenting with glomerulonephritis. Pediatr Nephrol 2003;18(5):454–6.
32. Lau CY, Mihalek AD, Wang J, et al. Pulmonary manifestations of the autoimmune lymphoproliferative syndrome. A retrospective study of a unique patient cohort. Ann Am Thorac Soc 2016;13(8):1279–88.
33. Miceli MC, Parnes JR. The roles of CD4 and CD8 in T cell activation. Semin Immunol 1991;3(3):133–41.
34. Fischer K, Voelkl S, Heymann J, et al. Isolation and characterization of human antigen-specific TCR alpha beta+ CD4(-)CD8- double-negative regulatory T cells. Blood 2005;105(7):2828–35.
35. Brandt D, Hedrich CM. TCRalphabeta(+)CD3(+)CD4(-)CD8(-) (double negative) T cells in autoimmunity. Autoimmun Rev 2018;17(4):422–30.
36. Tarbox JA, Keppel MP, Topcagic N, et al. Elevated double negative T cells in pediatric autoimmunity. J Clin Immunol 2014;34(5):594–9.
37. Dean GS, Anand A, Blofeld A, et al. Characterization of CD3+ CD4- CD8- (double negative) T cells in patients with systemic lupus erythematosus: production of IL-4. Lupus 2002;11(8):501–7.
38. Alunno A, Carubbi F, Bistoni O, et al. CD4(-)CD8(-) T-cells in primary Sjogren's syndrome: association with the extent of glandular involvement. J Autoimmun 2014;51:38–43.
39. Ling E, Shubinsky G, Press J. Increased proportion of CD3+CD4-CD8- double-negative T cells in peripheral blood of children with Behcet's disease. Autoimmun Rev 2007;6(4):237–40.

40. Leiding JW, Vogel TP, Santarlas VGJ, et al. Monogenic early-onset lymphoproliferation and autoimmunity: Natural history of STAT3 gain-of-function syndrome. J Allergy Clin Immunol 2023;151(4):1081–95.
41. Revel-Vilk S, Fischer U, Keller B, et al. Autoimmune lymphoproliferative syndrome-like disease in patients with LRBA mutation. Clin Immunol 2015; 159(1):84–92.
42. Li SX, Lv TT, Zhang CP, et al. Alteration of liver-infiltrated and peripheral blood double-negative T-cells in primary biliary cholangitis. Liver Int 2019;39(9): 1755–67.
43. Alunno A, Bistoni O, Bartoloni E, et al. IL-17-producing CD4-CD8- T cells are expanded in the peripheral blood, infiltrate salivary glands and are resistant to corticosteroids in patients with primary Sjogren's syndrome. Ann Rheum Dis 2013;72(2):286–92.
44. Crispin JC, Hedrich CM, Suarez-Fueyo A, et al. SLE-associated defects promote altered T cell function. Crit Rev Immunol 2017;37(1):39–58.
45. Crispin JC, Oukka M, Bayliss G, et al. Expanded double negative T cells in patients with systemic lupus erythematosus produce IL-17 and infiltrate the kidneys. J Immunol 2008;181(12):8761–6.
46. Ueyama A, Imura C, Fusamae Y, et al. Potential role of IL-17-producing CD4/CD8 double negative alphabeta T cells in psoriatic skin inflammation in a TPA-induced STAT3C transgenic mouse model. J Dermatol Sci 2017;85(1):27–35.
47. Shivakumar S, Tsokos GC, Datta SK. T cell receptor alpha/beta expressing double-negative (CD4-/CD8-) and CD4+ T helper cells in humans augment the production of pathogenic anti-DNA autoantibodies associated with lupus nephritis. J Immunol 1989;143(1):103–12.
48. Sieling PA, Porcelli SA, Duong BT, et al. Human double-negative T cells in systemic lupus erythematosus provide help for IgG and are restricted by CD1c. J Immunol 2000;165(9):5338–44.
49. Bowen RA, Dowdell KC, Dale JK, et al. Elevated vitamin B(1)(2) levels in autoimmune lymphoproliferative syndrome attributable to elevated haptocorrin in lymphocytes. Clin Biochem 2012;45(6):490–2.
50. Ermens AA, Vlasveld LT, Lindemans J. Significance of elevated cobalamin (vitamin B12) levels in blood. Clin Biochem 2003;36(8):585–90.
51. Fabre A, Marchal S, Barlogis V, et al. Clinical ASPECTS of STAT3 gain-of-function germline mutations: a systematic review. J Allergy Clin Immunol Pract 2019;7(6):1958–1969 e9.
52. Barzaghi F, Minniti F, Mauro M, et al. ALPS-like phenotype caused by ADA2 deficiency rescued by allogeneic hematopoietic stem cell transplantation. Front Immunol 2018;9:2767.
53. Sims JE, Smith DE. The IL-1 family: regulators of immunity. Nat Rev Immunol 2010;10(2):89–102.
54. Ihim SA, Abubakar SD, Zian Z, et al. Interleukin-18 cytokine in immunity, inflammation, and autoimmunity: biological role in induction, regulation, and treatment. Front Immunol 2022;13:919973.
55. Gangemi S, Merendino RA, Guarneri F, et al. Serum levels of interleukin-18 and s-ICAM-1 in patients affected by psoriasis: preliminary considerations. J Eur Acad Dermatol Venereol 2003;17(1):42–6.
56. Ciazynska M, Olejniczak-Staruch I, Sobolewska-Sztychny D, et al. The role of NLRP1, NLRP3, and AIM2 inflammasomes in psoriasis: review. Int J Mol Sci 2021;22(11). https://doi.org/10.3390/ijms22115898.

57. Furuya D, Yagihashi A, Komatsu M, et al. Serum interleukin-18 concentrations in patients with inflammatory bowel disease. J Immunother 2002;25(Suppl 1): S65–7.
58. Gualberto Cardoso PR, Diniz Lopes Marques C, de Melo Vilar K, et al. Interleukin-18 in brazilian rheumatoid arthritis patients: can leflunomide reduce it? Autoimmune Dis 2021;2021:6672987.
59. Colafrancesco S, Priori R, Alessandri C, et al. IL-18 serum level in adult onset still's disease: a marker of disease activity. Int J Inflam 2012;2012:156890.
60. Yasin S, Fall N, Brown RA, et al. IL-18 as a biomarker linking systemic juvenile idiopathic arthritis and macrophage activation syndrome. Rheumatology 2020; 59(2):361–6.
61. Romberg N, Al Moussawi K, Nelson-Williams C, et al. Mutation of NLRC4 causes a syndrome of enterocolitis and autoinflammation. Nat Genet 2014;46(10): 1135–9.
62. Canna SW, de Jesus AA, Gouni S, et al. An activating NLRC4 inflammasome mutation causes autoinflammation with recurrent macrophage activation syndrome. Nat Genet 2014;46(10):1140–6.
63. Wada T, Kanegane H, Ohta K, et al. Sustained elevation of serum interleukin-18 and its association with hemophagocytic lymphohistiocytosis in XIAP deficiency. Cytokine 2014;65(1):74–8.
64. Gabay C, Fautrel B, Rech J, et al. Open-label, multicentre, dose-escalating phase II clinical trial on the safety and efficacy of tadekinig alfa (IL-18BP) in adult-onset Still's disease. Ann Rheum Dis 2018;77(6):840–7.
65. Geerlinks AV, Dvorak AM, Consortium XDT. A case of XIAP Deficiency successfully managed with Tadekinig Alfa (rhIL-18BP). J Clin Immunol 2022;42(4): 901–3.
66. Dowdell KC, Niemela JE, Price S, et al. Somatic FAS mutations are common in patients with genetically undefined autoimmune lymphoproliferative syndrome. Blood 2010;115(25):5164–9.
67. Matson DR, Yang DT. Autoimmune lymphoproliferative syndrome: an overview. Arch Pathol Lab Med 2020;144(2):245–51.
68. Hafezi N, Zaki-Dizaji M, Nirouei M, et al. Clinical, immunological, and genetic features in 780 patients with autoimmune lymphoproliferative syndrome (ALPS) and ALPS-like diseases: a systematic review. Pediatr Allergy Immunol 2021;32(7):1519–32.
69. Lopez-Nevado M, Docampo-Cordeiro J, Ramos JT, et al. Next generation sequencing for detecting somatic FAs mutations in patients with autoimmune lymphoproliferative syndrome. Front Immunol 2021;12:656356.
70. Lo B, Ramaswamy M, Davis J, et al. A rapid ex vivo clinical diagnostic assay for fas receptor-induced T lymphocyte apoptosis. J Clin Immunol 2013;33(2): 479–88.
71. Boisson B, Casanova JL. TLR8 gain of function: a tall surprise. Blood 2021; 137(18):2420–2.
72. Lopez-Nevado M, Gonzalez-Granado LI, Ruiz-Garcia R, et al. Primary immune regulatory disorders with an autoimmune lymphoproliferative syndrome-like phenotype: immunologic evaluation, early diagnosis and management. Front Immunol 2021;12:671755.
73. Linsley PS, Brady W, Grosmaire L, et al. Binding of the B cell activation antigen B7 to CD28 costimulates T cell proliferation and interleukin 2 mRNA accumulation. J Exp Med 1991;173(3):721–30.

74. Tivol EA, Borriello F, Schweitzer AN, et al. Loss of CTLA-4 leads to massive lymphoproliferation and fatal multiorgan tissue destruction, revealing a critical negative regulatory role of CTLA-4. Immunity 1995;3(5):541–7.
75. Kuehn HS, Ouyang W, Lo B, et al. Immune dysregulation in human subjects with heterozygous germline mutations in CTLA4. Science 2014;345(6204):1623–7.
76. Verma N, Burns SO, Walker LSK, et al. Immune deficiency and autoimmunity in patients with CTLA-4 (CD152) mutations. Clin Exp Immunol 2017;190(1):1–7.
77. Schubert D, Bode C, Kenefeck R, et al. Autosomal dominant immune dysregulation syndrome in humans with CTLA4 mutations. Nat Med 2014;20(12):1410–6.
78. Schindler MK, Pittaluga S, Enose-Akahata Y, et al. Haploinsufficiency of immune checkpoint receptor CTLA4 induces a distinct neuroinflammatory disorder. J Clin Invest 2020;130(10):5551–61.
79. Krone KA, Winant AJ, Vargas SO, et al. Pulmonary manifestations of immune dysregulation in CTLA-4 haploinsufficiency and LRBA deficiency. Pediatr Pulmonol 2021;56(7):2232–41.
80. Kohatsu K, Suzuki T, Takimoto M, et al. Granulomatous interstitial nephritis with CTLA-4 haploinsufficiency: a case report. BMC Nephrol 2022;23(1):367.
81. Miyazaki H, Hoshi N, Kohashi M, et al. A case of autoimmune enteropathy with CTLA4 haploinsufficiency. Intest Res 2022;20(1):144–9.
82. Schwab C, Gabrysch A, Olbrich P, et al. Phenotype, penetrance, and treatment of 133 cytotoxic T-lymphocyte antigen 4-insufficient subjects. J Allergy Clin Immunol 2018;142(6):1932–46.
83. Siggs OM, Russell A, Singh-Grewal D, et al. Preponderance of CTLA4 variation associated with autosomal dominant immune dysregulation in the MYPPPY Motif. Front Immunol 2019;10:1544.
84. Mazzoni M, Dell'Orso G, Grossi A, et al. Underlying CTLA4 Deficiency in a patient with juvenile idiopathic arthritis and autoimmune lymphoproliferative syndrome features successfully treated with abatacept-A case report. J Pediatr Hematol Oncol 2021;43(8):e1168–72.
85. Lanz AL, Riester M, Peters P, et al. Abatacept for treatment-refractory pediatric CTLA4-haploinsufficiency. Clin Immunol 2021;229:108779.
86. Lo B, Zhang K, Lu W, et al. AUTOIMMUNE DISEASE. Patients with LRBA deficiency show CTLA4 loss and immune dysregulation responsive to abatacept therapy. Science 2015;349(6246):436–40.
87. Alroqi FJ, Charbonnier LM, Baris S, et al. Exaggerated follicular helper T-cell responses in patients with LRBA deficiency caused by failure of CTLA4-mediated regulation. J Allergy Clin Immunol 2018;141(3):1050–1059 e10.
88. Jamee M, Hosseinzadeh S, Sharifinejad N, et al. Comprehensive comparison between 222 CTLA-4 haploinsufficiency and 212 LRBA deficiency patients: a systematic review. Clin Exp Immunol 2021;205(1):28–43.
89. Rigaud S, Fondaneche MC, Lambert N, et al. XIAP deficiency in humans causes an X-linked lymphoproliferative syndrome. Nature 2006;444(7115):110–4.
90. Mudde ACA, Booth C, Marsh RA. Evolution of our understanding of XIAP deficiency. Front Pediatr 2021;9:660520.
91. Gerart S, Siberil S, Martin E, et al. Human iNKT and MAIT cells exhibit a PLZF-dependent proapoptotic propensity that is counterbalanced by XIAP. Blood 2013;121(4):614–23.
92. Damgaard RB, Nachbur U, Yabal M, et al. The ubiquitin ligase XIAP recruits LUBAC for NOD2 signaling in inflammation and innate immunity. Mol Cell 2012;46(6):746–58.

93. Knop J, Spilgies LM, Rufli S, et al. TNFR2 induced priming of the inflammasome leads to a RIPK1-dependent cell death in the absence of XIAP. Cell Death Dis 2019;10(10):700.
94. Speckmann C, Lehmberg K, Albert MH, et al. X-linked inhibitor of apoptosis (XIAP) deficiency: the spectrum of presenting manifestations beyond hemophagocytic lymphohistiocytosis. Clin Immunol 2013;149(1):133–41.
95. Chiang SCC, Owsley E, Panchal N, et al. Quercetin ameliorates XIAP deficiency-associated hyperinflammation. Blood 2022;140(7):706–15.
96. O'Shea JJ, Holland SM, Staudt LM. JAKs and STATs in immunity, immunodeficiency, and cancer. N Engl J Med 2013;368(2):161–70.
97. Hirano T, Ishihara K, Hibi M. Roles of STAT3 in mediating the cell growth, differentiation and survival signals relayed through the IL-6 family of cytokine receptors. Oncogene 2000;19(21):2548–56.
98. Bromberg J, Darnell JE Jr. The role of STATs in transcriptional control and their impact on cellular function. Oncogene 2000;19(21):2468–73.
99. Vogel TP, Leiding JW, Cooper MA, et al. STAT3 gain-of-function syndrome. Front Pediatr 2022;10:770077.
100. Cortes-Santiago N, Forbes L, Vogel TP, et al. Pulmonary histopathology findings in patients With STAT3 gain of function syndrome. Pediatr Dev Pathol 2021; 24(3):227–34.
101. Fabre A, Marchal S, Forbes LR, et al. STAT3 gain of function: a new kid on the block in interstitial lung diseases. Am J Respir Crit Care Med 2018;197(11): e22–3.
102. Milner JD, Vogel TP, Forbes L, et al. Early-onset lymphoproliferation and autoimmunity caused by germline STAT3 gain-of-function mutations. Blood 2015; 125(4):591–9.
103. Haapaniemi EM, Kaustio M, Rajala HL, et al. Autoimmunity, hypogammaglobulinemia, lymphoproliferation, and mycobacterial disease in patients with activating mutations in STAT3. Blood 2015;125(4):639–48.
104. Erdos M, Tsumura M, Kallai J, et al. Novel STAT-3 gain-of-function variant with hypogammaglobulinemia and recurrent infection phenotype. Clin Exp Immunol 2021;205(3):354–62.
105. Oliveira JB, Bidere N, Niemela JE, et al. NRAS mutation causes a human autoimmune lymphoproliferative syndrome. Proc Natl Acad Sci U S A 2007;104(21): 8953–8.
106. Niemela JE, Lu L, Fleisher TA, et al. Somatic KRAS mutations associated with a human nonmalignant syndrome of autoimmunity and abnormal leukocyte homeostasis. Blood 2011;117(10):2883–6.
107. Meyts I, Aksentijevich I. Deficiency of Adenosine Deaminase 2 (DADA2): updates on the phenotype, genetics, pathogenesis, and treatment. J Clin Immunol 2018;38(5):569–78.
108. Van Eyck L Jr, Hershfield MS, Pombal D, et al. Hematopoietic stem cell transplantation rescues the immunologic phenotype and prevents vasculopathy in patients with adenosine deaminase 2 deficiency. J Allergy Clin Immunol 2015; 135(1):283–287 e5.
109. Sayos J, Wu C, Morra M, et al. The X-linked lymphoproliferative-disease gene product SAP regulates signals induced through the co-receptor SLAM. Nature 1998;395(6701):462–9.
110. Hislop AD, Palendira U, Leese AM, et al. Impaired epstein-barr virus-specific CD8+ T-cell function in X-linked lymphoproliferative disease is restricted to SLAM family-positive B-cell targets. Blood 2010;116(17):3249–57.

111. Panchal N, Booth C, Cannons JL, et al. X-linked lymphoproliferative disease type 1: a clinical and molecular perspective. Front Immunol 2018;9:666.
112. Sullivan JL, Byron KS, Brewster FE, et al. Deficient natural killer cell activity in x-linked lymphoproliferative syndrome. Science 1980;210(4469):543–5.
113. Booth C, Gilmour KC, Veys P, et al. X-linked lymphoproliferative disease due to SAP/SH2D1A deficiency: a multicenter study on the manifestations, management and outcome of the disease. Blood 2011;117(1):53–62.
114. Elkaim E, Neven B, Bruneau J, et al. Clinical and immunologic phenotype associated with activated phosphoinositide 3-kinase delta syndrome 2: a cohort study. J Allergy Clin Immunol 2016;138(1):210–218 e9.
115. Coulter TI, Chandra A, Bacon CM, et al. Clinical spectrum and features of activated phosphoinositide 3-kinase delta syndrome: a large patient cohort study. J Allergy Clin Immunol 2017;139(2):597–606 e4.
116. Maccari ME, Abolhassani H, Aghamohammadi A, et al. Disease evolution and response to rapamycin in activated phosphoinositide 3-kinase delta syndrome: the european society for immunodeficiencies-activated phosphoinositide 3-kinase delta syndrome registry. Front Immunol 2018;9:543.
117. Rao VK, Webster S, Sediva A, et al. A randomized, placebo-controlled phase 3 trial of the PI3Kdelta inhibitor leniolisib for activated PI3Kdelta syndrome. Blood 2023;141(9):971–83.
118. Chun HJ, Zheng L, Ahmad M, et al. Pleiotropic defects in lymphocyte activation caused by caspase-8 mutations lead to human immunodeficiency. Nature 2002; 419(6905):395–9.
119. Chapel H, Cunningham-Rundles C. Update in understanding common variable immunodeficiency disorders (CVIDs) and the management of patients with these conditions. Br J Haematol 2009;145(6):709–27.
120. Ghafoor A, Joseph SM. Making a diagnosis of common variable immunodeficiency: a review. Cureus 2020;12(1):e6711.
121. Gereige JD, Maglione PJ. Current understanding and recent developments in common variable immunodeficiency associated autoimmunity. Front Immunol 2019;10:2753.
122. Cunningham-Rundles C. How I treat common variable immune deficiency. Blood 2010;116(1):7–15.

Genetic Defects in Early-Onset Inflammatory Bowel Disease

Atiye Olcay Bilgic Dagci, MD[a,*], Kelly Colleen Cushing, MD[b]

KEYWORDS

• Inflammatory bowel disease • Monogenic • Genetic • Early onset

KEY POINTS

- There are nearly 100 genes which have been linked to the development of monogenic inflammatory bowel disease.
- The pathogenesis of monogenic inflammatory bowel disease is multifactorial and includes defects in intestinal barrier function, phagocyte function, T and B cell function, and loss of regulatory mechanisms.
- Enhanced diagnostic approaches, which allow for detection of known and novel variants, will improve our understanding of early-onset inflammatory bowel disease, and may lead to improved precision medicine approaches in this patient population.

INTRODUCTION

Inflammatory bowel disease (IBD) is a group of complex, multifactorial disorders characterized by chronic inflammation of the gastrointestinal tract. The three subtypes of IBD are Crohn's disease, ulcerative colitis, and IBD-unclassified. IBD can present at any age and 25% of the total IBD population in the United States consists of pediatric-onset IBD patients.[1] Pathogenesis of IBD is not well understood. Various genetic, environmental, immunologic, and microbial factors associate with disease development and progression. IBD is considered a polygenic disease as evidenced by genome-wide association studies identifying over 240 risk loci.[2–4] However, several genetic defects have been identified to cause refractory IBD and IBD-like diseases by following Mendelian inheritance patterns. These diseases are described as monogenic IBD and they are more highly represented in patients presenting with very early-onset IBD (VEO-IBD), as compared with IBD diagnosed at an older age.[5] In this review, we

[a] Division of Pediatric Rheumatology, University of Michigan, C.S Mott Children's Hospital, 1500 East Medical Center Drive Medical Professional Building Floor 2, Ann Arbor, MI 48109-5718, USA; [b] Division of Gastroenterology, U-M Inflammatory Bowel Disease Program, University of Michigan, 3912 Taubman Center, 1500 East Medical Center Drive, SPC 5362, Ann Arbor, MI 48109-5362, USA
* Corresponding author.
E-mail address: bilgicda@med.umich.edu

Rheum Dis Clin N Am 49 (2023) 861–874
https://doi.org/10.1016/j.rdc.2023.06.006 rheumatic.theclinics.com
0889-857X/23/

will summarize the genetic contribution to the pathogenesis of IBD, with a focus on monogenic IBD, and outline the key points in diagnosis and management.

CLASSIFICATION OF INFLAMMATORY BOWEL DISEASE ACCORDING TO AGE GROUP

Patients diagnosed with IBD earlier than age 17 were defined as pediatric-onset IBD in the Montreal Classification (A1).[6] The Pediatric Paris modification of the Montreal Classification further subdivided pediatric-onset IBD into two groups: A1a (patients with onset <10 years) and A1b (patients from age 10 to <17 years of onset).[7]

Children who were diagnosed with IBD before age 6 were classified as VEO-IBD. Within this group, infantile (and toddler)-onset IBD represents children with a disease onset earlier than age 2 and neonatal IBD refers to patients who develop IBD in the first 28 days of life.[2,7]

EPIDEMIOLOGY

The incidence of pediatric-onset IBD was reported as 9.68/100,000 in a Canadian population-based cohort study.[8] VEO-IBD accounts for 15.4% for all pediatric IBD.[9] A retrospective cohort study from Canada estimated the incidence of inflammatory bowel disease in children aged 0 to 5 years at 2.1 per 100,000 and in children aged 6 to 10 years at 7.7 per 100,000.[10] Several studies reported the prevalence of monogenic IBD within pediatric IBD population between 3% and 13%.[11–13]

PATHOGENESIS OF MONOGENIC INFLAMMATORY BOWEL DISEASE

There is a growing number of causative monogenic variants of VEO-IBD. Most recently, Uhlig and colleagues reported a consensus gene list of 75 genes associated with monogenic IBD.[14] As sequencing technologies evolve and become readily available, an increasing number of genes linked to VEO-IBD have been discovered. Genetic defects cause impaired intestinal homeostasis via several mechanisms including abnormalities in barrier function, epithelial restitution, microbial defense, regulation of innate and adaptive immunity, cell recruitment, reactive oxygen species (ROS) generation, autophagy, apoptosis, endoplasmic reticulum stress, intracellular downstream signaling (ie, nuclear factor kappa light chain enhancer of activated B cells and janus kinase/signal transducers and activators of transcription), and antigen presentation (including dendritic cell activation).[15,16] These mechanisms can be categorized into 4 major groups[2,17,18] (**Fig. 1**).

1. Disruption in intestinal barrier function.
2. Reduced bacterial recognition and clearance by phagocytes.
3. Impaired development and function of the adaptive immune system (T and B cells).
4. Other autoimmune/autoinflammatory conditions causing loss of self-tolerance or hyperinflammation.

Table 1 outlines genes involved in the pathogenesis of monogenic IBD and their functional consequences.

Genes Associated with Disruption in Intestinal Barrier Function

The intestinal epithelium, composed of epithelial cells and tight junctions, forms a robust physical barrier between the luminal environment and the host immune system.[35,36] This barrier is important to promote tolerance to relatively harmless luminal exposures such as commensal bacteria or non-pathogenic food antigens. However, disruption of this barrier can lead to enhanced permeability to luminal contents, which can in turn lead to inappropriate activation of the host immune system.[37]

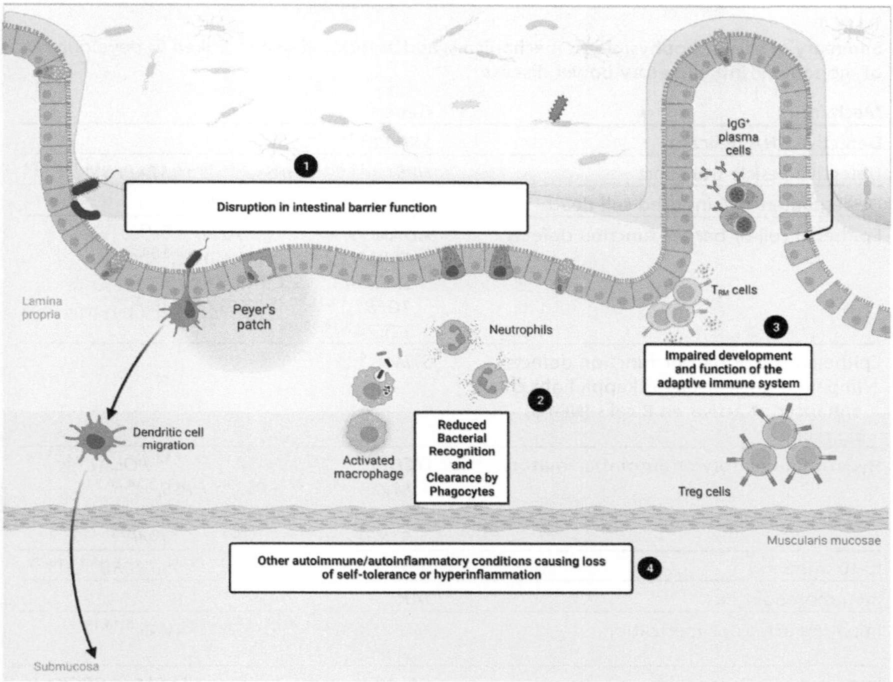

Fig. 1. Major causes of impaired intestinal homeostasis. Treg cells, T regulatory cells; TRM cells, tissue resident memory T cells. (Created with BioRender.com.)

Several gene mutations which affect barrier function have been implicated in the development of intestinal inflammation early in life. Loss of function mutations in the tetratricopeptide repeat domain 7 (*TTC7A*) gene was found in infants with VEO-IBD. Functional studies revealed a critical role in enterocyte homeostasis with decreased expression leading to aberrations in cell adhesion and increased apoptosis.[38] A gain of function mutation in *GUCY2* was identified in a Norwegian family, which resulted in markedly increased production of cyclic guanosine monophosphate . Several family members developed Crohn's disease thought to be related with proinflammatory effects of increased guanylate cyclase C signaling.[39] Deficiency of A disintegrin and metalloprotease 17 , which has been linked to a critical role in barrier function,[40] was found to cause multiorgan inflammatory disease in a 2011 case.[41] The skin and gut were the two organs predominantly affected, both organs with critical barrier functions which protect individuals from potentially harmful environmental pathogens. *FERMT1* encodes the protein kindlin-1, which is expressed in the intestinal epithelium and has been linked to a hemorrhagic ulcerative colitis-like colitis.[42] Mutations resulting of loss of function of SLC9A3, which is a sodium-hydrogen exchanger at the intestinal brush border, have also been linked to VEO-IBD.[43] Additional genes linked to intestinal inflammation via altered barrier function include *ALP1*, *SLC26A3*, *TGFB1*, and *TTC37*.[22]

Genes Associated with Reduced Bacterial Recognition and Clearance by Phagocytes

Mutations in genes which associate with chronic granulomatous diseases such as *CYBB*, *CYBA*, *NCF1*, *NCF2*, and *NCF4* have been linked to the development of chronic intestinal inflammation, which closely mimics Crohn's disease with more aggressive

Table 1
Summary of the pathophysiologic mechanisms, and associated genes, linked to development of monogenic inflammatory bowel disease

Mechanism	Gene
Defective RNA helicase	*SKIV2L*[5,14,19–22]
Defective vesicle transport	*HPS1*,[5,14,20–22] *HPS4*,[5,14,19–22] *STXBP3*[14,19,21,22]
Dysregulated TNF-induced cell death	*CASP8*,[5,14,21,22] *RIPK1*[5,14,21,22]
Epithelial cell or barrier function defects	*ADAM17*,[5,14,19–21,23] *ALPI*,[14,21,22] *FERMT1*,[5,14,20–22] *GUCY2C*,[5,14,20–22] *SLC26A3*,[22] *SLC9A3*,[5,14,21,22] *TGFB1*,[14,21,22,24] *TTC37*,[5,14,19–22] *TTC7A*[5,14,19–22]
Epithelial cell or barrier function defects; impaired nuclear factor kappa light chain enhancer of activated B cells (NF-κB) signaling	*STIM1*[14,19,21,22,25]
Hyperinflammatory or autoinflammatory	*ITCH*,[14,19,21,22] *NLRC4*,[14,19,21,22] *POLA1*,[14,21,22] *MVK*,[5,14,19–22] *HPS3*,[22] *HPS6*,[5,14,20,21] *MEFV*,[5,19–21] *PLCG2*,[5,14,19–21] *STXBP2*,[5,14,19–21] *SIRT1*,[22] *TYMP*[22]
IL-10 signaling	*IL10*,[5,14,19–22] *IL10RA*,[5,14,19–22] *IL10RB*[5,14,19–22]
Immunoregulation	*JAK1*[5]
Impaired actin polymerization	*ARPC1B*,[5,14,21,22] *DOCK2*,[22] *WAS*,[5,14,19–22] *WIPF1*[22]
Impaired NF-κB signaling	*BCL10*,[22] *IKBKG*,[5,14,19–22] *NFKBIA*,[22] *RBCK1*,[22] *RELA*,[22] *TNFAIP3*[14,21,22]
Leukocyte metabolism	*ADA2*,[22] *G6PC3*,[5,14,20–22] *LACC1*,[22] *SLC37A4*[5,14,20–22]
Leukocyte migration and activation	*ITGB2*[5,14,19–22]
Mesenchymal cells	*COL7A1*[5,14,20–22]
Mitochondrial function	*ANKZF1*[22,26]
NOD signaling	*TRIM22*,[5,14,21,22] *XIAP*[5,14,19–22]
Phagocyte defects	*CYBA*,[5,14,19–22] *CYBB*,[5,14,19–22] *CYBC1*,[22] *NCF1*,[5,14,20–22] *NCF2*,[5,14,19–22] *NCF4*,[5,14,19–22] *DUOX2*,[22,27,28] *NOX1*,[21,28,29] *NPC1*[5,14,21,22]
Prostaglandin production	*PLA2G4A*[21,30]
Prostaglandin transport	*SLCO2A1*,[5,14,21,22] *IRF2BP2*,[22] *NFAT5*,[19,22] *TRNT1*[14,21,22]
T cell, B cell, and complex function defects	*DOCK8*,[14,19–21] *DKC1*,[5,14,19–22] *PIK3CD*,[5,14,19,21,22] *RTEL1*,[5,14,19–22] *TGFBR1*,[5,14,21,22] *TGFBR2*,[5,14,21,22] *SH2D1A*[14,20,21]
T cell, B cell, and complex function defects: B cell differentiation	*AICDA*,[5,14,19–21] *PTEN*,[21,31] *ZBTB24*[5,14,21,32]
T cell, B cell, and complex function defects: dysregulation of the complement system	*MASP2*,[14,20–22] *CD55*,[5,14,21,22,33] *FCN3*[21,34]
T cell, B cell, and complex function defects: regulatory T cell function	*BACH2*,[22] *CTLA4*,[5,14,19,21,22] *FOXP3*,[5,14,19–22] *IL2RA*,[5,14,19–22] *IL2RB*,[14,19,21,22] *LRBA*,[5,14,19–22] *MALT1*,[5,14,21,22] *STAT1*,[5,14,19–22] *STAT3*[5,14,19,21,22]

(*continued on next page*)

Table 1
(*continued*)

Mechanism	Gene
T cell, B cell, and complex function defects: T- and B-lymphocyte defects	*BTK*,[5,14,19–22] *PIK3R1*[5,14,19–22]
T cell, B cell, and complex function defects: T cell activation	*CD40LG*,[5,14,19–22] *ICOS*[5,14,19–22]
T cell, B cell, and complex function defects: T cell development	*ADA*,[5,14,20–22] *CD3G*,[5,14,20–22] *DCLRE1C*,[5,14,20–22] *IL21*,[5,14,19–22] *IL2RG*,[5,14,20–22] *LIG4*,[5,14,19–22] *RAG1*,[14,21,22] *RAG2*,[5,14,20–22] *ZAP70*[5,14,20–22]

disease phenotypes (perianal, structuring disease).[44,45] The mechanism by which gastrointestinal injury occurs is presumed to be related to dysfunction of the nicotinamide adenine dinucleotide phosphate oxidase complex, which can lead to insufficient generation of ROS, impaired phagocyte function, and diminished capacity to protect against pathogens. However, the exact mechanisms that lead to intestinal inflammation are still unclear.[21] Defects in nucleotide-binding oligomerization domain (NOD) signaling, imparted by mutations in *XIAP* and *TRIM22*, also associate with monogenic IBD. NOD signaling has been shown to be important in bacterial recognition and processing. Interestingly, this pathway represents shared overlap with adult-onset IBD as NOD2 signaling is an established pathway of perturbation in this population.[46]

Genes Associated with Impaired Development and Function of the Adaptive Immune System

Many genes, which affect the function of the adaptive immune system, have been implicated in the development of monogenic IBD. While the innate immune system is responsible for the immediate immune response to pathogens, the adaptive immune system is responsible for longer term, higher specificity immune responses.[47] T and B lymphocytes are the cornerstone of the adaptive immune response. Antigen presenting cells (APCs) present antigens to T and B lymphocytes, which then stimulate antibody production (B lymphocytes) or cytokine release (T lymphocytes). Subsets of T lymphocytes can also have immune suppressive functions, which regulate autoimmunity (T regulatory cells). Any perturbation in the adaptive immune response can lead to overactivation of immune cells and associated tissue inflammation. Mutations in *ADA*, *CD3G*, *DCLRE1C*, *IL21*, *IL2RG*, *LIG4*, *RAG1*, *RAG2*, and *ZAP70* have been associated with aberrations in T cell development while mutations in *ICOS* and *CD40LG* affect T cell activation and mutations in *BACH2*, *CTLA4*, *FOXP3*, *IL2RA*, *IL2RB*, *LRBA*, *MALT1*, *STAT1*, and *STAT3* impact regulatory T cell function. Likewise, mutations in *AICDA* affect B cell differentiation. The wide range of genes which affect the adaptive immune responses highlights the complexity of the adaptive immune system.

Other Autoimmune/Autoinflammatory Conditions Causing Loss of Self-Tolerance or Hyperinflammation

Patients with this group of diseases could have a higher chance to present to a rheumatologist for an evaluation of unexplained fevers, arthritis, or constellation of persistent/recurrent symptoms, pertaining to multiple systems and laboratory evidence of systemic inflammation. Mevalonate kinase deficiency (*MVK* gene) characterized by recurrent fever, lymphadenopathy, polyarthralgia, rash, abdominal pain, diarrhea, blood in stool, chronic anemia, persistent leukocytosis, and C-reactive protein elevation should warrant further workup for IBD in patients with mevalonate kinase deficiency.[19,48] IBD could also be seen in patients with Familial Mediterranean Fever and Familial Cold Autoinflammatory Syndrome.[48,49]

STXBP2 mutations cause hemophagocytic lymphohistiocytosis, with a subset of patients also developing intestinal inflammation.[21] Inflammation is thought to be a result of impaired cytotoxicity and/or degranulation capabilities, which leads to impairment in antimicrobial activity.[50] Mutations in the gene *HPS* are associated with Hermansky-Pudlak syndrome, which is characterized by variety of phenotypes including but not limited to albinism, platelet dysfunction, immunodeficiency, lung disease, and intestinal inflammation.[5] The intestinal inflammation presents Crohn's-like with granulomatous enterocolitis and/or perianal disease. Interleukin (IL)-10 signaling is a critical signaling pathway, which suppresses inflammation and, thus, provides anti-inflammatory effects. Mutations in *IL10* or its receptor proteins (*IL10RA/IL10RB*) can, therefore, lead to proinflammatory effects with associated intestinal inflammation.[51]

CLINICAL FEATURES SUGGESTIVE OF MONOGENIC INFLAMMATORY BOWEL DISEASE

Early age of onset, positive family history, and consanguinity are strong predictors of a monogenic etiology. A systematic review by Nambu and colleagues reported infantile-onset IBD (from 28 days to younger than 2 years of age) was the most common age group among all monogenic IBD cases (28%).[52] In the same review, 63.4% of monogenic IBD presented before the age of 6 years.[52] They have also reported age distribution at the time of diagnosis stratified by underlying disorder. Many diseases including chronic granulomatous disease, immune dysregulation, polyendocrinopathy, enteropathy, X-linked syndrome, glycogen storage disease type 1b, XIAP, Wiscott-Aldrich syndrome (WAS)/WAS-like syndrome, and haploinsufficiency of A20 were diagnosed in patients with variable age groups.[53–61] However, most of the patients with TTC7A, IL-10 signaling colitis, and receptor-interacting protein kinase 1 deficiency presented with IBD within the first 6 months of age.[52] Although majority of children with monogenic IBD present before the age of 6 years, rare causative variants are detected later in life.[62] Familial guanylate cyclase 2C diarrhea syndrome and Hermansky-Pudlak syndrome were the two diseases distinguished from other conditions by having most cases develop IBD in adulthood.[52]

Extraintestinal manifestations including skin, dental, hair abnormalities (trichorrhexis nodosa, nail dystrophy, superficial skin abscesses, bullous epidermolysis, and eczematous skin lesions), endocrine dysfunctions (thyroiditis, type I diabetes mellitus), recurrent infections, autoimmune hemolytic anemia, hemophagocytic lymphohistiocytosis, lymphadenopathy, and hepatosplenomegaly should raise suspicion for monogenic IBD.[2,63] In addition to recurrent infections, infections with atypical organisms and intractable infections could also point toward single gene defects as a very broad range of types of immunodeficiencies can be associated with VEO-IBD.[64]

There are no specific histologic features that can distinguish IBD with or without a monogenic cause. However, several retrospective studies attempted to compare endoscopic findings of VEO-IBD with IBD developed later in life. Macroscopically predominantly isolated colonic distribution, presence of hemorrhagic mucosa, and microscopically presence of epithelial apoptosis, villous blunting, and eosinophilic infiltration were found in increased frequency in VEO-IBD cases.[65,66]

A single-center study based on whole-exome sequencing (WES) analyses of more than 1000 children reported that a greater proportion of children with monogenic IBD required surgery in comparison to cases of IBD not associated with a single variant.[12]

Another study investigating clinical phenotypes and outcomes of monogenic VEO-IBD found that ICU admissions at 3-year follow-up, stricturing, and penetrating disease were significantly more common in the monogenic disease group versus non-monogenic VEO-IBD.[67]

DIAGNOSTIC APPROACH

The diagnosis of IBD relies on a combination of history, physical and laboratory examination, esophagogastroduodenoscopy and colonoscopy with histology, and imaging of the small bowel. However, histology is the gold standard for diagnosis. Infectious, rheumatologic, and allergic conditions need to be considered in the differential diagnosis and should be ruled out before solidifying the diagnosis of IBD.[68] Once an IBD diagnosis is established, genetic testing should be considered in patients with clinical features suggestive of monogenic etiologies as described earlier. A detailed immune workup should complement the genetic studies, though most tests are not specific for monogenic IBD.[23] Evaluation of immune functions includes immunoglobulin levels, vaccine titers in response to vaccines, lymphocyte subsets, mitogen responses, and dihydrorhodamine fluorescence assay (to assess oxidative killing function of neutrophils). More specialized functional tests are available such as IL-10–mediated suppression of lipopolysaccharides-induced peripheral blood mononuclear cells to detect IL10RA and IL10RB defects. However, those tests can be reserved after detection of a pathogenic variant for functional confirmation.

Genomic diagnostics can provide valuable information guiding treatment choices such as selection of patients that would benefit from hematopoietic stem cell transplantation (HSCT) or identification of potential immunologic pathways that can be targeted by specific biologic therapies. HSCT was reported to be efficacious in patients with *IL10 R* mutations, whereas it was not found helpful in patients with epithelial defects.[69–72] IL-1 blockade had been used successfully in management of IBD related with mevalonate kinase deficiency,[73] *NLRC4*[74] and *NLRP3*[75] gene defects, and IL-10 receptor deficiency.[69,76] Similarly, IBD patients with lipopolysaccharide-responsive and beige-like anchor protein deficiency or *CTLA4* haploinsufficiency have shown to benefit from treatment with abatacept.[77–79]

Investigation for a monogenic cause in an IBD patient can begin with limited functional screening followed by genetic confirmation with candidate gene sequencing. However, this strategy is gradually being replaced by initial parallel genetic screening with next-generation sequencing and subsequent functional confirmation as the list of potential disease genes extending and each variant can be found associated with heterogenous extraintestinal phenotypes.[2,80] Targeted gene panel sequencing, exome sequencing, and genome sequencing have been utilized in detection of pathogenic mutations.[69] There are several commercially available and Clinical Laboratory Improvement Amendments (CLIA)-approved targeted gene panels (Mayo Clinic Laboratories, Children's Hospital of Philadelphia VEO-IBD genetic panel). These gene panels can provide high diagnostic accuracy for a subset of known genetic causes of IBD,[81,82] but do not have the have the potential to identify novel causal genetic variants in contrast to WES or whole-genome sequencing (WGS).[83] Therefore, targeted gene panels can be used for initial screening, and if results are unrevealing, WES can be performed subsequently.[14] With regards to choice of using singleton versus parent-child trio samples for WES, several studies reported higher diagnostic yield with trio sequencing.[84–86] Trio sequencing facilitates detection of *de novo* variants and allows phasing of compound heterozygous variants during interpretation.[87] Mutations outside of exons might impair normal splicing of exomes and these mutations can be missed by WES but can be captured by WGS.[88] Additionally, WGS provides more uniform coverage of the coding regions than WES and can detect copy number variants.[89] However, in routine clinical practice, the opportunities for computationally intensive investigation of multiple variants emerging from WGS are limited.[90,91]

Although potential of WES to identify causative novel mutations is promising, this technique produces extensive amounts of data that necessitate considerable bioinformatics for correct interpretation.[92] The American College of Medical Genetics and American College of Pathologists guidelines for the interpretation of sequence variants have been utilized by a substantial number of clinical laboratories.[93,94] The validation of candidate genetic variants builds upon previous evidence of their clinical relevance and functional impact. Public human variant databases (eg, gnomAD, Clinvar, ClinGen) are helpful resources in evaluating variant phenotype relations.[95,96]

SUMMARY

Although monogenic IBD constitutes a small subset of the VEO-IBD population, patients with these conditions have a severe course refractory to standard therapies more commonly than IBD patients without a single gene cause. Advent of genomic technologies provided better understanding of defective immunologic pathways which promoted opportunities for individualized treatment approaches. Detection of the monogenic cause and initiation of targeted treatment early in IBD course could anticipate and prevent complications leading to improved outcomes.

CLINICS CARE POINTS

- Single gene defects are reported in 3% to 13% of children with IBD.
- Early age of onset, positive family history, and consanguinity are strong predictors of a monogenic etiology.
- Genetic defects cause impaired intestinal homeostasis via several mechanisms including disruption in intestinal barrier function, reduced bacterial recognition and clearance by phagocytes, and impaired development and function of the adaptive immune system.
- There are a growing number of causative monogenic variants of VEO-IBD. Initial parallel genetic screening with next-generation sequencing followed by functional confirmation could be a favorable strategy while investigating for monogenic causes.

DISCLOSURE

A.O.B. Dagci and K.C. Cushing have no relevant financial or nonfinancial relationships to disclose.

REFERENCES

1. Moran CJ, Klein C, Muise AM, et al. Very early-onset inflammatory bowel disease: gaining insight through focused discovery. Inflamm Bowel Dis 2015;21(5):1166–75.
2. Uhlig HH, Schwerd T, Koletzko S, et al. The diagnostic approach to monogenic very early onset inflammatory bowel disease. Gastroenterology 2014;147(5):990–1007.e3.
3. Kelsen JR, Baldassano RN. The role of monogenic disease in children with very early onset inflammatory bowel disease. Curr Opin Pediatr 2017;29(5):566–71.

4. de Lange KM, Moutsianas L, Lee JC, et al. Genome-wide association study implicates immune activation of multiple integrin genes in inflammatory bowel disease. Nat Genet 2017;49(2):256–61.
5. Ouahed J, Spencer E, Kotlarz D, et al. Very Early Onset Inflammatory Bowel Disease: A Clinical Approach With a Focus on the Role of Genetics and Underlying Immune Deficiencies. Inflamm Bowel Dis 2020;26(6):820–42.
6. Silverberg MS, Satsangi J, Ahmad T, et al. Toward an integrated clinical, molecular and serological classification of inflammatory bowel disease: report of a Working Party of the 2005 Montreal World Congress of Gastroenterology. Can J Gastroenterol 2005;19(Suppl). A:5a-36a.
7. Levine A, Griffiths A, Markowitz J, et al. Pediatric modification of the Montreal classification for inflammatory bowel disease: the Paris classification. Inflamm Bowel Dis 2011;17(6):1314–21.
8. Benchimol EI, Bernstein CN, Bitton A, et al. Trends in Epidemiology of Pediatric Inflammatory Bowel Disease in Canada: Distributed Network Analysis of Multiple Population-Based Provincial Health Administrative Databases. Am J Gastroenterol 2017;112(7):1120–34.
9. Heyman MB, Kirschner BS, Gold BD, et al. Children with early-onset inflammatory bowel disease (IBD): analysis of a pediatric IBD consortium registry. J Pediatr 2005;146(1):35–40.
10. Benchimol EI, Mack DR, Nguyen GC, et al. Incidence, outcomes, and health services burden of very early onset inflammatory bowel disease. Gastroenterology 2014;147(4):803–13.e7 [quiz: e14-5].
11. Ashton JJ, Andreoletti G, Coelho T, et al. Identification of Variants in Genes Associated with Single-gene Inflammatory Bowel Disease by Whole-exome Sequencing. Inflamm Bowel Dis 2016;22(10):2317–27.
12. Crowley E, Warner N, Pan J, et al. Prevalence and Clinical Features of Inflammatory Bowel Diseases Associated With Monogenic Variants, Identified by Whole-Exome Sequencing in 1000 Children at a Single Center. Gastroenterology 2020;158(8):2208–20.
13. Lega S, Pin A, Arrigo S, et al. Diagnostic Approach to Monogenic Inflammatory Bowel Disease in Clinical Practice: A Ten-Year Multicentric Experience. Inflamm Bowel Dis 2020;26(5):720–7.
14. Uhlig HH, Charbit-Henrion F, Kotlarz D, et al. Clinical Genomics for the Diagnosis of Monogenic Forms of Inflammatory Bowel Disease: A Position Paper From the Paediatric IBD Porto Group of European Society of Paediatric Gastroenterology, Hepatology and Nutrition. J Pediatr Gastroenterol Nutr 2021;72(3):456–73.
15. Khor B, Gardet A, Xavier RJ. Genetics and pathogenesis of inflammatory bowel disease. Nature 2011;474(7351):307–17.
16. Ashton JJ, Ennis S, Beattie RM. Early-onset paediatric inflammatory bowel disease. Lancet Child Adolesc Health 2017;1(2):147–58.
17. Kelsen JR, Sullivan KE, Rabizadeh S, et al. North American Society for Pediatric Gastroenterology, Hepatology, and Nutrition Position Paper on the Evaluation and Management for Patients With Very Early-onset Inflammatory Bowel Disease. J Pediatr Gastroenterol Nutr 2020;70(3):389–403.
18. Conrad MA, Kelsen JR. Genomic and Immunologic Drivers of Very Early-Onset Inflammatory Bowel Disease. Pediatr Dev Pathol 2019;22(3):183–93.
19. Kelsen JR, Russo P, Sullivan KE. Early-Onset Inflammatory Bowel Disease. Immunol Allergy Clin North Am 2019;39(1):63–79.
20. Batura V, Muise AM. Very early onset IBD: novel genetic aetiologies. Curr Opin Allergy Clin Immunol 2018;18(6):470–80.

21. Ouahed JD. Understanding inborn errors of immunity: A lens into the pathophysiology of monogenic inflammatory bowel disease. Front Immunol 2022;13:1026511.
22. Bolton C, Smillie CS, Pandey S, et al. An Integrated Taxonomy for Monogenic Inflammatory Bowel Disease. Gastroenterology 2022;162(3):859–76.
23. de Mesquita MB, Shouval DS. Evaluation of very early-onset inflammatory bowel disease. Curr Opin Gastroenterol 2020;36(6):464–9.
24. Levine AE, Zheng HB, Suskind DL. Linking Genetic Diagnosis to Therapeutic Approach in Very Early Onset Inflammatory Bowel Disease: Pharmacologic Considerations. Paediatr Drugs 2022;24(3):207–16.
25. Liang X, Xie J, Liu H, et al. STIM1 Deficiency In Intestinal Epithelium Attenuates Colonic Inflammation and Tumorigenesis by Reducing ER Stress of Goblet Cells. Cellular and molecular gastroenterology and hepatology 2022;14(1):193–217.
26. van Haaften-Visser DY, Harakalova M, Mocholi E, et al. Ankyrin repeat and zinc-finger domain-containing 1 mutations are associated with infantile-onset inflammatory bowel disease. J Biol Chem 2017;292(19):7904–20.
27. Kyodo R, Takeuchi I, Narumi S, et al. Novel biallelic mutations in the DUOX2 gene underlying very early-onset inflammatory bowel disease: A case report. Clin Immunol 2022;238:109015.
28. Hayes P, Dhillon S, O'Neill K, et al. Defects in NADPH Oxidase Genes NOX1 and DUOX2 in Very Early Onset Inflammatory Bowel Disease. Cellular and molecular gastroenterology and hepatology 2015;1(5):489–502.
29. Hsu NY, Nayar S, Gettler K, et al. NOX1 is essential for TNFα-induced intestinal epithelial ROS secretion and inhibits M cell signatures. Gut 2023;72(4):654–62.
30. Brooke MA, Longhurst HJ, Plagnol V, et al. Cryptogenic multifocal ulcerating stenosing enteritis associated with homozygous deletion mutations in cytosolic phospholipase A2-α. Gut 2014;63(1):96–104.
31. Heindl M, Händel N, Ngeow J, et al. Autoimmunity, intestinal lymphoid hyperplasia, and defects in mucosal B-cell homeostasis in patients with PTEN hamartoma tumor syndrome. Gastroenterology 2012;142(5):1093–6.e6.
32. Conrad MA, Dawany N, Sullivan KE, et al. Novel ZBTB24 Mutation Associated with Immunodeficiency, Centromere Instability, and Facial Anomalies Type-2 Syndrome Identified in a Patient with Very Early Onset Inflammatory Bowel Disease. Inflamm Bowel Dis 2017;23(12):2252–5.
33. Chongsrisawat V, Suratannon N, Chatchatee P, et al. Novel CD55 Mutation Associated With Severe Small Bowel Ulceration Mimicking Inflammatory Bowel Disease in a Pair of Siblings. Inflamm Bowel Dis 2022;28(9):1458–61.
34. Babaha F, Abolhassani H, Hamidi Esfahani Z, et al. A new case of congenital ficolin-3 deficiency with primary immunodeficiency. Expet Rev Clin Immunol 2020;16(7):733–8.
35. Hooper LV, Macpherson AJ. Immune adaptations that maintain homeostasis with the intestinal microbiota. Nat Rev Immunol 2010;10(3):159–69.
36. Maloy KJ, Powrie F. Intestinal homeostasis and its breakdown in inflammatory bowel disease. Nature 2011;474(7351):298–306.
37. Mehandru S, Colombel JF. The intestinal barrier, an arbitrator turned provocateur in IBD. Nat Rev Gastroenterol Hepatol 2021;18(2):83–4.
38. Avitzur Y, Guo C, Mastropaolo LA, et al. Mutations in tetratricopeptide repeat domain 7A result in a severe form of very early onset inflammatory bowel disease. Gastroenterology 2014;146(4):1028–39.
39. Fiskerstrand T, Arshad N, Haukanes BI, et al. Familial diarrhea syndrome caused by an activating GUCY2C mutation. N Engl J Med 2012;366(17):1586–95.

40. Murthy A, Shao YW, Narala SR, et al. Notch activation by the metalloproteinase ADAM17 regulates myeloproliferation and atopic barrier immunity by suppressing epithelial cytokine synthesis. Immunity 2012;36(1):105–19.
41. Blaydon DC, Biancheri P, Di WL, et al. Inflammatory skin and bowel disease linked to ADAM17 deletion. N Engl J Med 2011;365(16):1502–8.
42. Kern JS, Herz C, Haan E, et al. Chronic colitis due to an epithelial barrier defect: the role of kindlin-1 isoforms. J Pathol 2007;213(4):462–70.
43. Janecke AR, Heinz-Erian P, Yin J, et al. Reduced sodium/proton exchanger NHE3 activity causes congenital sodium diarrhea. Hum Mol Genet 2015;24(23): 6614–23.
44. Dhillon SS, Fattouh R, Elkadri A, et al. Variants in nicotinamide adenine dinucleotide phosphate oxidase complex components determine susceptibility to very early onset inflammatory bowel disease. Gastroenterology 2014;147(3):680–9.e2.
45. Denson LA, Jurickova I, Karns R, et al. Clinical and Genomic Correlates of Neutrophil Reactive Oxygen Species Production in Pediatric Patients With Crohn's Disease. Gastroenterology 2018;154(8):2097–110.
46. Cho JH, Abraham C. Inflammatory bowel disease genetics: Nod2. Annu Rev Med 2007;58:401–16.
47. Netea MG, Schlitzer A, Placek K, et al. Innate and Adaptive Immune Memory: an Evolutionary Continuum in the Host's Response to Pathogens. Cell Host Microbe 2019;25(1):13–26.
48. Bianco AM, Girardelli M, Tommasini A. Genetics of inflammatory bowel disease from multifactorial to monogenic forms. World J Gastroenterol 2015;21(43): 12296–310.
49. Egritas O, Dalgic B. Infantile colitis as a novel presentation of familial Mediterranean fever responding to colchicine therapy. J Pediatr Gastroenterol Nutr 2011; 53(1):102–5.
50. Zhao XW, Gazendam RP, Drewniak A, et al. Defects in neutrophil granule mobilization and bactericidal activity in familial hemophagocytic lymphohistiocytosis type 5 (FHL-5) syndrome caused by STXBP2/Munc18-2 mutations. Blood 2013; 122(1):109–11.
51. Zhu L, Shi T, Zhong C, et al. IL-10 and IL-10 Receptor Mutations in Very Early Onset Inflammatory Bowel Disease. Gastroenterology Res 2017;10(2):65–9.
52. Nambu R, Warner N, Mulder DJ, et al. A Systematic Review of Monogenic Inflammatory Bowel Disease. Clin Gastroenterol Hepatol 2022;20(4):e653–63.
53. Chen N, Zhang ZY, Liu DW, et al. The clinical features of autoimmunity in 53 patients with Wiskott-Aldrich syndrome in China: a single-center study. Eur J Pediatr 2015;174(10):1311–8.
54. Dupuis-Girod S, Medioni J, Haddad E, et al. Autoimmunity in Wiskott-Aldrich syndrome: risk factors, clinical features, and outcome in a single-center cohort of 55 patients. Pediatrics 2003;111(5 Pt 1):e622–7.
55. LaBere B, Gutierrez MJ, Wright H, et al. Chronic Granulomatous Disease With Inflammatory Bowel Disease: Clinical Presentation, Treatment, and Outcomes From the USIDNET Registry. J Allergy Clin Immunol Pract 2022;10(5):1325–33.e5.
56. Okou DT, Mondal K, Faubion WA, et al. Exome sequencing identifies a novel FOXP3 mutation in a 2-generation family with inflammatory bowel disease. J Pediatr Gastroenterol Nutr 2014;58(5):561–8.
57. Volz MS, Nassir M, Treese C, et al. Inflammatory bowel disease (IBD)-like disease in a case of a 33-year old man with glycogenosis 1b. BMC Gastroenterol 2015; 15:45.

58. Yamaguchi T, Ihara K, Matsumoto T, et al. Inflammatory bowel disease-like colitis in glycogen storage disease type 1b. Inflamm Bowel Dis 2001;7(2):128–32.
59. Sanderson IR, Bisset WM, Milla PJ, et al. Chronic inflammatory bowel disease in glycogen storage disease type 1B. J Inherit Metab Dis 1991;14(5):771–6.
60. Speckmann C, Lehmberg K, Albert MH, et al. X-linked inhibitor of apoptosis (XIAP) deficiency: the spectrum of presenting manifestations beyond hemophagocytic lymphohistiocytosis. Clin Immunol 2013;149(1):133–41.
61. Aeschlimann FA, Laxer RM. Haploinsufficiency of A20 and other paediatric inflammatory disorders with mucosal involvement. Curr Opin Rheumatol 2018; 30(5):506–13.
62. Nambu R, Muise AM. Advanced Understanding of Monogenic Inflammatory Bowel Disease. Front Pediatr 2020;8:618918.
63. Nameirakpam J, Rikhi R, Rawat SS, et al. Genetics on early onset inflammatory bowel disease: An update. Genes Dis 2020;7(1):93–106.
64. Kelsen JR, Sullivan KE. Inflammatory Bowel Disease in Primary Immunodeficiencies. Curr Allergy Asthma Rep 2017;17(8):57.
65. Conrad MA, Carreon CK, Dawany N, et al. Distinct Histopathological Features at Diagnosis of Very Early Onset Inflammatory Bowel Disease. J Crohns Colitis 2019;13(5):615–25.
66. Paul T, Birnbaum A, Pal DK, et al. Distinct phenotype of early childhood inflammatory bowel disease. J Clin Gastroenterol 2006;40(7):583–6.
67. Collen LV, Kim DY, Field M, et al. Clinical Phenotypes and Outcomes in Monogenic Versus Non-monogenic Very Early Onset Inflammatory Bowel Disease. J Crohns Colitis 2022;16(9):1380–96.
68. Levine A, Koletzko S, Turner D, et al. ESPGHAN revised porto criteria for the diagnosis of inflammatory bowel disease in children and adolescents. J Pediatr Gastroenterol Nutr 2014;58(6):795–806.
69. Uhlig HH, Muise AM. Clinical Genomics in Inflammatory Bowel Disease. Trends Genet 2017;33(9):629–41.
70. Engelhardt KR, Shah N, Faizura-Yeop I, et al. Clinical outcome in IL-10- and IL-10 receptor-deficient patients with or without hematopoietic stem cell transplantation. J Allergy Clin Immunol 2013;131(3):825–30.
71. Kotlarz D, Beier R, Murugan D, et al. Loss of interleukin-10 signaling and infantile inflammatory bowel disease: implications for diagnosis and therapy. Gastroenterology 2012;143(2):347–55.
72. Babcock SJ, Flores-Marin D, Thiagarajah JR. The genetics of monogenic intestinal epithelial disorders. Hum Genet 2022. https://doi.org/10.1007/s00439-022-02501-5.
73. Bader-Meunier B, Martins AL, Charbit-Henrion F, et al. Mevalonate Kinase Deficiency: A Cause of Severe Very-Early-Onset Inflammatory Bowel Disease. Inflamm Bowel Dis 2021;27(11):1853–7.
74. Canna SW, de Jesus AA, Gouni S, et al. An activating NLRC4 inflammasome mutation causes autoinflammation with recurrent macrophage activation syndrome. Nat Genet 2014;46(10):1140–6.
75. Raymond KN, Martin JED. Cryopyrin-associated periodic syndrome with inflammatory bowel disease: A case study. JGH Open 2021;5(5):629–31.
76. Shouval DS, Biswas A, Kang YH, et al. Interleukin 1β Mediates Intestinal Inflammation in Mice and Patients With Interleukin 10 Receptor Deficiency. Gastroenterology 2016;151(6):1100–4.
77. Kiykim A, Ogulur I, Dursun E, et al. Abatacept as a Long-Term Targeted Therapy for LRBA Deficiency. J Allergy Clin Immunol Pract 2019;7(8):2790–800.e15.

78. Maggiore R, Grossi A, Fioredda F, et al. Unusual Late-onset Enteropathy in a Patient With Lipopolysaccharide-responsive Beige-like Anchor Protein Deficiency. J Pediatr Hematol Oncol 2020;42(8):e768–71.
79. Lee S, Moon JS, Lee CR, et al. Abatacept alleviates severe autoimmune symptoms in a patient carrying a de novo variant in CTLA-4. J Allergy Clin Immunol 2016;137(1):327–30.
80. Kammermeier J, Lamb CA, Jones KDJ, et al. Genomic diagnosis and care co-ordination for monogenic inflammatory bowel disease in children and adults: consensus guideline on behalf of the British Society of Gastroenterology and British Society of Paediatric Gastroenterology, Hepatology and Nutrition. Lancet Gastroenterol Hepatol 2023;8(3):271–86.
81. Petersen BS, August D, Abt R, et al. Targeted Gene Panel Sequencing for Early-onset Inflammatory Bowel Disease and Chronic Diarrhea. Inflamm Bowel Dis 2017;23(12):2109–20.
82. Kammermeier J, Drury S, James CT, et al. Targeted gene panel sequencing in children with very early onset inflammatory bowel disease–evaluation and prospective analysis. J Med Genet 2014;51(11):748–55.
83. Petersen BS, Fredrich B, Hoeppner MP, et al. Opportunities and challenges of whole-genome and -exome sequencing. BMC Genet 2017;18(1):14.
84. Clark MM, Stark Z, Farnaes L, et al. Meta-analysis of the diagnostic and clinical utility of genome and exome sequencing and chromosomal microarray in children with suspected genetic diseases. NPJ Genom Med 2018;3:16.
85. Liu Z, Zhu L, Roberts R, et al. Toward Clinical Implementation of Next-Generation Sequencing-Based Genetic Testing in Rare Diseases: Where Are We? Trends Genet 2019;35(11):852–67.
86. Retterer K, Juusola J, Cho MT, et al. Clinical application of whole-exome sequencing across clinical indications. Genet Med 2016;18(7):696–704.
87. Kingsmore SF, Cakici JA, Clark MM, et al. A Randomized, Controlled Trial of the Analytic and Diagnostic Performance of Singleton and Trio, Rapid Genome and Exome Sequencing in Ill Infants. Am J Hum Genet 2019;105(4):719–33.
88. Belkadi A, Bolze A, Itan Y, et al. Whole-genome sequencing is more powerful than whole-exome sequencing for detecting exome variants. Proc Natl Acad Sci U S A 2015;112(17):5473–8.
89. Murdock DR, Rosenfeld JA, Lee B. What Has the Undiagnosed Diseases Network Taught Us About the Clinical Applications of Genomic Testing? Annu Rev Med 2022;73:575–85.
90. Taylor JC, Martin HC, Lise S, et al. Factors influencing success of clinical genome sequencing across a broad spectrum of disorders. Nat Genet 2015;47(7):717–26.
91. Sullivan JA, Schoch K, Spillmann RC, et al. Exome/Genome Sequencing in Undiagnosed Syndromes. Annu Rev Med 2023;74:489–502.
92. Tegtmeyer D, Seidl M, Gerner P, et al. Inflammatory bowel disease caused by primary immunodeficiencies-Clinical presentations, review of literature, and proposal of a rational diagnostic algorithm. Pediatr Allergy ImmunolAug 2017;28(5):412–29.
93. Richards S, Aziz N, Bale S, et al. Standards and guidelines for the interpretation of sequence variants: a joint consensus recommendation of the American College of Medical Genetics and Genomics and the Association for Molecular Pathology. Genet Med 2015;17(5):405–24.

94. Niehaus A, Azzariti DR, Harrison SM, et al. A survey assessing adoption of the ACMG-AMP guidelines for interpreting sequence variants and identification of areas for continued improvement. Genet Med 2019;21(8):1699–701.
95. MacArthur DG, Manolio TA, Dimmock DP, et al. Guidelines for investigating causality of sequence variants in human disease. Nature 2014;508(7497):469–76.
96. Gudmundsson S, Singer-Berk M, Watts NA, et al. Variant interpretation using population databases: Lessons from gnomAD. Hum Mutat 2022;43(8):1012–30.

Mechanisms and Emerging Therapies for Treatment of Seizures in Pediatric Autoimmune Encephalitis and Autoinflammatory/Autoimmune-Associated Epilepsy

Milena M. Andzelm, MD, PhD[a], Coral M. Stredny, MD[a,b,*]

KEYWORDS

- Autoimmune encephalitis • FIRES • Rasmussen syndrome
- Anti-NMDAR encephalitis • Anti-MOG-associated disease
- Autoimmune-associated epilepsy

KEY POINTS

- Acute symptomatic seizures secondary to autoimmune encephalitis are often highly responsive to immunotherapy, whereas those in chronic autoimmune-associated epilepsies tend to be refractory to multimodal therapy.
- Expert consensus guidelines suggest treatments targeting the innate immune system in patients with cryptogenic new-onset refractory status epilepticus and febrile infection-related epilepsy syndrome based on available evidence.
- Despite the inflammatory nature, Rasmussen syndrome tends to be only partially responsive to immunotherapy and it is therefore typically reserved for patients not deemed to be surgical candidates.
- Children with systemic autoimmune diseases, including systemic lupus erythematosus, Parry Romberg syndrome, and celiac, are at higher risk for seizures and epilepsy than the general population.

INTRODUCTION

Although first proposed over a century ago,[1,2] in the past few decades, there has been an increasing appreciation of the role of the immune system and inflammation in

[a] Program in Neuroimmunology, Department of Neurology, Boston Children's Hospital, Harvard Medical School, Boston, MA, USA; [b] Division of Epilepsy and Neurophysiology, Department of Neurology, Boston Children's Hospital, Harvard Medical School, Boston, MA, USA
* Corresponding author. 300 Longwood Avenue, Boston, MA 02115.
E-mail address: coral.stredny@childrens.harvard.edu

Rheum Dis Clin N Am 49 (2023) 875–893
https://doi.org/10.1016/j.rdc.2023.06.010
rheumatic.theclinics.com

seizure generation and epilepsy.[3] While the pathogenesis is not fully understood, greater mechanistic insight is accumulating and with this comes more targeted therapies. In pediatrics, autoimmune-related seizures most often present acutely in the context of autoimmune encephalitis (AE), but an ongoing predilection for seizures can be a feature of chronic autoinflammatory/autoimmune-associated epilepsies and systemic autoimmune diseases.[12] In this review, the authors discuss the various presentations of immune-mediated seizures in children, as well as the underlying pathophysiology and mechanisms behind emerging therapies.

PATHOPHYSIOLOGIC HYPOTHESES UNDERLYING IMMUNE-MEDIATED SEIZURE PROPAGATION

One area of interest focuses largely on inflammation-dependent changes in neuronal excitability. In particular, interleukin (IL)-1β, tumor necrosis factor, and IL-6, as well as the danger signal high-mobility group box 1, have been found to have dual effects in neurons of increasing excitability and decreasing inhibition to decrease seizure threshold.[4,5] Beyond intrinsic neuronal excitability, these cytokines also have pleiotropic ictogenic effects, including the ability to regulate glutamate, the blood-brain barrier, and astrocyte functions.[4] Although most of these studies have been performed in rodent seizure models, some have been extended to patient brain tissue[6] and helped usher in a wave of targeted cytokine therapies that are increasingly recognized to have potential efficacy in seizure treatment, particularly in AE and new-onset refractory status epilepticus (NORSE) and febrile infection–related epilepsy syndrome (FIRES).[7,8]

Beyond cytokines and soluble mediators, there are a diversity of other mechanisms that may produce seizures, including B-cell and autoantibody-mediated processes. As an illustrative example, in anti-N-methyl-D-aspartate receptor encephalitis (NMDARE), the autoantibody recognizes the glycine-binding NR1 subunit, leading to cross-linking and internalization and decreased NMDAR currents. Similar mechanisms by which antibodies bind directly to receptors yielding hyperexcitability and dysfunction exist in other cell-surface antibody-mediated encephalitides.[9]

Finally, via a variety of mechanisms, T-cell–mediated inflammation yields neuronophagia (destruction of neural cells by phagocytes) and gliosis, and this structural injury may further perpetuate refractory seizures.[10] These mechanisms underpin autoimmune-associated epilepsy syndromes, namely Rasmussen syndrome (RS), as well as disorders with intraneuronal antibody positivity, such as glutamic acid decarboxylase 65 (GAD65)-associated epilepsy. As such, intraneuronal antibodies are thought to be a biomarker of the disease in most instances but are not clearly pathogenic as are their cell-surface counterparts.[9]

DISTINGUISHING ACUTE SYMPTOMATIC SEIZURES AND AUTOIMMUNE-ASSOCIATED EPILEPSY

Many inflammation-associated seizures occur in an acute or subacute fashion in cases of AE, and most often do not lead to a long-standing predisposition for seizures, that is, epilepsy. This is an important distinction, as immunomodulation rather than chronic antiseizure medications (ASMs) is both a faster and more effective treatment in such instances.[11] Thus, efforts have been made to distinguish between acute symptomatic seizures secondary to AE versus autoimmune-associated epilepsy,[12] the latter of which represents rare but deleterious conditions that tend to be refractory to multimodal therapy, including immunomodulation. RS, GAD65-associated epilepsy, and likely the chronic stage of NORSE/FIRES represent autoinflammatory/autoimmune-associated epilepsies.[12]

SEIZURES IN AUTOIMMUNE ENCEPHALITIS

NMDARE and myelin oligodendrocyte glycoprotein antibody-associated disease (MOGAD) are the most common causes of AE in children.[13] Seizures are frequently encountered in the context of AE, where they are more common in children than adults and seen in at least 70% of the children presenting with NMDARE, for instance.[14] Overall, the risk of enduring epilepsy in patients with AE secondary to cell-surface antigens is low, with nearly 90% of patients with leucine-rich glioma inactivated 1 (LGI1), NMDAR, and gamma-aminobutyric acid beta receptor [$(GABA)_BR$] encephalitis becoming seizure free in one study. Importantly, seizures came under control sooner with immunotherapy compared with ASMs (4 vs 8.5 weeks, respectively).[11] In adult studies, the presence of status epilepticus (SE), temporal epileptiform discharges, periodic epileptiform discharges, persistent epileptiform discharges on follow-up electroencephalogram (EEG), development of hippocampal sclerosis, and delay in immunotherapy initiation were found to be predictors of epilepsy.[9,15,16]

As such, early identification, diagnosis, and immunotherapy initiation are crucial. Recently, pediatric-specific criteria were proposed for the diagnosis of AE.[17] The criteria suggest that at least two of the following symptoms should onset over $\leq$3 months: new focal neurologic symptoms, cognitive changes, regression, psychiatric symptoms, movement disorder, abnormal EEG or seizures. When initial clinical features are met in a patient with a positive paraclinical test (cerebral spinal fluid [CSF] pleocytosis, MRI T2/fluid-attenuated inversion recovery [FLAIR] hyperintensities, or inflammatory pathology on brain biopsy) and exclusion of mimics, a therapeutic trial is generally appropriate pending antibody results. Choice and duration of maintenance immunotherapy may depend on the specific antibody identified, but acute, first-line treatments are similar (**Tables 1** and **2**). Consensus guidelines for NMDARE[18] and MOGAD[20] provide comprehensive treatment pathways; other cell-surface antibodies are rare and lack formal treatment guidelines but similar paradigms are often applied.

Cortical Encephalitis secondary to MOGAD

Antibodies targeting MOG found on the myelin sheaths of neuronal axons have been identified in the past decade as representing a distinct neuroimmunologic disorder that is particularly frequent in pediatrics. It can present with varying phenotypes, commonly acute disseminated encephalomyelitis (ADEM), optic neuritis, transverse myelitis, or non-ADEM cortical encephalitis. Diagnosis is based on the presence of a typical aforementioned clinical phenotype and serum MOG positivity with titer typically $\geq$ 1:100 on cell-based assay or lower titer with additional supportive clinical/MRI features.[21] ADEM is the most common presenting phenotype in children younger than 10 years, representing an often monophasic, acute onset of multifocal neurologic symptoms, encephalopathy, and multifocal T2/FLAIR lesions on brain MRI.[21,22] Additionally, in a large pediatric cohort, MOGAD accounted for 34% of patients with non-ADEM encephalitis, more common than all other antibodies combined (33%).[22] Seizures are present in most with non-ADEM encephalitis, including SE in some.[22–24] Isolated seizures have been reported in some children preceding the subsequent development of MOGAD-related MRI lesions. Risk of ongoing epilepsy in MOGAD is not well studied but estimated at 3% to 13% in 2 studies.[25,26]

Consensus guidelines suggest acute treatment with intravenous (IV) methylprednisolone and moving to IV immunoglobulin (IVIG) and/or plasma exchange if incomplete

Table 1
Acute and prolonged first-line immunotherapy in autoimmune encephalitis and autoimmune-associated epilepsies

Therapy	Dosing	Caveats of Use
Methylprednisolone[a]	IV 20–30 mg/kg (max 1000 mg) daily for 3–5 days; may continue 1–3 days/month for prolonged first-line therapy	May worsen psychotic symptoms
IVIG	IV 2 g/kg divided over 2–5 days; may continue 1-2 g/kg divided over 1–2 days monthly for prolonged first-line therapy	If plasma exchange considered, would defer IVIG until its completion
Plasma Exchange	Typically 5–7 exchanges over 7–14 days	Patients with psychiatric symptoms may have difficulty tolerating central catheter; may remove other important medications, including ASMs

[a] Oral prednisone (1–2 mg/kg/day [max 60 mg] and slowly weaned) and oral dexamethasone (20 mg/m^2/day divided twice daily [max 12 mg/dose] for 3 days; may continue for 3 days every 4 weeks for prolonged first-line treatment) are occasionally used as alternative steroid regimens.
Data from Stingl 2018, Bruijstens 2020, and Nosadini 2021.[18–20]

Table 2
Second-line and maintenance immunotherapies in autoimmune encephalitis

Therapy	Dosing	Mechanism of Action
Rituximab[b,c]	IV 375–750 mg/m^2 (max 1000 mg) on day 0 and 14 OR IV 375 mg/m^2 (max 1000 mg) weekly x 4 weeks; redosing may be considered after 6 months or upon B cell repopulation	Anti-CD20
Cyclophosphamide[c]	IV 500–1000 mg/m^2 (max 1500 mg) every month for 3–6 months	Alkylating agent
Tocilizumab[d]	<30 kg: IV 12 mg/kg (max 800 mg) every 4 weeks ≥30 kg: IV 8 mg/kg (max 800 mg) every 4 weeks	IL-6 receptor antagonist
Mycophenolate mofetil[a,b]	PO 600 mg/m^2/dose (max 1000 mg) twice daily as goal dose	Purine synthesis inhibitor
Azathioprine[a,b]	PO 2–2.5 mg/kg (max 150 mg) once daily as goal dose	Purine synthesis inhibitor

[a] Considered for maintenance therapy in patients with NMDARE not improving on rituximab, cyclophosphamide, and/or tocilizumab.
[b] Typical maintenance immunotherapy options in MOGAD.
[c] Typical options for second-line immunotherapy in NMDARE.
[d] Option for escalation second-line immunotherapy in NMDARE
Data from Stingl 2018, Bruijstens 2020, and Nosadini 2021.[18,19,20]

recovery. Steroids are often slowly weaned over up to 3 months given concern for early relapse with more abrupt weans, but data are conflicting. Many guidelines suggest initiating maintenance immunotherapy only after the first relapse, although it can be considered after the initial event in a patient with poor response to first-line immunotherapy. Common maintenance or prolonged first-line therapy regimens include mycophenolate mofetil or azathioprine, rituximab, or monthly IVIG.[20]

Patients tend to be quite responsive to steroids, with good or full recovery in 70% to 95%, although outcomes can vary.[27] Relapse rates also vary widely in different studies and seem to be consistently more common in older patients. Persistent positivity of serum anti-MOG is associated with a higher relapse rate (38% vs 13%).[28]

Anti-NMDA Receptor Encephalitis

Seizures are frequent in NMDARE, occurring in at least 70% of children[14,29,30] and being the presenting symptom in approximately 35%.[14] Diagnosis is confirmed when a patient presents with at least 2 core neuropsychiatric symptoms, including seizures, movement disorder, change in speech, dysautonomia or central hypoventilation, behavior change or cognitive decline, and/or decreased level of consciousness and CSF NMDAR antibody positivity.[17] NMDARE represents one of the few autoimmune encephalitides that is often paraneoplastic in older children, with 6% of females younger than 12 years and 52% of females older than 12 years having an associated tumor, most often an ovarian teratoma.[14]

Per published guidelines, treatment with IV methylprednisolone is suggested, moving to IVIG and/or plasma exchange within 1 week if response is inadequate. Rituximab is recommended within 2 weeks for cases refractory to first-line treatment, with cyclophosphamide then considered if improvement is not seen in 1 to 3 months. Tocilizumab is an alternate or escalation second-line therapy for those not responding to rituximab and cyclophosphamide. Prolonged first-line or maintenance immunotherapy with monthly steroids or IVIG or mycophenolate mofetil is also often initiated, with duration dependent on response.[18]

Outcomes are generally favorable, with 70% to 80% of patients experiencing good outcomes (modified Rankin scale score 0–2) at 2 years, although persisting cognitive deficits are likely more prevalent. Earlier time to immunotherapy is associated with better outcomes. Approximately 15% of patients experience a relapse, and these are generally milder than initial presentation. Immunotherapy is associated with decreased risk of relapse.[14]

Anti-LGI1 and CASPR2–associated conditions

Antibodies against LGI1 and contactin-associated protein-like-(CASPR)2 are rare in children and not typically associated with limbic encephalitis or Morvan syndrome seen in adults. One recent review[31] identified 37 pediatric cases, of which the median age of onset was 9 years. Approximately half of patients had seizures, but none with faciobrachial dystonic seizures classically described in LGI1-associated limbic encephalitis in adults. In addition, more than half of the patients with CASPR2 antibodies displayed epilepsy or epileptic encephalopathies. Many patients with isolated epilepsy did not receive immunotherapy, and on follow-up, 43% had ongoing seizures.

Anti-GABA$_A$ Receptor Encephalitis

Children with anti-gamma-aminobutyric acid alpha (GABA$_A$) receptor encephalitis frequently present with seizures, mostly generalized and often with SE.[32,33] MRI typically shows multifocal T2/FLAIR hyperintensities. Therefore, the combination of SE and multifocal T2/FLAIR hyperintensities should prompt consideration of this cause as $GABA_A$ receptor antibodies are still not present on commercially available antibody panels.[32] In a review of children with anti-$GABA_A$ receptor encephalitis, over half had incomplete recovery.[33]

Limbic Encephalitis secondary to cell-surface antigens: $GABA_B$, mGluR5, and Amphiphysin

Although rare, limbic encephalitis marked by seizures and cognitive impairment is a typical presentation of $GABA_B$, metabotropic glutamate receptor subtype 5 (mGluR5), and amphiphysin antibodies when present in children.[33] MRI may show mesial temporal MRI changes or T2/FLAIR hyperintensities in varying locations outside the limbic system. Specifically in mGluR5 encephalitis, seizures are often generalized, associated with Hodgkin lymphoma, and extra-limbic symptoms and MRI findings can be seen.[34]

Anti-Glycine Receptor–associated conditions

The majority of children with glycine receptor (GlyR) antibodies present with seizures (60%), which are often temporal. Another presentation associated with GlyR antibodies is stiff-person syndrome (SPS) or progressive encephalomyelitis with myoclonus.[33]

Anti-GAD65–associated conditions

GAD65 antibodies are unique compared to those described earlier in that they target an intracellular antigen and, in contrast to cell-surface antibodies, are not believed to be directly pathogenic. Rather, GAD65-associated disease is thought to be primarily T-cell mediated.[10] Clinical presentations include SPS, cerebellar ataxia, and epilepsy often with limbic encephalitis. In one study of 212 children and adults with GAD65 antibodies,[35] epilepsy was seen in approximately 30%, being focal in 90% and localized to the temporal lobe in more than 60%. Musicogenic seizures triggered by listening to certain types of music have been associated with GAD65 antibodies.[36] Diagnosis is established by high-titer serum GAD65 and CSF GAD65 positivity. Low-titer serum GAD65 antibodies are less specific for neurologic autoimmunity and are seen in diabetes and thyrogastric disorders as well as healthy controls.[37] Patients with GAD65 antibody–related epilepsy often have medically and surgically refractory epilepsy.[35]

AUTOIMMUNE-ASSOCIATED SEIZURES WITHOUT SYNDROMIC ENCEPHALITIS

In addition to antibody-positive encephalitides, there are patients who present with suspected autoimmune-mediated epilepsy without encephalitis. There are several clinical prediction tools predominantly studied in adult cohorts to assist in identifying such patients, although they have limitations particularly in children, including lack of non-antibody biomarkers incorporated into the model such as cytokines. Nonetheless, some clinical features in a patient with new-onset focal epilepsy that should prompt consideration of an autoimmune/inflammatory cause include cognitive, autonomic, behavior, or speech changes, systemic autoimmune or autoinflammatory disease, and absence of other epilepsy risk factors.[38,39] In such cases, a trial of immunotherapy with IV methylprednisolone (30 mg/kg/dose [max 1000 mg] daily x 3 to 5 days and then once weekly x 4 to 6 weeks) or IVIG (2 g/kg over 2–5 days and then 1 g/kg every 4 weeks $\times$ 3 months) is often considered.[40]

NORSE/FIRES

Definitions and Cause

According to recent consensus definitions, NORSE describes new-onset refractory SE in a previously neurologically healthy patient without a structal lesion or metabolic/toxic etiology. FIRES, a subtype of NORSE, occurs when a fever is present 1-14 days prior and may be absent at the time of seizure onset.[41] Although there are no age restrictions, in published cohorts, NORSE tends to occur in adults and FIRES in school-aged children.[42,43] Patients typically present with focal seizures that progress to SE over days and remain refractory to ASMs and first-line immunotherapy in most cases.[44] An underlying cause is identified in only 50% of patients, with AE being most common in adults[43] and infectious encephalitis and genetic epilepsies in children.[45] The remaining cases are considered cryptogenic.

Diagnostic Considerations

These patients require a full workup for autoimmune, infectious, and genetic causes including MRI, continuous EEG monitoring, serum and CSF analysis, body imaging for tumor screen and whole exome sequencing.[46] Notably, FIRES and hemophagocytic lymphohistiocytosis (HLH) have been shown to co-occur, so a clinical decompensation with multisystem organ involvement should prompt consideration of screening for HLH.[47]

Pathogenesis

Although the pathophysiology is not fully understood, a recent Delphi procedure reaffirmed the consensus that inflammatory and postinfectious immune activation is likely to contribute to the development of cryptogenic NORSE/FIRES.[46] Upregulation of serum and intrathecal cytokines is seen, including IL-1β, IL-6, C-X-C motif ligand (CXCL)8, CXCL9, and CXCL10.[48–50] Although SE from other causes can also result in elevation of serum/CSF cytokines, a unique profile is seen in NORSE, including elevation of CSF IL-1β and serum CXCL8, C-C motif ligand (CCL)2, and macrophage inflammatory protein-1 alpha.[49] In addition, 2 studies have suggested association with the RN2 allele and other noncoding variants in *IL1RN*, the gene that encodes IL-1 receptor, in some patients with FIRES compared with controls.[50,51]

Treatment

Although retrospective and uncontrolled, some studies suggest that earlier treatment with second-line immunotherapy may be associated with shorter hospitalization and duration of mechanical ventilation.[52] Thus, expert consensus guidelines suggest prompt, aggressive treatment.[46] Initially, the pathway calls for management of possible infections and seizures per local SE guidelines for the first 48 to 72 hours as a diagnostic workup ensues. If no cause is identified and response to conventional seizure management is incomplete within 72 hours, IV methylprednisolone or IVIG is typically initiated, with the option to use plasma exchange, although this should not delay second-line therapies (see **Table 1**). Within 1 week of SE onset, if still poorly responsive, the ketogenic diet is recommended as well as the concurrent initiation of either rituximab if autoimmune encephalitis is suspected or anakinra or tocilizumab if cryptogenic (**Table 3**).[46]

The use of anakinra in FIRES stemmed from initial animal models[57] and a subsequent case report.[58] Its use was then reported in a retrospective international cohort of 25 children and associated with decreased duration of hospital stay and mechanical ventilation. Anakinra was stopped in one patient secondary to infection. Notably, 3 patients experienced drug reaction with eosinophilia and systemic symptoms (DRESS) potentially attributable to anakinra, although many ASMs used concurrently can also cause DRESS.[52] The largest series of tocilizumab use in NORSE found that 6 of 7 patients had resolution of SE after 1 to 2 doses, and one patient with preexisting sepsis died.[54] In addition, a recent series of 6 patients with FIRES reported the use of

Table 3
Second-line and maintenance immunotherapies in NORSE/FIRES

Therapy	Dosing	Outcomes
Rituximab	IV 375–750 mg/m² (max 1000 mg) on day 0 and 14; OR IV 375 mg/m² (max 1000 mg) weekly x 4 weeks	30% with good functional outcome[53]
Anakinra	IV/subcutaneous (SQ) 3–5 mg/kg/day initial dose; 4–9 mg/kg/day final dose; at least 2 week trial[52]	>50% seizure reduction in 11/15 patients with EEG data; earlier initiation was associated with shorter mechanical ventilation, intensive care unit and hospital length of stay[52]
Tocilizumab	<30 kg: IV 12 mg/kg (max 800 mg) every 4 weeks ≥30 kg: IV 8 mg/kg (max 800 mg) every 4 weeks[a]	6/7 adults with SE cessation[54]
Ketogenic diet	Ketosis as measured by serum beta-hydroxybutyric acid	60%–75% with SE cessation[55,56]

[a] Dosing not well established in NORSE/FIRES and typically extrapolated from other disorders.
Data from Wickstrom 2022, Lai 2020, and Nosadini 2021.[46,52]

intrathecal dexamethasone, yielding ability to wean continuous infusions and seizure reduction in 50%, although further studies are needed and this has not yet included in consensus treatment guidelines.[59] Compared with medications, the ketogenic diet is perhaps more efficacious in NORSE/FIRES[55] and may have a direct anti-inflammatory effect on the IL-1 pathway and decrease inflammasome activity.[60] Overall, data are currently limited to retrospective case reports and small series, and larger, controlled studies are needed to understand efficacy and safety profiles of these novel immunotherapies in NORSE/FIRES.

Outcomes

Most patients with NORSE/FIRES experience neurodevelopmental decline and chronic epilepsy, and the mortality rate approximates 10% to 25% in children.[42,43,61,62] In a cohort treated with anakinra in the acute phase (initiated 2–3 weeks after onset), all 25 children developed drug-resistant epilepsy[52]; in another cohort of 6 patients treated with anakinra (initiated within median of 11 days), all had cognitive decline.[63] Together, this presentation and subsequent clinical course have led to FIRES being described as an acute encephalopathy followed by a developmental epileptic encephalopathy.[64] Outcomes in those with NORSE/FIRES secondary to AE may be better.[14] Controlled studies are needed to understand best treatments and long-term outcomes, although such trials are challenging in this rare and heterogeneous disease.

RASMUSSEN SYNDROME

Epidemiology

Rasmussen encephalitis, now preferably termed Rasmussen syndrome (RS), is a rare childhood epilepsy marked by progressive cerebral hemiatrophy, focal epilepsy, and hemiplegia first identified in the 1950s.[65] Its incidence is estimated to be 1:5 million,[66] and median age of onset is 6 years, with greater than 80% onset in children.[69,70]

Pathogenesis and Pathology

In RS, there is increasing evidence suggesting T cell–based inflammation is a driving force of pathology, although the innate immune system also seems to be involved, particularly early in the disease. Initially, microglial nodules form, where Toll-like receptors 3 and 7 are upregulated, which is hypothesized to promote activation of the inflammasome and T-cell migration.[71,72] Sequencing of T-cell receptors has shown clonal expansion of T cells in the brain,[73] particularly of CD8+ T cells, with shared clones between patients.[74] Interferon gamma (IFNγ)-producing T cells infiltrate the central nervous system,[75,76] and elevated IFNγ and chemokines suggest an early Th1 immune response.[77] Infiltrating cytotoxic T cells have been further shown to cause apoptosis in neurons[79] as well as astrocytes.[80] Finally, peripheral blood mononuclear cells isolated from patients with RS can produce RS-like pathology when injected into mice.[81] In this model, injecting α4 integrin–blocking antibody early limited T-cell infiltration, and this, as well as IVIG treatment, improved seizure frequency. Intriguingly, in that model, the pathology is bihemispheric, and the unihemispheric nature in patients remains unclear, although yet-to-be identified somatic variants and/or ipsilateral perinatal complications or facial autoimmune conditions may be potential contributors to the unilaterality.[82] In addition, several examples of dual pathology have been identified with focal cortical dysplasia co-occurring on the affected side.[83,84]

Histologically, RS specimens show initial T-cell infiltration with perivascular cuffs, astrogliosis, and microglial activation that progressively worsens with accompanying neuronophagia, with final late stages marked by cortical degeneration and cavitation and severe neuronal loss.[85]

Clinical Presentation and Diagnostic Considerations

Patients generally present with focal seizures of unilateral onset that become progressively more refractory, and many develop epilepsia partialis continua (EPC), or continuous myoclonic jerks often isolated to a distal arm and/or leg with maintained awareness. The clinical diagnostic criteria were established in 2005[86] and revised in 2013,[78] which include the typical seizure presentation with progressive hemiplegia and often language decline, EEG with unilateral slowing, epileptiform discharges, and/or seizures, MRI with cortical atrophy and T2/FLAIR hyperintesity, and/or consistent histopathology if biopsy is obtained. In addition to meeting diagnostic criteria, mimics should be excluded before making the diagnosis, including serum and CSF investigations for autoimmune encephalitis, indolent infections, systemic rheumatologic or vasculitic diseases, and consideration of genetic testing.[67]

RS progresses through 3 stages. First, patients have rare seizures and mild hemiparesis, followed by an acute stage marked by frequent focal seizures, EPC, progressive hemiparesis, and cognitive decline. The chronic or residual phase yields permanent neurologic deficits with ongoing but decreased seizures.[69,70]

Atypical features including atrophy that precedes the development of seizures[87] or very rarely bilateral RS have been reported.[88] There is additionally a variant in which onset is later in adolescence and early adulthood, and these patients experience slower deterioration and overall better outcomes.[89]

Treatment Approach

Despite the established inflammatory nature, immunotherapy often has limited efficacy in seizure management and may slow but not halt disease progression. Patients remain largely refractory to ASMs.[68] Hemispherectomy is typically the most effective seizure treatment, with seizure freedom rates approximating 70%,[90,91] although this rate may decrease with further time from surgery.[92] However, hemispherectomy invariably results in weakness, particularly of the contralateral fine finger movements, and potentially language decline, depending on laterality and age. Immunotherapy is often reserved for patients with later onset, mild functional impairment and/or milder seizure burden who are less likely to be surgical candidates. Immunomodulation can have more efficacy in slowing functional decline rather than seizure control, and as such, a "pyrrhic victory" has been described in which immunotherapy may leave patients with more preserved function but ongoing refractory epilepsy, yielding the decision of if/when to proceed to hemispherectomy even more challenging and potentially delaying it to an age where outcomes could be less favorable.[66,68]

Immunomodulation

Given mouse model data,[81] there is consideration that early immunomodulating treatment may be particularly beneficial, although a prompt diagnosis of RS remains challenging given lack of early biomarkers and treatment initiation is therefore often delayed.

Regarding acute or first-line immunotherapies (see **Table 1**), in a recent systematic review, about 70% of published patients responded to corticosteroids primarily measured as improved seizure frequency,[93] but long-term side effects and waning efficacy limit chronic treatment.[94] IVIG was found to reduce seizures in 30%[93] and can be efficacious in slowing cortical atrophy and motor decline compared with historical controls.[66] Plasma exchange likely has a limited role in RS.[93]

First-line immunotherapies may serve as a bridge to maintenance and second-line immunotherapies as summarized in **Table 4**, although there is limited data to guide use. Considering all published studies, improved seizure control is noted with azathioprine (70%), rituximab (60%), and adalimumab (50%). IVIG and tacrolimus are less likely to control seizures but may slow disease progression in terms of motor decline and MRI atrophy.[93] Other immunosuppressive agents such as anakinra, natalizumab, cyclophosphamide, and mitoxantrone have been studied in case reports with some potential efficacy but are not regularly used in many centers.[99–101] Particularly the latter 2 are limited by cumulative toxicity.[93] Additional controlled studies comparing efficacy of these and novel treatments are needed, and there are no current consensus guidelines on immunomodulation in RS.

SEIZURES IN SYSTEMIC AUTOIMMUNE DISORDERS

Apart from specific autoimmune-associated epilepsies, it is notable that autoimmune disease in general increases seizure risk and even more so in children (odds ratio [OR] 5.2).[3] Although a comprehensive description of the links between epilepsy and systemic autoimmune disease is beyond the scope of this article, the authors review seizures seen in systemic lupus erythematosus (SLE), Parry-Romberg syndrome (PRS), and celiac disease.

Systemic Lupus Erythematosus

Children with SLE are at increased risk of seizures (OR 22).[3] Predominantly described in adult cohorts, seizures are more likely to occur at SLE onset and are associated with disease activity and younger age. Hydroxychloroquine has been found to be relatively protective against seizures.[102,103] In one adult study, 76% of seizures resolved without ASMs.[102] In another, seizures recurred in 1.3% of patients, and this was specifically associated with antiphospholipid syndrome (APLS).[104] Diagnostic workup

Table 4
Second-line and maintenance immunotherapies in Rasmussen Syndrome

Therapy	Dosing	Outcomes
IVIG[a]	IV 1–2 g/kg divided over 1–2 days every 4 weeks	When IVIG or tacrolimus were compared with historical controls, treated patients had slower rates of functional decline and MRI atrophy; none of those with refractory epilepsy at onset experienced seizure control with immunotherapy. The study was not powered to determine superiority of either treatment.[66]
Tacrolimus	Initial goal serum level 12–15 ng/mL, decreased to 5–8 ng/mL maintenance in one study[66]	Tacrolimus was associated with increased side effects compared to IVIG, with 2 patients discontinuing therapy due to infection.[66]
Azathioprine	PO 1.5 mg/kg/day as goal dose[95]	Sustained seizure improvement in 89% after weaning steroids; delayed but did not prevent functional decline and had no effect on cognitive decline compared to controls [95]
Mycophenolate mofetil	PO 600 mg/m^2/dose (max 1000 mg) twice daily as goal dose	Case reports with seizure improvement and slowed neurologic decline in some; no effect in others[93,96]
Rituximab	IV 375–750 mg/m^2 (max 1000 mg) on day 0 and 14; OR IV 375 mg/m^2 (max 1000 mg) weekly x 4 weeks; redosing may be considered after 6 months or upon B cell repopulation	In a series, 6/9 patients experienced improved seizures/EPC; 6/9 stable or improved motor function; 5/9 stable MRI[97]
Adalimumab	SC 24 mg/m^2 (max 40 mg) every 2 weeks[98]	5/11 patients with improved seizures, 3 of whom neurologically stabilized; benefit seen in later onset, slowly progressive form[98]

[a] Prolonged first-line immunotherapy with IVIG is often considered.
Data from Nosadini 2021.[18]

should include MRI, CSF evaluation, assessing for antiphospholipid syndrome, and correlation with systemic SLE disease activity at the time of seizure onset to differentiate seizures attributable to neuropsychiatric SLE (NPSLE) versus other causes, such as infection or malignancy.[105] In recent diagnostic and treatment consensus guidelines for pediatric SLE, when a patient has recurrent seizures, a trial of ASMs is likely indicated and once NPSLE manifestations are confirmed and thought to be inflammatory in nature, treatment with immunosuppression is suggested.[106] In addition, antiplatelet therapy/anticoagulation should be appropriately considered if APLS is identified.[105]

Parry Romberg Syndrome

PRS exists along a spectrum from localized scleroderma subtly seen on the forehead to a hemifacial atrophy that rarely involves up to the full hemibody or can even be bilateral. A recent systematic review confirmed that most cases (80%) start in children.[107] Neuroimaging is abnormal in 60% to 90% and can be ipsilateral to systemic scleroderma but no strong colateralization has been demonstrated.[107,108] Reported rates of seizures range broadly, from approximately 20% to 85%.[107–109] Those with seizures are more likely to have ipsilateral white matter disease and hemispheric atrophy.[108] Seizures may also be a presenting symptom of PRS, seen in nearly 20% of one cohort.[107] When it could be identified, seizure semiology was most often unilateral focal motor, and approximately 15% to 40% of patients had refractory epilepsy.[105,109] EPC has also been reported.[109] ASMs in addition to immunomodulation are often used for treatment of seizures in PRS, and epilepsy surgery is pursued in some.[109] Notably, there are cases of PRS and RS either coexisting or the intracranial manifestations of PRS closely mimicking RS.[110]

Celiac Disease

A recent metanalysis demonstrated that epilepsy is nearly 2 times more prevalent in patients with celiac disease.[111] Occipital epilepsy with bilateral occipital calcifications has been described in children with celiac disease, most often with onset in the first decade of life. Seizures are typically focal, and an epileptic encephalopathy may ensue in some. The epilepsy syndrome can precede gastrointestinal manifestations, so an index of suspicion and appropriate diagnostics should be pursued particularly if MRI calcifications are seen.[112] Initiation of a gluten-free diet may be an effective management strategy, and there is suggestion that earlier initiation can yield better outcomes.[112–114]

SUMMARY

Emerging knowledge of pathophysiologic mechanisms behind seizure generation has led to increased targeted therapeutics (eg, rituximab, IL-1 and IL-6 inhibitors) in the treatment of acute seizures secondary to autoimmunity or autoinflammation as well as chronic autoimmune/autoinflammatory-associated epilepsies. Those with acute symptomatic seizures as seen in AE and SLE may have the best treatment response, whereas patients with chronic autoimmune/autoinflammatory-associated epilepsies tend to be refractory to multimodal treatment, including immunomodulation. Further research to delineate the most efficacious treatment strategy, as well as how to distinguish these seizures from alternative causes to initiate specific treatment early, is needed.

DISCLOSURE

C. Stredny receives grant support from the Pediatric Epilepsy Research Foundation, United States. She is a member of the Medical and Scientific Advisory Board of the NORSE Institute. M.M. Andzelm is funded through the National Institutes of Health, United States/NINDS through the CH/BIDMC/Harvard Medical School Neurology Resident Research Education Program, 5R25NS070682-13.

All treatments discussed represent off-label uses. Dosing and medications should be individualized to the patient and considered in the specific clinical context by the treating physician.

CLINICS CARE POINTS

- Care should be used to distinguish seizures in the setting of autoimmune encephalitis from chronic epilepsy, as the majority respond better and faster to immunomodulation compared to anti-seizure medication.
- Early recognition and treatment of autoimmune encephalitis may yield improved outcomes; preliminary data are encouraging, but additional studies are needed to understand if early and aggressive immunomodulation may also improve outcomes in Rasmussen syndrome and new-onset refractory status epilepticus.
- Thorough diagnostic evaluation is essential in new-onset refractory status epilepticus and febrile infection-related epilepsy syndrome to identify a potential etiology, target treatment, and inform prognosis.
- Immunotherapy should be used cautiously in patients with Rasmussen syndrome, as it may slow progression of the disease with relatively less effect on seizure control and subsequently delay hemispherectomy to an age when outcomes may be less favorable.

REFERENCES

1. Delezenne C. Sérums néurotoxiques. Ann Inst Pasteur 1900;14:686–704.
2. Ettlinger G, Lowrie MB. An immunological factor in epilepsy. Lancet 1976; 1(7974):1386.
3. Ong MS, Kohane IS, Cai T, et al. Population-level evidence for an autoimmune etiology of epilepsy. JAMA Neurol 2014;71(5):569–74.
4. Villasana-Salazar B, Vezzani A. Neuroinflammation microenvironment sharpens seizure circuit. Neurobiol Dis 2023;178:106027.
5. Vezzani A, Viviani B. Neuromodulatory properties of inflammatory cytokines and their impact on neuronal excitability. Neuropharmacology 2015;96(PA):70–82.
6. Roseti C, van Vliet EA, Cifelli P, et al. GABAA currents are decreased by IL-1β in epileptogenic tissue of patients with temporal lobe epilepsy: implications for ictogenesis. Neurobiol Dis 2015;82:311–20.
7. van Vliet EA, Aronica E, Vezzani A, et al. Review: Neuroinflammatory pathways as treatment targets and biomarker candidates in epilepsy: emerging evidence from preclinical and clinical studies. Neuropathol Appl Neurobiol 2018;44(1): 91–111.
8. Vezzani A, Balosso S, Ravizza T. Neuroinflammatory pathways as treatment targets and biomarkers in epilepsy. Nat Rev Neurol 2019;15(8):459–72.
9. Geis C, Planagumà J, Carreño M, et al. Autoimmune seizures and epilepsy. J Clin Invest 2019;129(3):926–40.
10. Wesselingh R, Broadley J, Buzzard K, et al. Prevalence, risk factors, and prognosis of drug-resistant epilepsy in autoimmune encephalitis. Epilepsy Behav 2022;132. https://doi.org/10.1016/j.yebeh.2022.108729.
11. De Bruijn MAAM, Van Sonderen A, Van Coevorden-Hameete MH, et al. Evaluation of seizure treatment in anti-LGI1, anti-NMDAR, and anti-GABABR encephalitis. Neurology 2019;92(19):E2185–96.
12. Steriade C, Britton J, Dale RC, et al. Acute symptomatic seizures secondary to autoimmune encephalitis and autoimmune-associated epilepsy: Conceptual definitions. Epilepsia 2020;61(7):1341–51.
13. Armangue T, Olivé-Cirera G, Martínez-Hernandez E, et al. Associations of paediatric demyelinating and encephalitic syndromes with myelin oligodendrocyte

glycoprotein antibodies: a multicentre observational study. Lancet Neurol 2020; 19(3):234–46.
14. Titulaer MJ, McCracken L, Gabilondo I, et al. Treatment and prognostic factors for long-term outcome in patients with anti-NMDA receptor encephalitis: an observational cohort study. Lancet Neurol 2013;12(2):157–65.
15. Gifreu A, Falip M, Sala-Padró J, et al. Risk of Developing Epilepsy after Autoimmune Encephalitis. Brain Sci 2021;11(9):1182.
16. Zhong R, Zhang X, Chen Q, et al. Acute Symptomatic Seizures and Risk of Epilepsy in Autoimmune Encephalitis: A Retrospective Cohort Study. Front Immunol 2022;13:710.
17. Cellucci T, Van Mater H, Graus F, et al. Clinical approach to the diagnosis of autoimmune encephalitis in the pediatric patient. Neurology - Neuroimmunology Neuroinflammation. 2020;7(2):663.
18. Nosadini M, Thomas T, Eyre M, et al. International Consensus Recommendations for the Treatment of Pediatric NMDAR Antibody Encephalitis. Neurology(R) neuroimmunology & neuroinflammation. 2021;8(5). https://doi.org/10.1212/NXI.0000000000001052.
19. Stingl C, Cardinale K, Mater H Van. An Update on the Treatment of Pediatric Autoimmune Encephalitis Compliance with Ethical Standards Human and Animal Rights and Informed Consent HHS Public Access. Curr Treatm Opt Rheumatol 2018;4(1):14–28.
20. Bruijstens AL, Wendel EM, Lechner C, et al. E.U. paediatric MOG consortium consensus: Part 5 - Treatment of paediatric myelin oligodendrocyte glycoprotein antibody-associated disorders. Eur J Paediatr Neurol 2020;29:41–53.
21. Krupp LB, Tardieu M, Amato MP, et al. International Pediatric Multiple Sclerosis Study Group criteria for pediatric multiple sclerosis and immune-mediated central nervous system demyelinating disorders: revisions to the 2007 definitions. Mult Scler 2013;19(10):1261–7.
22. Banwell B, Bennett JL, Marignier R, et al. Diagnosis of myelin oligodendrocyte glycoprotein antibody-associated disease: International MOGAD Panel proposed criteria. Lancet Neurol 2023;22(3):268–82.
23. Wegener-Panzer A, Cleaveland R, Wendel EM, et al. Clinical and imaging features of children with autoimmune encephalitis and MOG antibodies. Neurol Neuroimmunol Neuroinflamm 2020;7(4):731.
24. Vega E, Arrambide G, Olivé G, et al. Non-ADEM encephalitis in patients with myelin oligodendrocyte glycoprotein antibodies: a systematic review. Eur J Neurol 2023;30(5):1515–27.
25. Ramanathan S, Mohammad S, Tantsis E, et al. Research paper: Clinical course, therapeutic responses and outcomes in relapsing MOG antibody-associated demyelination. J Neurol Neurosurg Psychiatry 2018;89(2):127.
26. Zhou J, Lu X, Zhang Y, et al. Follow-up study on Chinese children with relapsing MOG-IgG-associated central nervous system demyelination. Mult Scler Relat Disord 2019;28:4–10.
27. Bruijstens AL, Breu M, Wendel EM, et al. E.U. paediatric MOG consortium consensus: Part 4 - Outcome of paediatric myelin oligodendrocyte glycoprotein antibody-associated disorders. Eur J Paediatr Neurol 2020;29:32–40.
28. Waters P, Fadda G, Woodhall M, et al. Serial Anti–Myelin Oligodendrocyte Glycoprotein Antibody Analyses and Outcomes in Children With Demyelinating Syndromes. JAMA Neurol 2020;77(1):82–93.

29. Shen CH, Fang GL, Yang F, et al. Seizures and risk of epilepsy in anti-NMDAR, anti-LGI1, and anti-GABA B R encephalitis. Ann Clin Transl Neurol 2020;7(8): 1392–9.
30. Zhang J, Sun J, Zheng P, et al. Clinical Characteristics and Follow-Up of Seizures in Children With Anti-NMDAR Encephalitis. Front Neurol 2022;12:2455.
31. Nosadini M, Toldo I, Tascini B, et al. LGI1 and CASPR2 autoimmunity in children: Systematic literature review and report of a young girl with Morvan syndrome. J Neuroimmunol 2019;335. https://doi.org/10.1016/J.JNEUROIM.2019.577008.
32. Spatola M, Petit-Pedrol M, Simabukuro MM, et al. Investigations in GABA A receptor antibody-associated encephalitis. Neurology 2017;88(11):1012–20.
33. Ancona C, Masenello V, Tinnirello M, et al. Autoimmune Encephalitis and Other Neurological Syndromes With Rare Neuronal Surface Antibodies in Children: A Systematic Literature Review. Front Pediatr 2022;10. https://doi.org/10.3389/FPED.2022.866074.
34. Spatola M, Sabater L, Planagumà J, et al. Encephalitis with mGluR5 antibodies. Neurology 2018;90(22):e1964–72.
35. Budhram A, Sechi E, Flanagan EP, et al. Clinical spectrum of high-titre GAD65 antibodies. J Neurol Neurosurg Psychiatry 2021;92(6):645–54.
36. Smith KM, Zalewski NL, Budhram A, et al. Musicogenic epilepsy: Expanding the spectrum of glutamic acid decarboxylase 65 neurological autoimmunity. Epilepsia 2021;62(5):e76–81.
37. Walikonis JE, Lennon VA. Radioimmunoassay for glutamic acid decarboxylase (GAD65) autoantibodies as a diagnostic aid for stiff-man syndrome and a correlate of susceptibility to type 1 diabetes mellitus. Mayo Clin Proc 1998;73(12): 1161–6.
38. de Bruijn MAAM, Bastiaansen AEM, Mojzisova H, et al. Antibodies Contributing to Focal Epilepsy Signs and Symptoms Score. Ann Neurol 2021;89(4):698–710.
39. McGinty RN, Handel A, Moloney T, et al. Clinical features which predict neuronal surface autoantibodies in new-onset focal epilepsy: implications for immunotherapies. J Neurol Neurosurg Psychiatry 2021;92(3):291–4.
40. Toledano M, Britton JW, McKeon A, et al. Utility of an immunotherapy trial in evaluating patients with presumed autoimmune epilepsy. Neurology 2014;82(18): 1578.
41. Hirsch LJ, Gaspard N, van Baalen A, et al. Proposed consensus definitions for new-onset refractory status epilepticus (NORSE), febrile infection-related epilepsy syndrome (FIRES), and related conditions. Epilepsia 2018;59(4):739–44.
42. Kramer U, Chi CS, Lin KL, et al. Febrile infection-related epilepsy syndrome (FIRES): pathogenesis, treatment, and outcome: a multicenter study on 77 children. Epilepsia 2011;52(11):1956–65.
43. Gaspard N, Foreman BP, Alvarez V, et al. New-onset refractory status epilepticus: Etiology, clinical features, and outcome. Neurology 2015;85(18):1604–13.
44. Farias-Moeller R, Bartolini L, Staso K, et al. Early ictal and interictal patterns in FIRES: The sparks before the blaze. Epilepsia 2017;58(8):1340–8.
45. Lattanzi S, Leitinger M, Rocchi C, et al. Unraveling the enigma of new-onset refractory status epilepticus: a systematic review of aetiologies. Eur J Neurol 2022; 29(2):626.
46. Wickstrom R, Taraschenko O, Dilena R, et al. International consensus recommendations for management of New Onset Refractory Status Epilepticus (NORSE) including Febrile Infection-Related Epilepsy Syndrome (FIRES): Summary and Clinical Tools. Epilepsia 2022. https://doi.org/10.1111/EPI.17391.

47. Farias-Moeller R, LaFrance-Corey R, Bartolini L, et al. Fueling the FIRES: Hemophagocytic lymphohistiocytosis in febrile infection-related epilepsy syndrome. Epilepsia 2018;59(9):1753–63.
48. Sakuma H, Tanuma N, Kuki I, et al. Intrathecal overproduction of proinflammatory cytokines and chemokines in febrile infection-related refractory status epilepticus. J Neurol Neurosurg Psychiatry 2015;86(7):820–2.
49. Hanin A, Cespedes J, Huttner A, et al. Neuropathology of New-Onset Refractory Status Epilepticus (NORSE). J Neurol 2023;20:1–15.
50. Clarkson BDS, LaFrance-Corey RG, Kahoud RJ, et al. Functional deficiency in endogenous interleukin-1 receptor antagonist in patients with febrile infection-related epilepsy syndrome. Ann Neurol 2019;85(4):526.
51. Saitoh M, Kobayashi K, Ohmori I, et al. Cytokine-related and sodium channel polymorphism as candidate predisposing factors for childhood encephalopathy FIRES/AERRPS. J Neurol Sci 2016;368:272–6.
52. Lai YC, Muscal E, Wells E, et al. Anakinra usage in febrile infection related epilepsy syndrome: an international cohort. Ann Clin Transl Neurol 2020;7(12): 2467–74.
53. Cabezudo-García P, Mena-Vázquez N, Ciano-Petersen NL, et al. Functional outcomes of patients with NORSE and FIRES treated with immunotherapy: A systematic review. Neurologia 2022. https://doi.org/10.1016/J.NRLENG.2022.03.004.
54. Jun JS, Lee ST, Kim R, et al. Tocilizumab treatment for new onset refractory status epilepticus. Ann Neurol 2018;84(6):940–5.
55. Schoeler NE, Simpson Z, Zhou R, et al. Dietary Management of Children With Super-Refractory Status Epilepticus: A Systematic Review and Experience in a Single UK Tertiary Centre. Front Neurol 2021;12. https://doi.org/10.3389/FNEUR.2021.643105.
56. Nabbout R, Mazzuca M, Hubert P, et al. Efficacy of ketogenic diet in severe refractory status epilepticus initiating fever induced refractory epileptic encephalopathy in school age children (FIRES). Epilepsia 2010;51(10):2033–7.
57. Vezzani A, Moneta D, Conti M, et al. Powerful anticonvulsant action of IL-1 receptor antagonist on intracerebral injection and astrocytic overexpression in mice. Proc Natl Acad Sci U S A 2000;97(21):11534–9.
58. Kenney-Jung DL, Vezzani A, Kahoud RJ, et al. Febrile infection-related epilepsy syndrome treated with anakinra. Ann Neurol 2016;80(6):939–45.
59. Horino A, Kuki I, Inoue T, et al. Intrathecal dexamethasone therapy for febrile infection-related epilepsy syndrome. Ann Clin Transl Neurol 2021;8(3):645.
60. Youm YH, Nguyen KY, Grant RW, et al. The ketone metabolite beta-hydroxybutyrate blocks NLRP3 inflammasome-mediated inflammatory disease. Nat Med 2015;21(3):263–9.
61. Sculier C, Barcia Aguilar C, Gaspard N, et al. Clinical presentation of new onset refractory status epilepticus in children (the pSERG cohort). Epilepsia 2021; 62(7):1629–42.
62. Wu J, Lan X, Yan L, et al. A retrospective study of 92 children with new-onset refractory status epilepticus. Epilepsy Behav 2021;125. https://doi.org/10.1016/J.YEBEH.2021.108413.
63. Shrestha A, Wood EL, Berrios-Siervo G, et al. Long-term neuropsychological outcomes in children with febrile infection-related epilepsy syndrome (FIRES) treated with anakinra. Front Neurol 2023;14. https://doi.org/10.3389/FNEUR.2023.1100551.

64. Specchio N, Wirrell EC, Scheffer IE, et al. International League Against Epilepsy classification and definition of epilepsy syndromes with onset in childhood: Position paper by the ILAE Task Force on Nosology and Definitions. Epilepsia 2022;63(6):1398–442.
65. Rasmussen T, Olszewski J, Lloyd-Smith D. Focal seizures due to chronic localized encephalitis. Neurology 1958;8(6):435–45.
66. Bien CG, Tiemeier H, Sassen R, et al. Rasmussen encephalitis: incidence and course under randomized therapy with tacrolimus or intravenous immunoglobulins. Epilepsia 2013;54(3):543–50.
67. Bien CG, Elger CE, Leitner Y, et al. Slowly progressive hemiparesis in childhood as a consequence of Rasmussen encephalitis without or with delayed-onset seizures. Eur J Neurol 2007;14(4):387–90.
68. Varadkar S, Bien CG, Kruse CA, et al. Rasmussen's encephalitis: clinical features, pathobiology, and treatment advances. Lancet Neurol 2014;13(2): 195–205.
69. Oguni H, Andermann F, Rasmussen TB. The syndrome of chronic encephalitis and epilepsy. A study based on the MNI series of 48 cases. Adv Neurol 1992; 57:419–33.
70. Bien CG, Widman G, Urbach H, et al. The natural history of Rasmussen's encephalitis. Brain 2002;125(Pt 8):1751–9.
71. Tröscher AR, Wimmer I, Quemada-Garrido L, et al. Microglial nodules provide the environment for pathogenic T cells in human encephalitis. Acta Neuropathol 2019;137(4):619–35.
72. Wiendl H, Gross CC, Bauer J, et al. Fundamental mechanistic insights from rare but paradigmatic neuroimmunological diseases. Nat Rev Neurol 2021;17(7): 433–47.
73. Dandekar S, Wijesuriya H, Geiger T, et al. Shared HLA Class I and II Alleles and Clonally Restricted Public and Private Brain-Infiltrating alphabeta T Cells in a Cohort of Rasmussen Encephalitis Surgery Patients. Front Immunol 2016;7:608.
74. Schneider-Hohendorf T, Mohan H, Bien CG, et al. CD8(+) T-cell pathogenicity in Rasmussen encephalitis elucidated by large-scale T-cell receptor sequencing. Nat Commun 2016;7:11153.
75. Kreutzfeldt M, Bergthaler A, Fernandez M, et al. Neuroprotective intervention by interferon-gamma blockade prevents CD8+ T cell-mediated dendrite and synapse loss. J Exp Med 2013;210(10):2087–103.
76. Al Nimer F, Jelcic I, Kempf C, et al. Phenotypic and functional complexity of brain-infiltrating T cells in Rasmussen encephalitis. Neurol Neuroimmunol Neuroinflamm 2018;5(1):e419.
77. Owens GC, Huynh MN, Chang JW, et al. Differential expression of interferon-gamma and chemokine genes distinguishes Rasmussen encephalitis from cortical dysplasia and provides evidence for an early Th1 immune response. J Neuroinflammation 2013;10:56.
78. Olson HE, Lechpammer M, Prabhu SP, et al. Clinical application and evaluation of the Bien diagnostic criteria for Rasmussen encephalitis. Epilepsia 2013; 54(10):1753–60.
79. Bien CG, Bauer J, Deckwerth TL, et al. Destruction of neurons by cytotoxic T cells: a new pathogenic mechanism in Rasmussen's encephalitis. Ann Neurol 2002;51(3):311–8.
80. Bauer J, Elger CE, Hans VH, et al. Astrocytes are a specific immunological target in Rasmussen's encephalitis. Ann Neurol 2007;62(1):67–80.

81. Kebir H, Carmant L, Fontaine F, et al. Humanized mouse model of Rasmussen's encephalitis supports the immune-mediated hypothesis. J Clin Invest 2018; 128(5):2000–9.
82. Fauser S, Elger CE, Woermann F, et al. Rasmussen encephalitis: Predisposing factors and their potential role in unilaterality. Epilepsia 2022;63(1):108–19.
83. Takei H, Wilfong A, Malphrus A, et al. Dual pathology in Rasmussen's encephalitis: a study of seven cases and review of the literature. Neuropathology 2010;30(4):381–91.
84. Gilani A, Kleinschmidt-DeMasters BK. How frequent is double pathology in Rasmussen encephalitis? Clin Neuropathol 2020;39(2):55–63.
85. Pardo CA, Vining EPG, Guo L, et al. The Pathology of Rasmussen Syndrome: Stages of Cortical Involvement and Neuropathological Studies in 45 Hemispherectomies. Epilepsia 2004;45(5):516–26.
86. Bien CG, Granata T, Antozzi C, et al. Pathogenesis, diagnosis and treatment of Rasmussen encephalitis: A European consensus statement. Brain 2005;128(3): 454–71.
87. Bien CG, Urbach H, Deckert M, et al. Diagnosis and staging of Rasmussen's encephalitis by serial MRI and histopathology. Neurology 2002;58(2):250–7.
88. Tobias SM, Robitaille Y, Hickey WF, et al. Bilateral Rasmussen encephalitis: postmortem documentation in a five-year-old. Epilepsia 2003;44(1):127–30.
89. Dupont S, Gales A, Sammey S, et al. Late-onset Rasmussen Encephalitis: A literature appraisal. Autoimmun Rev 2017;16(8):803–10.
90. Pulsifer MB, Brandt J, Salorio CF, et al. The Cognitive Outcome of Hemispherectomy in 71 Children. Epilepsia 2004;45(3):243–54.
91. Kossoff EH, Vining EPG, Pillas DJ, et al. Hemispherectomy for intractable unihemispheric epilepsy Etiology vs outcome. Neurology 2003;61(7):887–90.
92. Sundar SJ, Lu E, Schmidt ES, et al. Seizure Outcomes and Reoperation in Surgical Rasmussen Encephalitis Patients. Neurosurgery 2022;91(1):93–102.
93. Lagarde S, Boucraut J, Bartolomei F. Medical treatment of Rasmussen's Encephalitis: A systematic review. Rev Neurol (Paris) 2022;178(7):675–91.
94. Bahi-Buisson N, Villanueva V, Bulteau C, et al. Long term response to steroid therapy in Rasmussen encephalitis. Seizure 2007;16(6):485–92.
95. Pellegrin S, Baldeweg T, Pujar S, et al. Immunomodulation With Azathioprine Therapy in Rasmussen Syndrome: A Multimodal Evaluation. Neurology 2021; 96(2):e267–79.
96. Orsini A, Foiadelli T, Carli N, et al. Rasmussen's encephalitis: From immune pathogenesis towards targeted-therapy. Seizure 2020;81:76–83.
97. Jagtap SA, Patil S, Joshi A, et al. Rituximab in Rasmussen's encephalitis: A single center experience and review of the literature. Epilepsy Behav Rep 2022;19. https://doi.org/10.1016/J.EBR.2022.100540.
98. Lagarde S, Villeneuve N, Trebuchon A, et al. Anti-tumor necrosis factor alpha therapy (adalimumab) in Rasmussen's encephalitis: An open pilot study. Epilepsia 2016;57(6):956–66.
99. Bittner S, Simon OJ, Göbel K, et al. Rasmussen encephalitis treated with natalizumab. Neurology 2013;81(4):395–7.
100. Stabile A, Deleo F, Didato G, et al. Adult-onset Rasmussen encephalitis treated with mitoxantrone. Eur J Neurol 2018;25(12):e125–6.
101. Mochol M, Taubøll E, Sveberg L, et al. Seizure control after late introduction of anakinra in a patient with adult onset Rasmussen's encephalitis. Epilepsy Behav Rep 2021;16. https://doi.org/10.1016/J.EBR.2021.100462.

102. Hanly JG, Urowitz MB, Su L, et al. Seizure disorders in systemic lupus erythematosus results from an international, prospective, inception cohort study. Ann Rheum Dis 2012;71(9):1502–9.
103. Andrade RM, Alarcón GS, González LA, et al. Seizures in patients with systemic lupus erythematosus: data from LUMINA, a multiethnic cohort (LUMINA LIV). Ann Rheum Dis 2008;67(6):829–34.
104. Appenzeller S, Cendes F, Costallat LTL. Epileptic seizures in systemic lupus erythematosus. Neurology 2004;63(10):1808–12.
105. Fanouriakis A, Kostopoulou M, Alunno A, et al. 2019 update of the EULAR recommendations for the management of systemic lupus erythematosus. Ann Rheum Dis 2019;78(6):736–45.
106. Groot N, De Graeff N, Avcin T, et al. European evidence-based recommendations for diagnosis and treatment of childhood-onset systemic lupus erythematosus: the SHARE initiative. Ann Rheum Dis 2017;76(11):1788–96.
107. Hixon AM, Christensen E, Hamilton R, et al. Epilepsy in Parry-Romberg syndrome and linear scleroderma en coup de sabre: Case series and systematic review including 140 patients. Epilepsy Behav 2021;121(Pt A). https://doi.org/10.1016/J.YEBEH.2021.108068.
108. De la Garza-Ramos C, Jain A, Montazeri SA, et al. Brain Abnormalities and Epilepsy in Patients with Parry-Romberg Syndrome. AJNR Am J Neuroradiol 2022;43(6):850–6.
109. Rocha R, Kaliakatsos M. Epilepsy in paediatric patients with Parry-Romberg syndrome: A review of the literature. Seizure 2020;76:89–95.
110. Longo D, Paonessa A, Specchio N, et al. Parry-Romberg syndrome and Rasmussen encephalitis: possible association. Clinical and neuroimaging features. J Neuroimaging 2011;21(2):188–93.
111. Julian T, Hadjivassiliou M, Zis P. Gluten sensitivity and epilepsy: a systematic review. J Neurol 2019;266(7):1557–65.
112. Taylor I, Scheffer IE, Berkovic SF. Occipital epilepsies: identification of specific and newly recognized syndromes. Brain 2003;126(Pt 4):753–69.
113. Hernández MA, Colina G, Ortigosa L. Epilepsy, cerebral calcifications and clinical or subclinical coeliac disease. Course and follow up with gluten-free diet. Seizure 1998;7(1):49–54.
114. Gobbi G, Ambrosetto P, Zaniboni MG, et al. Celiac disease, posterior cerebral calcifications and epilepsy. Brain Dev 1992;14(1):23–9.

Molecular Pathways in the Pathogenesis of Systemic Juvenile Idiopathic Arthritis

Grant S. Schulert, MD, PhD[a,*], Christoph Kessel, PhD[b]

KEYWORDS

• Macrophage activation syndrome • Autoinflammation • Neutrophil • IL-18

KEY POINTS

- Recent findings in systemic juvenile idiopathic arthritis (sJIA) have expanded the understanding of both the early innate immune response and adaptive immune cells involved in disease pathogenesis.
- Active sJIA is marked by extremely high levels of IL-18, neutrophil activation and expansion, and activation of monocytes with a mixed polarization phenotype and features of macrophage differentiation.
- Several recent studies have highlighted key roles for lymphocytes including γδT cells, Th1 and Th17 cells, T peripheral helper cells, and B cells.
- Further discoveries in sJIA pathogenesis may support new treatments including cytokine blockade and lymphocyte targeting.

INTRODUCTION

Systemic juvenile idiopathic arthritis (sJIA, Still disease) is a rare childhood arthropathy that is thought to represent a continuous disease spectrum with adult-onset Still disease (AOSD) (**Fig. 1**).[1,2] Although the terminology implies the disease to represent a systemic variant of juvenile idiopathic arthritis (JIA), recent studies have indicated a unique genetic architecture in sJIA is in line with its distinct clinical spectrum.[3]

At onset, the clinical presentation of sJIA is frequently dominated by features reminiscent of monogenic autoinflammatory periodic fever syndromes, including quotidian spiking fever accompanied by erythematous rash, while arthritis at onset is variably present. Further, hepatosplenomegaly, lymphadenopathy, and/or serositis are clinical hallmarks that separate sJIA from other JIA subtypes.[4] SJIA can be complicated by

[a] Division of Rheumatology, Department of Pediatrics, Cincinnati Children's Hospital Medical Center, University of Cincinnati College of Medicine, 3333 Burnet Avenue, MLC 4010, Cincinnati, OH 45229, USA; [b] Department of Pediatric Rheumatology and Immunology, Translational Inflammation Research, University Children's Hospital, Muenster, Germany
* Corresponding author.
E-mail address: Grant.schulert@cchmc.org

Rheum Dis Clin N Am 49 (2023) 895–911
https://doi.org/10.1016/j.rdc.2023.06.007 rheumatic.theclinics.com

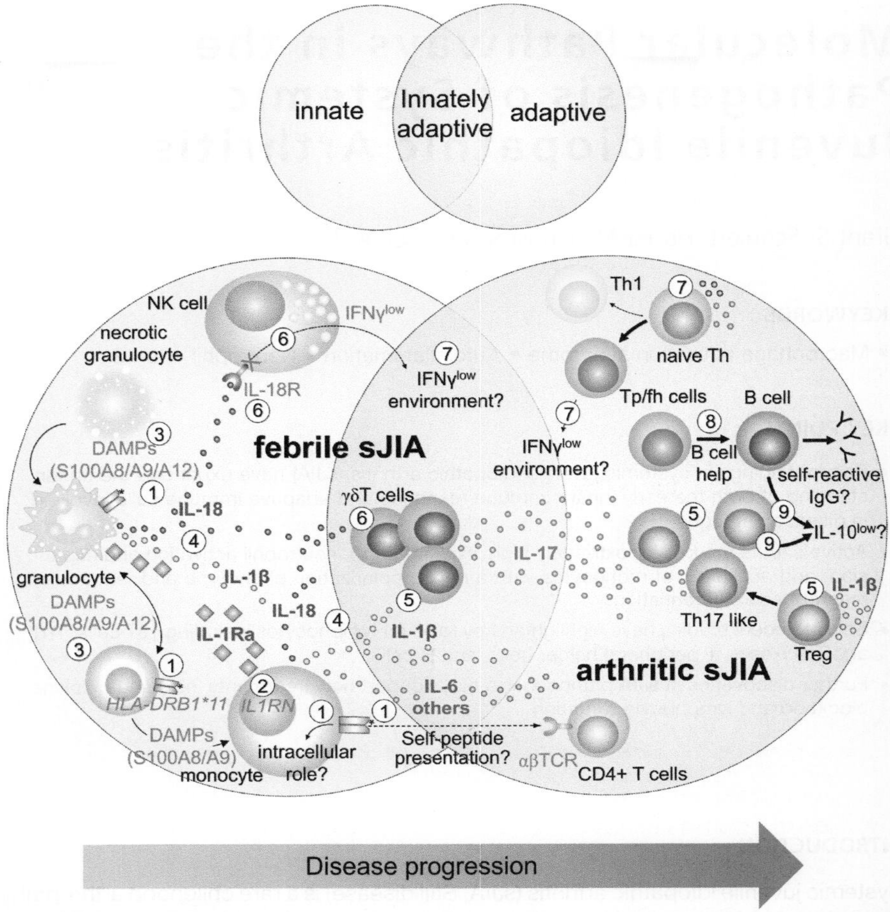

Fig. 1. Key innate and adaptive pathologic processes involved in acute/febrile and chronic/arthritic sJIA. (1) At a genetic level HLA-DRB1*11 has been identified as the strongest single risk factor for sJIA. Its precise mechanistic implication is still elusive. (2) Polymorphisms in the IL1RN gene have been suggested to associate with sJIA as well as response to treatment: low-expressing alleles may result in suboptimal IL-1Ra levels and could thus predispose for sJIA, whereas individuals carrying high-expressing alleles can also develop sJIA but are at risk for nonresponse to IL-1 targeting drugs. (3) SJIA granulocytes are expanded and activated, including overexpressing S100 proteins (A8/A9 and A12) at both the gene and protein level. When released from stressed or dying/necrotizing cells, these can operate as DAMPs, also termed alarmins, and trigger sterile inflammatory immune activation via toll-like receptor 4. (4) Such sterile inflammatory innate immune cell activation triggers release of proinflammatory cytokines such as IL-1β and IL-18. At the single-cell level, sJIA granulocytes also overexpress IL-18 versus its endogenous inhibitor IL-18 binding protein. (5) IL-1β can trigger IL-17 expression from γδT cells and reprogram sJIA Tregs toward T helper (Th) 17-like cells. (6) Although excessive IL-18 can promote T cell proliferation (including γδT), it fails to trigger IFN-γ expression from NK cells, due to a defective IL-18R. (7) Together with preferential differentiation of naïve Th cells toward inflammatory follicular/peripheral T helper (Tp/fh) cells, this IL-18 resistance may result in an environment with suboptimal IFNγ levels, further promoting T cell IL-17 expression. (8) Activated sJIA Th and Tp/fh cells can drive B cell plasmablast generation, and during chronic inflammation, patients with sJIA may accumulate self-reactive IgG. (9) Patients with sJIA also show reduced regulatory B cells and low-level regulatory cytokine expression from B and/or Tregs, particularly IL-10.

macrophage activation syndrome (MAS), a life-threatening hyperferritinemic cytokine storm condition,[5,6] as well as potentially fatal pulmonary complications.[5,7]

At the cellular and molecular level, the dominance of an innate immunity driven pathologic condition involving excessive expression of inflammasome components, damage associated molecular pattern molecules (DAMPs) and IL-1 family cytokines as well as increased IL-1 signaling further underpin analogies with monogenic autoinflammatory disorders. Therapeutic IL-1 blockade (recombinant IL-1 receptor antagonist, anakinra; IL-1β-targeting monoclonal antibody, canakinumab) can significantly improve disease outcomes[8] and current data point toward high efficacy of first-line anakinra therapy during the systemic disease phase.[9–11]

Importantly, if untreated or treatment-refractory, sJIA can progress toward a chronic destructive arthritis, that—in its clinical presentation—more resembles an autoimmunity-driven phenotype.[5,12] Indeed, a genetic association of sJIA with the major histocompatibility complex (MHC) class II specific allele, *HLA-DRB1*11*,[13] as well as alterations in adaptive immune cell signatures[14–16] and IL-17A–expressing T cells,[17,18] support the prevalence of an autoimmune component in sJIA.[12,19] The biphasic disease course in sJIA has fueled considerations on a window-of-opportunity for therapeutic intervention in order to achieve optimal clinical outcome. In this review, we summarize the latest data and evidence for both innate and adaptive immune mechanisms that seem relevant in sJIA pathology, and how the overall rapid increase in disease understanding can advance diagnostic approaches as well as targeted treatment strategies. Our review focuses on sJIA pathology and does not address (recurrent) MAS because this has been extensively reviewed elsewhere.[5,6,20]

INNATE IMMUNITY IN SYSTEMIC JUVENILE IDIOPATHIC ARTHRITIS

As noted above, sJIA is distinctive among the subtypes of JIA for prominent systemic features that are rather reminiscent of those seen in the monogenic periodic fever syndromes, in which mutations affecting innate immune pathways lead to recurrent fevers and other signs of multisystem inflammation. The discovery of these molecular mechanisms led to the concept of autoinflammation, in which inflammatory disease is driven not by autoantibodies or autoreactive lymphocytes as in autoimmunity but by spontaneous, inappropriate, or uncontrolled innate immune activation.[21] sJIA is similarly characterized by a lack of specific autoantibodies but high levels of proinflammatory cytokines that are principally but not exclusively produced by innate immune effector cells, most notably IL-1, IL-6, and IL-18.

IL-1 is a pleiotropic cytokine that is a central regulator of fever, activates vascular endothelial cells, stimulates destruction of bone and cartilage and orchestrates expression of numerous other inflammatory mediators, most prominently IL-6 as a primary proxy of IL-1(β) signaling. Of note, specific polymorphisms in the IL1RN gene, identified in sJIA patients, resulting in lower IL-1Ra expression are associated with an increased risk for disease development.[22] However, the strength of this association varies by population and remains controversial.[23,24] Nevertheless, a prominent role for IL-1 signaling in sJIA pathogenesis has been proposed,[8] and a mouse model of arthritis due to knockout of IL1RN (encoding the IL-1 receptor antagonist) manifests clinical features resembling those of sJIA.[25] Most strikingly, therapeutic treatment that neutralizes IL-1 proved highly clinically efficacious. IL-6 is a key driver of the acute phase response, which is clinically seen in sJIA. In contrast to IL-1β, elevated circulating IL-6 is more easily detected in the serum of children with sJIA, and levels are associated with active disease and track with fever spikes.[26–28] Inhibition of IL-6 through the monoclonal antibody tocilizumab is also highly effective. Although the role of IL-18 in sJIA and its complications are not fully understood (see later discussion), its marked elevation is a distinctive and possibly diagnostic feature of this disorder.

In contrast to the autoinflammatory periodic fever syndromes, the genetic basis of sJIA has remained elusive but is generally not considered to be monogenic. One exception to this is rare patients with biallelic mutations in *LACC1*, which were first identified in several consanguineous families with multiple children with an sJIA phenotype.[29] *LACC1* encodes FAMIN, a key regulator of macrophage metabolism including lipid flux, glycolysis, and energy generation that control several key inflammatory functions including inflammasome activation.[30] Large genome-wide association studies performed in more common sporadic sJIA have made several important discoveries toward understanding disease pathogenesis. First, genetic loci with genome-wide significance in polyarticular JIA, rheumatoid arthritis, and other classic autoimmune disorders are largely absent from patient with sJIA,[3] supporting that there are fundamental differences in disease etiology. Second, the single strongest association in sJIA is within the human leukocyte antigen (HLA) region, specifically with the MHC class II allele *HLA-DRB1*11*, which suggests that this disorder may not be "purely" autoinflammatory[13,19] (see later dicussion). Finally, 23 loci were identified with suggestive associations with sJIA but these mapped largely to poorly characterized genomic regions.[3] Together these genetic studies support a model wherein sJIA has a fundamentally different pathogenesis from other forms of JIA and may involve more innate immune mechanisms. In contrast, although comprehensive genomic studies of AOSD are lacking, the striking clinical, pathologic, and immunologic similarities between this and sJIA strongly suggest that these exist on the same disease continuum.[31–33]

Role of Innate Cells

Patients with sJIA demonstrate activation and expansion of granulocytes and myeloid cells during active disease, and several lines of evidence support a key pathogenic role for these cells.

Neutrophils in sJIA—Early studies in both sJIA and AOSD demonstrated high levels of circulating neutrophils in active disease.[34,35] A prospective study of newly diagnosed patients with sJIA found marked elevation in neutrophil counts, which rapidly normalized on initiation of anakinra treatment.[36] This neutrophilia was associated with high levels of neutrophil-related proteins including S100A8/A9, matrix metalloprotease (MMP)-8 and MMP-9, and intercellular adhesion molecule 1 (ICAM-1).[36–38] Neutrophils in active sJIA also show a highly activated, proinflammatory transcriptional signature including activation of surface receptors, inflammasome components, and IL-1 family members.[36,39] These neutrophils demonstrate a hypersegmented phenotype with decreased CD62 L expression.[36,39] There are also increased levels of low-density granulocytes in active sJIA and AOSD[40,41] as well as evidence for enhanced formation of neutrophil extraceullar traps (NETs) NETosis.[42] Interestingly, although immature and hypersegmented neutrophils are largely absent during clinically inactive disease, neutrophils from children with sJIA show a persistently active phenotype, including increased release of S100 proteins and a continued proinflammatory gene expression changes,[39] which could support a role for neutrophils in mediating disease chronicity and risk of flare.

Although there is no fully representative animal model of sJIA, chronic inflammation in interferon gamma knock-out (IFNg-KO) mice due to Freund's complete adjuvant induces a clinical state of neutrophilia, systemic inflammation, organomegaly, anemia, and arthritis.[43] Treatment with granulocyte-colony stimulating factor neutralizing antibody blocked maturation of neutrophils and lead to near complete resolution of arthritis.[44] Together, this supports neutrophil activation as a central inflammatory mediator in sJIA.

Monocytes and macrophages in sJIA—Patients with active, new-onset sJIA can show a peripheral monocytosis,[45] although less commonly and dramatically compared with neutrophil activation.[36] However phenotypically, monocytes in sJIA demonstrate profound transcriptional and functional activation. Myeloid cells can adopt distinct functional polarization phenotypes based on their inflammatory microenvironment, which although originally proposed to be a binary process of "classic" proinflammatory M1 and alternative M2 phenotypes is now considered more diverse, nuanced, and dynamic.[46] During active sJIA, monocytes show a mixed polarization profile, with upregulation of genes involved in both classical and alternative activation, and surface expression of numerous activation markers including CD40, CD80, CD163, and CD206.[47] Isolated monocytes from patients with active disease (indicated by elevated serum ferritin) showed a transcriptional pattern of overlapping polarization states,[48] as well as a microRNA profile including elevated miR-125a-5p.[49] In vitro, overexpression of miR-125a-5p drives monocytes and macrophages toward a polarization phenotype resembling the profile observed in sJIA.[49]

Bulk gene expression studies of peripheral blood mononuclear cells also demonstrated upregulation of genes involved in monocyte and macrophage differentiation.[50] Indeed, several studies have suggested that monocytes in sJIA have features of cells pushed toward macrophage differentiation, including high circulating levels of CD163,[51] downregulation of the aryl hydrocarbon receptor,[52] and increased the expression of microRNA of the miR-17-92 cluster.[53] Functionally, sJIA monocytes also differentiated in vitro with a skew toward macrophages compared with dendritic cells[52] and showed reduced histone H3 amino terminus proteolytic cleavage that primes chromatin for macrophage differentiation.[54] Functionally, monocytes in sJIA also demonstrate altered responsiveness to cytokine signaling, including increased responsiveness to interferon gamma (IFNγ).[55,56] Notably, although a strong IFNγ signature is largely absent during active sJIA, it is strongly linked to the emergence of MAS.[57,58] Isolated monocytes from patients with sJIA and bone marrow macrophages during MAS showed an increased expression of tripartite motrif containing 8 (TRIM8), a positive regulator of IFNγ signaling, and in vitro inhibition of TRIM8 reduced IFNγ responsiveness.[48] Together, these findings of skewed myeloid differentiation and hyperresponsiveness are intriguing and may provide mechanisms to explain the strong association between sJIA and MAS.

Role of Toll-like Receptor (TLR) Signaling in Systemic Juvenile Idiopathic Arthritis

DAMPs or alarmins that are preferentially released from stressed, damaged, or dying cells (outside apoptosis) are thought to have a prominent role in sJIA pathogenesis.[37,38,58,59] Indeed, serum levels of S100A8/A9 (MRP8/14) or S100A12 (EN-RAGE, MRP6), mainly expressed by monocytes and granulocytes, serve as excellent mechanistic biomarkers to support the diagnosis and to monitor response to treatment.[37,38,60,61] S100A8/A9 and S100A12, particularly when present in homodimeric (S100A8)[62] or hexameric (S100A12)[63] quaternary structure, have been demonstrated to bind and signal through toll-like receptor 4 (TLR4) and thus can trigger sterile inflammatory activation of target cells.[62–64] Yet, even though there are compelling mechanistic data on these proteins' general proinflammatory role, their specific implication in sJIA pathophysiology remains to be demonstrated.

ADAPTIVE IMMUNITY IN SYSTEMIC JUVENILE IDIOPATHIC ARTHRITIS

A key criterion for diagnosis of sJIA is the absence of specific autoimmunity. However, the observed association with the MHC class II allele *HLA-DRB1*11* has fueled speculations on an underappreciated contribution of adaptive immunity in sJIA pathology.[13,19] The specific cytokine environment generated by (over)activation of innate immune cells in sJIA has the potential to also prime and activate cells of adaptive immunity, namely T and B cells. IL-18 has historically been named "IFNγ-inducing factor" due to its strong capacity to activate particularly cytotoxic T cells.[65] Moreover, IL-1β signaling in CD4+ memory T cells stabilizes cytokine transcripts to enable productive and rapid effector functions and thus operates as a licensing signal to permit effector cytokine production across Th1, Th2, and Th17 lineages.[66] IL-1 supports antibody production in the context of vaccination,[67–70] where germinal center intrinsic IL-1β signaling to follicular T helper (Tfh) cells, results in IL-4 and IL-21 production that enables B cell plasmablast generation and immunoglobulin expression.[71] Here, we will discuss the currently available evidence for key roles of adaptive immune cells in sJIA pathogenesis.

ROLE OF "INNATELY" ADAPTIVE IMMUNE CELLS

Natural killer (NK) as well as T cells expressing the γδ T cell receptor (γδT cells) represent a unique subset of immune cells, which are thought to bridge innate and adaptive immunity because they feature effector functions and characteristics of both.[72,73]

NK cells—More than 20 years ago, both NK and γδT cells were reported to be decreased in percentage and absolute numbers in sJIA peripheral blood when compared with matched healthy controls, which separated sJIA from oligoarticular and polyarticular JIA.[74] However, whether a decrease in peripheral NK cell frequency is a robust hallmark of sJIA as well as AOSD immunology has remained a matter of controversy.[75] Several studies report NK cells in sJIA as dysfunctional in terms of cytotoxicity and/or cytotoxic protein expression[76,77] (in-depth reviewed by Vandenhaute and colleagues[75]). However, at least some of these data seem confounded by decreased NK cell numbers in samples; when correcting for this, NK cell cytotoxicity normalized.[76] Along similar lines, both RNAseq as well as protein expression data demonstrated normal to increased expression of perforin as well as granzyme A and B in isolated sJIA NK cells.[76] However, in CD56^{bright} NK cells, the same study[76] reported a decreased expression of granzyme K on both transcriptional as well as protein levels, which may translate into defective killing of autologous activated T cells as observed in different disease contexts such as multiple sclerosis.[78] Although such functional implications still warrant experimental proof in patients with sJIA, the IFNγ-KO mouse model of sJIA[43] recapitulates an NK cytotoxicity defect and suggests defective NK cell control over inflammatory monocytes contributes to the sJIA-like symptoms in this model.

The underlying cause for a cytotoxicity defect of sJIA NK cells remains largely unknown. Currently available experimental evidence suggests a hyporesponsiveness of sJIA NK cells toward highly overexpressed IL-18, which is due to defective phosphorylation of the IL-18 receptor.[76,79] Importantly, this may be transient and a function of prolonged exposure to IL-6, as treatment with anti-IL-6 receptor targeting antibodies (ie, tocilizumab) restores NK cell cytotoxicity.[80]

γδT cells—Several studies demonstrated decreased γδT cell numbers in sJIA.[14,18,45,74] Using a machine learning approach, changes in γδT cell frequency was also identified as a prime immunologic marker in sJIA.[14] Decrease in peripheral γδTs was particularly evident in samples obtained during active disease or flare,[18,45] suggesting γδT cells leave the periphery and to migrate into inflamed tissues to drive local inflammation.[18,45] This may resemble cell trafficking as also reported in psoriasis, where γδT cells have a prominent role in pathogenesis.[81]

Importantly, sJIA γδT cells have been observed to overexpress IL-17A per cell,[18] although overall numbers of circulating IL-17+ γδT cells remained unchanged compared with controls.[17,18] It has been suggested that the sJIA inflammatory environment, characterized by high levels of IL-1β and IL-18, specifically primes γδT cells for IL-17 overexpression.[18] Indeed, γδ T cell IL-17A expression is particularly sensitive to IL-1β signaling,[18,82] whereas IL-18 can drive cell proliferation.[18,83] The critical role of IL-1β signaling for IL-17 expression from γδT cells has also been demonstrated in mice developing IL-17-dependent spontaneous arthritis due to the lack of endogenous IL-1 receptor antagonist (IL-1RA, *Il1rn*$^{-/-}$).[84,85] Strikingly, γδT cells have also been critically implicated in disease pathology of the sJIA mouse model described above. In these animals, γδT cell numbers in draining lymph nodes as well as their IL-17 expression were strongly increased and the disease phenotype could be corrected by neutralization of IL-23,[43] which—in concert with IL-1β—is the main driver of peripheral γδT cellular IL-17A expression.[86]

Role of CD4+ T cells in Systemic Juvenile Idiopathic Arthritis

Different CD4+ T helper (Th) phenotypes have been described in association with sJIA. Here, we will focus on Th1 and Th17 cells, with their main effector molecules IFNγ and IL-17A, as well as a more recently described inflammatory Th cell subset, T peripheral helper (Tph) cells, which support B cell differentiation within inflamed tissue.

Th1 cells—Th1 cells in sJIA have been observed to express lower levels of IFNγ compared with controls,[18] which recapitulates earlier reports on low IFNγ release from sJIA peripheral blood mononuclear cells (PBMCs) stimulated with anti-CD3/CD28 or Phorbol-12-myristat-13-acetat.[87] Importantly, current data point toward a dichotomous role for IFNγ in the sJIA-specific continuum of inflammation. Cytokine levels in active sJIA without features of MAS indicated either no[57,58,88] or only partial elevation[58,89] of IFNγ or CXCL9 (as surrogate of IFNγ signaling) and the previously described sJIA mouse model requires absence of IFNγ to recapitulate sJIA disease features.[43,90] IFNγ-signaling may even protect from sJIA progression because it has been shown to inhibit IL-1 signaling in PBMCs.[89] This is in marked contrast to its prominent role in MAS (as extensively reviewed elsewhere[91]).

Th17 cells—Along with its prominent role in γδT cell IL-17 expression, IL-1β—together with IL-6—is crucial in driving naive Th cell differentiation toward a Th17 cell phenotype.[92–94] Similar to Th1 cells, Th17 cells have been reported either unchanged[14,17,18] or were found in higher proportions in the peripheral blood of patients with sJIA compared with pediatric age-matched controls,[15] and increased IL-17A serum levels have been reported among active versus inactive sJIA patients or controls.[18] Importantly, a recent study investigating T cell polarization in sJIA reported an expanded population of activated regulatory T cells (Tregs) in acute and chronic sJIA that was not observed in healthy controls or in children with oligoarticular or polyarticular JIA.[17] In acute sJIA, these Tregs expressed IL-17A and demonstrated a gene expression signature reflecting Th17 polarization. In more chronic sJIA, the Th17 transcriptional signature was instead identified in T effector cells but did not translate in elevated IL-17A release. Similar to γδT cell IL-17 expression,[18] the observed Th17 polarization was abrogated in patients responding to IL-1 blockade.[17] Thus, it can be speculated that the specific cytokine environment in sJIA may potentially drive both an evolving Th17 polarization of Tregs as well as γδT cell IL-17 expression and expansion.

Tph cells—T follicular helper (Tfh) cells reside within lymphoid organs and provide help within B cell follicles in germinal centers to promote B cell survival, differentiation, and (high-affinity) antibody production.[95] In contrast, the more recently discovered subset of Tph cells does not require lymphoid organs and can drive corresponding plasmablast generation within peripheral inflamed tissue.[96] Tphs or activated Tph-like cells have already been reported to accumulate in the joints of anti-nuclear antibody (ANA)-positive and oligoarticular JIA patients[97,98] and to promote local B cell differentiation,[97] which might reflect the particular autoimmune response in the joints of ANA-positive patients with JIA.[97] A recent study reported that in sJIA, the differentiation of naïve peripheral Th cells was skewed toward a Tph/Tfh phenotype particularly in more established disease.[16] Interestingly, independent data deposited with a deep-phenotyping flow cytometry analysis of systemic and nonsystemic JIA patients' samples as well as other inflammatory conditions demonstrates enhanced frequencies of circulating CD4+CXCR5+ Tfh cells in active sJIA.[14]In line with this, *BCL6* as a master transcription factor for Tf/ph differentiation[99–101] was highly overexpressed in retrospective analyses of sJIA whole blood RNA sequencing data,[16,102] and whole transcriptome transcription factor motif enrichment analyses previously found Bcl-6 to be among the most prominent binding motifs in sJIA immune cells.[103]

Role of CD8+ T cells in Systemic Juvenile Idiopathic Arthritis

CD8+ T cells encompass cytotoxic T lymphocytes that, similar to NK cells, express lytic enzymes such as perforin or granzymes. The initial study that demonstrated defects in the lytic machinery of sJIA NK cells also made similar observations for CD8+ T cells from patients with sJIA.[77] More recently, De Matteis and colleagues reported a unique CD8+ T cell subset ($CD38^{high}$/$HLA\text{-}DR^{+}$) with an effector memory phenotype and the capability to produce elevated levels of IFNγ and TNF to be increased in active versus inactive sJIA but collectively their frequency was far lower than observed in MAS or secondary hemophagocytic lymphohistiocytosis (sHLH). To date it is unclear whether these cells may have a pathomechanistic role in sJIA outside of a MAS context.

Role of B cells and (Auto)antibodies in Systemic Juvenile Idiopathic Arthritis

Autoantibodies as the main effector molecules of a self-reactive B cells represent the immunologic hallmark of classic autoimmunity, and thus absence of known antibody signatures (most prominently rheumatoid factor) is a key criterion when establishing sJIA diagnosis. Yet, a recent study reports distinct IgG-self-reactivity profiles from patients with sJIA compared with healthy children.[16] The antigens that were observed to strongly reacted to sJIA patients' serum include some with reported major roles in immunity (eg, *PLCG1*, *DOCK2*) and collagen metabolism (*LUM*, *PEPD*). Further, the very same study included a post hoc analysis of a previous data set[14] that found a significant fraction of patients with sJIA with positive antinuclear antibodies, which was linked to longer median disease duration.[16] This echoes independent findings on the development of both ANAs and rheumatoid factor in patients with arthritic sJIA during the course of disease.[104] Together, these studies suggest that patients with longstanding, chronic sJIA may accumulate specific autoantibodies.

At present, no specific B cell phenotypes or other functional data can be linked with these observations on autoantibody levels. Yet, it has been demonstrated that in vitro activated and differentiated naïve sJIA Th cells could drive plasmablast generation from allogenic memory B cells.[16] Further, ex vivo deep-phenotyping data indicate an inverse correlation of Tfh frequencies in sJIA and circulating memory B cell numbers, which may indicate elevated Tfh levels in disease to promote enhanced memory B cell differentiation.[14] However, aside from establishing antibody responses, B cells can also have a regulatory function during inflammation.[105–108] Regulatory B cells have been reported to produce IL-10 and thereby suppress Th cell proliferation as well as their differentiation into Th1 and Th17 subsets, and rather drive their conversion into Tregs.[105] Importantly, in patients with sJIA, lower frequencies of IL-10–producing regulatory B cells as well as overall IL-10 to inflammatory cytokine ratios have been observed compared with healthy controls.[109] In concordance with these data, defective IL-10 production particularly among B cells has been reported from the sJIA mouse model on a IFN$\gamma^{-/-}$ background, and IL-10 depletion resulted in chronic inflammation with clinical and hematologic features mimicking sJIA.[109]

TRANSLATING ADVANCES IN DISEASE PATHOGENESIS TO NEW TREATMENT APPROACHES

As noted above, the introduction of biologic therapy targeting IL-1 and IL-6 transformed the clinical management of sJIA. However, although many patients demonstrate high-level responses to these therapies, with resolution of fever, arthritis, and systemic symptoms, others have a more refractory course. Although the incidence of refractory sJIA is unclear, it may include 20% to 33% of children.[5] In addition, recent descriptions of sJIA-LD in association with biologic use,[110,111] as well as concerns for potential drug reactions,[112] has emphasized the need for new therapeutic approaches.[113] Discoveries in sJIA pathogenesis in recent years have suggested several potential avenues to consider, including additional cytokine drivers, signaling pathways, and cellular players such as T lymphocytes.

The robust clinical responses seen in targeting IL-1 and IL-6 in sJIA could support an approach of neutralizing additional inflammatory cytokines. The most distinctive cytokine elevation seen in sJIA is IL-18, which is seen to be near-universal but more common in patients with active disease, history of MAS or SJIA-LD, and particularly active MAS.[88,111,114,115] Several strategies for neutralizing IL-18 are in the development or clinical trials, including recombinant human IL-18 binding protein (tadekinig alpha[116,117]), monoclonal antibodies against IL-18 (NCT01035645), and a bispecific antibody neutralizing IL-1 and IL-18.[118] As an alternative strategy to block cytokine signaling, janus kinase (JAK) inhibitors are increasingly used in autoimmune and autoinflammatory disorders. Tofacitinib is currently FDA approved for polyarticular course JIA (including sJIA), whereas other JAK inhibitors have been reported efficacious in case reports[119–121] and are in clinical trials (NCT03000439).

The emerging understanding of the role of T cells in sJIA has led to a reconsideration of the role of medications used for more typical autoimmune disorders such as polyarticular JIA. TNF inhibitors are highly efficacious in other forms of JIA, and notably registration trials of such agents typically included patients with sJIA and active arthritis. Abatacept is a fusion protein including the extracellular domain of CTLA4, which binds to T cells to prevent costimulation and activation. Such treatment could prevent the activation of proinflammatory T cell subsets described above, and indeed patients with sJIA included in clinical trials of abatacept had similar responses to other patients with JIA.[122,123] The central role for IL-17A in driving such T cell responses could also support modulation of this pathway. Secukinumab directly targets IL-17A and has recently been shown safe and effective in children with juvenile psoriatic arthritis and enthesitis-related arthritis.[124] Finally, recent study has highlighted important roles of the mechanistic target of rapamycin (mTOR) pathway in sJIA. Data from the *Il1rn−/−* mouse model for sJIA demonstrated preferential monocytic activation of mTORC1, and transcriptomic sJIA patient data revealed decreased expression of respective inhibitors (TSC1/2) and a mTORC1 gene signature.[25] In mice, mTORC1 inhibition or monocyte depletion ameliorated inflammation, whereas *Tsc2* deletion was sufficient to induce disease and exacerbate aMAS-like phenotype. Removal of *TSC2* from human monocytes resulted in phenocopy of these effects. Collectively, these findings suggest mTORC1 as potential drugable target.[25] The broad efficacy of such novel treatment approaches is currently unknown but demonstrate how new research into disease pathogenesis may directly drive rational treatment approaches for refractory sJIA.

CLINICS CARE POINTS

- While many patient with SJIA demonstrate high-lvele responses to anti-IL-1 or IL-6 biologic thearpy, up to 20-30% have refractory disease courses.
- New insights into innate immune responses in SJIA may support targeting IL-18 or interferon pathways as emerging therapeutic strategies.
- Newly defined roles for lymphocyte populations in SJIA could also support targeting these cell populations in refactory disease courses.

DISCLOSURES

Dr G.S. Schulert has received consulting fees from Swedish Orphan Biovitrum (SOBI) and research support from IpiNovyx. Dr C. Kessel has received consulting and speaking fees from Novartis and SOBI and receives research support from Novartis, Switzerland. Dr G.S. Schulert is supported by the National Institutes of Health, United States (NIH, R01 AR079524). Dr C. Kessel's study is supported by the German Research Foundation (DFG, grant number KE 2026 1/3). Drs G.S. Schulert and C. Kessel are also supported by a Childhood Arthritis and Rheumatology Research Alliance, United States (CARRA)/Pediatric Rheumatology European Society (PReS) Collaborative Research Award.

REFERENCES

1. Petty RE, Southwood TR, Manners P, et al. International League of Associations for Rheumatology classification of juvenile idiopathic arthritis: second revision, Edmonton, 2001. J Rheumatol 2004;31(2):390–2.
2. Nirmala N, Brachat A, Feist E, et al. Gene-expression analysis of adult-onset Still's disease and systemic juvenile idiopathic arthritis is consistent with a continuum of a single disease entity. Pediatr Rheumatol Online J 2015;13:50.
3. Ombrello MJ, Arthur VL, Remmers EF, et al. Genetic architecture distinguishes systemic juvenile idiopathic arthritis from other forms of juvenile idiopathic arthritis: clinical and therapeutic implications. Ann Rheum Dis 2017;76(5): 906–13.
4. Pardeo M, Bracaglia C, De Benedetti F. Systemic juvenile idiopathic arthritis: New insights into pathogenesis and cytokine directed therapies. Best Pract Res Clin Rheumatol 2017;31(4):505–16.
5. Erkens R, Esteban Y, Towe C, et al. Pathogenesis and Treatment of Refractory Disease Courses in Systemic Juvenile Idiopathic Arthritis: Refractory Arthritis, Recurrent Macrophage Activation Syndrome and Chronic Lung Disease. Rheum Dis Clin North Am 2021;47(4):585–606.
6. Crayne CB, Albeituni S, Nichols KE, et al. The Immunology of Macrophage Activation Syndrome. Front Immunol 2019;10:119.

7. Kimura Y, Weiss JE, Haroldson KL, et al. Pulmonary Hypertension and Other Potentially Fatal Pulmonary Complications in Systemic Juvenile Idiopathic Arthritis. Arthrit Care Res 2013;65(5):745–52.
8. Pascual V, Allantaz F, Arce E, et al. Role of interleukin-1 (IL-1) in the pathogenesis of systemic onset juvenile idiopathic arthritis and clinical response to IL-1 blockade. J Exp Med 2005;201(9):1479–86.
9. Nigrovic PA, Mannion M, Prince FHM, et al. Anakinra as First-Line Disease-Modifying Therapy in Systemic Juvenile Idiopathic Arthritis Report of Forty-Six Patients From an International Multicenter Series. Arthritis Rheum-Us 2011;63(2): 545–55.
10. Vastert SJ, de Jager W, Noordman BJ, et al. Effectiveness of First-Line Treatment With Recombinant Interleukin-1 Receptor Antagonist in Steroid-Naive Patients With New-Onset Systemic Juvenile Idiopathic Arthritis Results of a Prospective Cohort Study. Arthritis Rheumatol 2014;66(4):1034–43.
11. Ter Haar NM, van Dijkhuizen EHP, Swart JF, et al. Treat-to-target using first-line recombinant interleukin-1 receptor antagonist monotherapy in new-onset systemic juvenile idiopathic arthritis: results from a five year follow-up study. Arthritis Rheumatol 2019;71(7):1163–73.
12. Nigrovic PA. Review: is there a window of opportunity for treatment of systemic juvenile idiopathic arthritis? Arthritis Rheumatol 2014;66(6):1405–13.
13. Ombrello MJ, Remmers EF, Tachmazidou I, et al. HLA-DRB1*11 and variants of the MHC class II locus are strong risk factors for systemic juvenile idiopathic arthritis. Proc Natl Acad Sci U S A 2015;112(52):15970–5.
14. Van Nieuwenhove E, Lagou V, Van Eyck L, et al. Machine learning identifies an immunological pattern associated with multiple juvenile idiopathic arthritis subtypes. Ann Rheum Dis 2019;78(5):617–28.
15. Omoyinmi E, Hamaoui R, Pesenacker A, et al. Th1 and Th17 cell subpopulations are enriched in the peripheral blood of patients with systemic juvenile idiopathic arthritis. Rheumatology 2012;51(10):1881–6.
16. Kuehn J, Schleifenbaum S, Hendling M, et al. Aberrant naive CD4+ T cell differentiation in systemic juvenile idiopathic arthritis is committed to B cell help. Arthritis Rheumatol 2022;75(5):826–41.
17. Henderson LA, Hoyt KJ, Lee PY, et al. Th17 reprogramming of T cells in systemic juvenile idiopathic arthritis. JCI Insight 2020;5(6).
18. Kessel C, Lippitz K, Weinhage T, et al. Pro-inflammatory cytokine environments can drive IL-17 over-expression by gammadeltaT cells in systemic juvenile idiopathic arthritis. Arthritis Rheumatol 2017;69(7):1480–94.
19. Nigrovic PA. Autoinflammation and autoimmunity in systemic juvenile idiopathic arthritis. P Natl Acad Sci USA 2015;112(52):15785–6.
20. Grom AA, Horne A, De Benedetti F. Macrophage activation syndrome in the era of biologic therapy. Nat Rev Rheumatol 2016;12(5):259–68.
21. Masters SL, Simon A, Aksentijevich I, et al. Horror autoinflammaticus: the molecular pathophysiology of autoinflammatory disease (*). Annu Rev Immunol 2009; 27:621–68.
22. Arthur VL, Shuldiner E, Remmers EF, et al. IL1RN Variation Influences Both Disease Susceptibility and Response to Recombinant Human Interleukin-1 Receptor Antagonist Therapy in Systemic Juvenile Idiopathic Arthritis. Arthritis Rheumatol 2018;70(8):1319–30.
23. Hinze C, Fuehner S, Kessel C, et al. Impact of IL1RN Variants on Response to Interleukin-1 Blocking Therapy in Systemic Juvenile Idiopathic Arthritis. Arthritis Rheumatol 2020;72(3):499–505.

24. Pardeo M, Rossi MN, Marafon DP, et al. Early Treatment and IL1RN Single-Nucleotide Polymorphisms Affect Response to Anakinra in Systemic Juvenile Idiopathic Arthritis. Arthritis Rheumatol 2021;73(6):1053–61.
25. Huang Z, You X, Chen L, et al. mTORC1 links pathology in experimental models of Still's disease and macrophage activation syndrome. Nat Commun 2022; 13(1):6915.
26. Muller K, Herner EB, Stagg A, et al. Inflammatory cytokines and cytokine antagonists in whole blood cultures of patients with systemic juvenile chronic arthritis. Br J Rheumatol 1998;37(5):562–9.
27. Pignatti P, Vivarelli M, Meazza C, et al. Abnormal regulation of interleukin 6 in systemic juvenile idiopathic arthritis. J Rheumatol 2001;28(7):1670–6.
28. Reiff A. The use of anakinra in juvenile arthritis. Curr Rheumatol Rep 2005;7(6): 434–40.
29. Wakil SM, Monies DM, Abouelhoda M, et al. Association of a mutation in LACC1 with a monogenic form of systemic juvenile idiopathic arthritis. Arthritis Rheumatol 2015;67(1):288–95.
30. Cader MZ, Boroviak K, Zhang Q, et al. C13orf31 (FAMIN) is a central regulator of immunometabolic function. Nat Immunol 2016;17(9):1046–56.
31. Inoue N, Shimizu M, Tsunoda S, et al. Cytokine profile in adult-onset Still's disease: Comparison with systemic juvenile idiopathic arthritis. Clin Immunol 2016;169:8–13.
32. Nigrovic PA, Colbert RA, Holers VM, et al. Biological classification of childhood arthritis: roadmap to a molecular nomenclature. Nat Rev Rheumatol 2021;17(5): 257–69.
33. Nigrovic PA, Martinez-Bonet M, Thompson SD. Implications of juvenile idiopathic arthritis genetic risk variants for disease pathogenesis and classification. Curr Opin Rheumatol 2019;31(5):401–10.
34. Choi JH, Suh CH, Lee YM, et al. Serum cytokine profiles in patients with adult onset Still's disease. J Rheumatol 2003;30(11):2422–7.
35. Gattorno M, Piccini A, Lasiglie D, et al. The pattern of response to anti-interleukin-1 treatment distinguishes two subsets of patients with systemic-onset juvenile idiopathic arthritis. Arthritis Rheum 2008;58(5):1505–15.
36. Ter Haar NM, Tak T, Mokry M, et al. Reversal of Sepsis-Like Features of Neutrophils by Interleukin-1 Blockade in Patients With Systemic-Onset Juvenile Idiopathic Arthritis. Arthritis Rheumatol 2018;70(6):943–56.
37. Frosch M, Ahlmann M, Vogl T, et al. The myeloid-related proteins 8 and 14 complex, a novel ligand of toll-like receptor 4, and interleukin-1beta form a positive feedback mechanism in systemic-onset juvenile idiopathic arthritis. Arthritis Rheum 2009;60(3):883–91.
38. Wittkowski H, Frosch M, Wulffraat N, et al. S100A12 is a novel molecular marker differentiating systemic-onset juvenile idiopathic arthritis from other causes of fever of unknown origin. Arthritis Rheum 2008;58(12):3924–31.
39. Brown RA, Henderlight M, Do T, et al. Neutrophils From Children With Systemic Juvenile Idiopathic Arthritis Exhibit Persistent Proinflammatory Activation Despite Long-Standing Clinically Inactive Disease. Front Immunol 2018;9:2995.
40. Liu Y, Xia C, Chen J, et al. Elevated circulating pro-inflammatory low-density granulocytes in adult-onset Still's disease. Rheumatology 2021;60(1):297–303.
41. Ramanathan K, Glaser A, Lythgoe H, et al. Neutrophil activation signature in juvenile idiopathic arthritis indicates the presence of low-density granulocytes. Rheumatology 2018;57(3):488–98.

42. Ahn MH, Han JH, Chwae YJ, et al. Neutrophil Extracellular Traps May Contribute to the Pathogenesis in Adult-onset Still Disease. J Rheumatol 2019;46(12): 1560–9.
43. Avau A, Mitera T, Put S, et al. Systemic juvenile idiopathic arthritis-like syndrome in mice following stimulation of the immune system with freund's complete adjuvant: Regulation by interferon-γ. Arthritis Rheumatol 2014;66(5):1340–51.
44. Malengier-Devlies B, Bernaerts E, Ahmadzadeh K, et al. Role for Granulocyte Colony-Stimulating Factor in Neutrophilic Extramedullary Myelopoiesis in a Murine Model of Systemic Juvenile Idiopathic Arthritis. Arthritis Rheumatol 2022; 74(7):1257–70.
45. Macaubas C, Nguyen K, Deshpande C, et al. Distribution of circulating cells in systemic juvenile idiopathic arthritis across disease activity states. Clin Immunol 2010;134(2):206–16.
46. Xue J, Schmidt SV, Sander J, et al. Transcriptome-based network analysis reveals a spectrum model of human macrophage activation. Immunity 2014; 40(2):274–88.
47. Macaubas C, Nguyen KD, Peck A, et al. Alternative activation in systemic juvenile idiopathic arthritis monocytes. Clin Immunol 2012;142(3):362–72.
48. Schulert GS, Pickering AV, Do T, et al. Monocyte and bone marrow macrophage transcriptional phenotypes in systemic juvenile idiopathic arthritis reveal TRIM8 as a mediator of IFN-gamma hyper-responsiveness and risk for macrophage activation syndrome. Ann Rheum Dis 2021;80(5):617–25.
49. Schulert GS, Fall N, Harley JB, et al. Monocyte MicroRNA Expression in Active Systemic Juvenile Idiopathic Arthritis Implicates MicroRNA-125a-5p in Polarized Monocyte Phenotypes. Arthritis Rheumatol 2016;68(9):2300–13.
50. Fall N, Barnes M, Thornton S, et al. Gene expression profiling of peripheral blood from patients with untreated new-onset systemic juvenile idiopathic arthritis reveals molecular heterogeneity that may predict macrophage activation syndrome. Arthritis Rheum 2007;56(11):3793–804.
51. Bleesing J, Prada A, Siegel DM, et al. The diagnostic significance of soluble CD163 and soluble interleukin-2 receptor alpha-chain in macrophage activation syndrome and untreated new-onset systemic juvenile idiopathic arthritis. Arthritis Rheum 2007;56(3):965–71.
52. Cepika AM, Banchereau R, Segura E, et al. A multidimensional blood stimulation assay reveals immune alterations underlying systemic juvenile idiopathic arthritis. J Exp Med 2017;214(11):3449–66.
53. Takellapti D, Niu XL, Do T, et al. Changes in MiR-17-92 Cluster Expression Link Systemic Juvenile Idiopathic Arthritis, Monocyte-to-Macrophage Differentiation, and Interferon Regulation. Arthritis Rheumatol 2019;71.
54. Cheung P, Schaffert S, Chang SE, et al. Repression of CTSG, ELANE and PRTN3-mediated histone H3 proteolytic cleavage promotes monocyte-to-macrophage differentiation. Nat Immunol 2021;22(6):711–22.
55. Sikora KA, Fall N, Thornton S, et al. The limited role of interferon-gamma in systemic juvenile idiopathic arthritis cannot be explained by cellular hyporesponsiveness. Arthritis Rheum 2012;64(11):3799–808.
56. Macaubas C, Wong E, Zhang Y, et al. Altered signaling in systemic juvenile idiopathic arthritis monocytes. Clin Immunol 2016;163:66–74.
57. Bracaglia C, de Graaf K, Pires Marafon D, et al. Elevated circulating levels of interferon-gamma and interferon-gamma-induced chemokines characterise patients with macrophage activation syndrome complicating systemic juvenile idiopathic arthritis. Ann Rheum Dis 2017;76(1):166–72.

58. Kessel C, Fall N, Grom A, et al. Definition and validation of serum biomarkers for optimal differentiation of hyperferritinaemic cytokine storm conditions in children: a retrospective cohort study. Lancet Rheumatol 2021;3(8):E563–73.
59. Kessel C, Holzinger D, Foell D. Phagocyte-derived S100 proteins in autoinflammation: putative role in pathogenesis and usefulness as biomarkers. Clin Immunol 2013;147(3):229–41.
60. Park C, Miranda-Garcia M, Berendes R, et al. MRP8/14 serum levels as diagnostic markers for systemic juvenile idiopathic arthritis in children with prolonged fever. Rheumatology 2022;61(7):3082–92.
61. Holzinger D, Frosch M, Kastrup A, et al. The Toll-like receptor 4 agonist MRP8/14 protein complex is a sensitive indicator for disease activity and predicts relapses in systemic-onset juvenile idiopathic arthritis. Ann Rheum Dis 2012; 71(6):974–80.
62. Vogl T, Stratis A, Wixler V, et al. Autoinhibitory regulation of S100A8/S100A9 alarmin activity locally restricts sterile inflammation. J Clin Invest 2018;128(5): 1852–66.
63. Kessel C, Fuehner S, Zell J, et al. Calcium and zinc tune autoinflammatory toll-like receptor 4 signaling by S100A12. J Allergy Clin Immunol 2018;142(4): 1370–3.e8.
64. Armaroli G, Verweyen E, Pretzer C, et al. Monocyte-Derived Interleukin-1beta As the Driver of S100A12-Induced Sterile Inflammatory Activation of Human Coronary Artery Endothelial Cells: Implications for the Pathogenesis of Kawasaki Disease. Arthritis Rheumatol 2019;71(5):792–804.
65. Kohno K, Kataoka J, Ohtsuki T, et al. IFN-gamma-inducing factor (IGIF) is a costimulatory factor on the activation of Th1 but not Th2 cells and exerts its effect independently of IL-12. J Immunol 1997;158(4):1541–50.
66. Jain A, Song R, Wakeland EK, et al. T cell-intrinsic IL-1R signaling licenses effector cytokine production by memory CD4 T cells. Nat Commun 2018;9(1): 3185.
67. Li H, Nookala S, Re F. Aluminum hydroxide adjuvants activate caspase-1 and induce IL-1beta and IL-18 release. J Immunol 2007;178(8):5271–6.
68. Nakae S, Asano M, Horai R, et al. Interleukin-1 beta, but not interleukin-1 alpha, is required for T-cell-dependent antibody production. Immunology 2001;104(4): 402–9.
69. Nakae S, Asano M, Horai R, et al. IL-1 enhances T cell-dependent antibody production through induction of CD40 ligand and OX40 on T cells. J Immunol 2001; 167(1):90–7.
70. Staats HF, Ennis FA. IL-1 is an effective adjuvant for mucosal and systemic immune responses when coadministered with protein immunogens. J Immunol 1999;162(10):6141–7.
71. Ritvo PG, Churlaud G, Quiniou V, et al. T(fr) cells lack IL-2Ralpha but express decoy IL-1R2 and IL-1Ra and suppress the IL-1-dependent activation of T(fh) cells. Sci Immunol 2017;2(15).
72. Vivier E, Raulet DH, Moretta A, et al. Innate or adaptive immunity? The example of natural killer cells. Science 2011;331(6013):44–9.
73. Ferreira LM. Gammadelta T cells: innately adaptive immune cells? Int Rev Immunol 2013;32(3):223–48.
74. Wouters CH, Ceuppens JL, Stevens EA. Different circulating lymphocyte profiles in patients with different subtypes of juvenile idiopathic arthritis. Clin Exp Rheumatol 2002;20(2):239–48.

75. Vandenhaute J, Wouters CH, Matthys P. Natural Killer Cells in Systemic Autoinflammatory Diseases: A Focus on Systemic Juvenile Idiopathic Arthritis and Macrophage Activation Syndrome. Front Immunol 2019;10:3089.
76. Put K, Vandenhaute J, Avau A, et al. Inflammatory Gene Expression Profile and Defective Interferon-gamma and Granzyme K in Natural Killer Cells From Systemic Juvenile Idiopathic Arthritis Patients. Arthritis Rheumatol 2017;69(1):213–24.
77. Wulffraat NM, Rijkers GT, Elst E, et al. Reduced perforin expression in systemic juvenile idiopathic arthritis is restored by autologous stem-cell transplantation. Rheumatology 2003;42(2):375–9.
78. Jiang W, Chai NR, Maric D, et al. Unexpected role for granzyme K in CD56bright NK cell-mediated immunoregulation of multiple sclerosis. J Immunol 2011;187(2):781–90.
79. de Jager W, Vastert SJ, Beekman JM, et al. Defective phosphorylation of interleukin-18 receptor beta causes impaired natural killer cell function in systemic-onset juvenile idiopathic arthritis. Arthritis Rheum 2009;60(9):2782–93.
80. Cifaldi L, Prencipe G, Caiello I, et al. Inhibition of natural killer cell cytotoxicity by interleukin-6: implications for the pathogenesis of macrophage activation syndrome. Arthritis Rheumatol 2015;67(11):3037–46.
81. Laggner U, Di Meglio P, Perea GK, et al. Identification of a novel proinflammatory human skin-homing V gamma 9V delta 2 T cell subset and its role in the pathogenesis of psoriasis. J Invest Dermatol 2011;131:S1.
82. Lalor SJ, Dungan LS, Sutton CE, et al. Caspase-1-processed cytokines IL-1beta and IL-18 promote IL-17 production by gammadelta and CD4 T cells that mediate autoimmunity. J Immunol 2011;186(10):5738–48.
83. Li W, Kubo S, Okuda A, et al. Effect of IL-18 on expansion of gammadelta T cells stimulated by zoledronate and IL-2. J Immunother 2010;33(3):287–96.
84. Horai R, Nakajima A, Habiro K, et al. TNF-alpha is crucial for the development of autoimmune arthritis in IL-1 receptor antagonist-deficient mice. J Clin Invest 2004;114(11):1603–11.
85. Ikeda S, Saijo S, Murayama MA, et al. Excess IL-1 Signaling Enhances the Development of Th17 Cells by Downregulating TGF-beta-Induced Foxp3 Expression. J Immunol 2014;192(4):1449–58.
86. Papotto PH, Goncalves-Sousa N, Schmolka N, et al. IL-23 drives differentiation of peripheral gammadelta17 T cells from adult bone marrow-derived precursors. EMBO Rep 2017;18(11):1957–67.
87. Raziuddin S, Bahabri S, Al-Dalaan A, et al. A mixed Th1/Th2 cell cytokine response predominates in systemic onset juvenile rheumatoid arthritis: Immunoregulatory IL-10 function. Clin Immunol Immunopathol 1998;86(2):192–8.
88. Weiss ES, Girard-Guyonvarc'h C, Holzinger D, et al. Interleukin-18 diagnostically distinguishes and pathogenically promotes human and murine macrophage activation syndrome. Blood 2018;131(13):1442–55.
89. Put K, Avau A, Brisse E, et al. Cytokines in systemic juvenile idiopathic arthritis and haemophagocytic lymphohistiocytosis: tipping the balance between interleukin-18 and interferon-gamma. Rheumatology 2015;54(8):1507–17.
90. Malengier-Devlies B, Decaesteker T, Dekoster K, et al. Lung Functioning and Inflammation in a Mouse Model of Systemic Juvenile Idiopathic Arthritis. Front Immunol 2021;12:642778.
91. De Benedetti F, Prencipe G, Bracaglia C, et al. Targeting interferon-gamma in hyperinflammation: opportunities and challenges. Nat Rev Rheumatol 2021;17(11):678–91.

92. Deknuydt F, Bioley G, Valmori D, et al. IL-1 beta and IL-2 convert human Treg into T(H)17 cells. Clin Immunol 2009;131(2):298–307.
93. Zhou LA, Ivanov II, Spolski R, et al. IL-6 programs TH-17 cell differentiation by promoting sequential engagement of the IL-21 and IL-23 pathways. Nat Immunol 2007;8(9):967–74.
94. Ferraccioli G, Bracci-Laudiero L, Alivernini S, et al. Interleukin-1beta and interleukin-6 in arthritis animal models: roles in the early phase of transition from acute to chronic inflammation and relevance for human rheumatoid arthritis. Mol Med 2010;16(11–12):552–7.
95. Liu X, Nurieva RI, Dong C. Transcriptional regulation of follicular T-helper (Tfh) cells. Immunol Rev 2013;252(1):139–45.
96. Yoshitomi H, Ueno H. Shared and distinct roles of T peripheral helper and T follicular helper cells in human diseases. Cell Mol Immunol 2021;18(3):523–7.
97. Fischer J, Dirks J, Klaussner J, et al. Effect of Clonally Expanded PD-1(high) CXCR5-CD4+ Peripheral T Helper Cells on B Cell Differentiation in the Joints of Patients With Antinuclear Antibody-Positive Juvenile Idiopathic Arthritis. Arthritis Rheumatol 2022;74(1):150–62.
98. Jule AM, Hoyt KJ, Wei K, et al. Th1 polarization defines the synovial fluid T cell compartment in oligoarticular juvenile idiopathic arthritis. JCI Insight 2021;6(18).
99. Johnston RJ, Poholek AC, DiToro D, et al. Bcl6 and Blimp-1 are reciprocal and antagonistic regulators of T follicular helper cell differentiation. Science 2009; 325(5943):1006–10.
100. Nurieva RI, Chung Y, Martinez GJ, et al. Bcl6 mediates the development of T follicular helper cells. Science 2009;325(5943):1001–5.
101. Yu D, Rao S, Tsai LM, et al. The transcriptional repressor Bcl-6 directs T follicular helper cell lineage commitment. Immunity 2009;31(3):457–68.
102. Mo A, Marigorta UM, Arafat D, et al. Disease-specific regulation of gene expression in a comparative analysis of juvenile idiopathic arthritis and inflammatory bowel disease. Genome Med 2018;10(1):48.
103. Hugle B, Schippers A, Fischer N, et al. Transcription factor motif enrichment in whole transcriptome analysis identifies STAT4 and BCL6 as the most prominent binding motif in systemic juvenile idiopathic arthritis. Arthritis Res Ther 2018; 20(1):98.
104. Hugle B, Hinze C, Lainka E, et al. Development of positive antinuclear antibodies and rheumatoid factor in systemic juvenile idiopathic arthritis points toward an autoimmune phenotype later in the disease course. Pediatr Rheumatol Online J 2014;12:28.
105. Flores-Borja F, Bosma A, Ng D, et al. CD19+CD24hiCD38hi B cells maintain regulatory T cells while limiting TH1 and TH17 differentiation. Sci Transl Med 2013;5(173). 173ra123.
106. Hayashi M, Yanaba K, Umezawa Y, et al. IL-10-producing regulatory B cells are decreased in patients with psoriasis. J Dermatol Sci 2016;81(2):93–100.
107. Hayashi M, Yanaba K, Umezawa Y, et al. Corrigendum to "IL-10-producing regulatory B cells are decreased in patients with psoriasis". J Dermatol Sci 2017; 86(1):79 [J. Dermatol. Sci. 81 (2016) 93-100].
108. Wang WW, Yuan XL, Chen H, et al. CD19(+)CD24(hi)CD38(hi)Bregs involved in downregulate helper T cells and upregulate regulatory T cells in gastric cancer. Oncotarget 2015;6(32):33486–99.
109. Imbrechts M, Avau A, Vandenhaute J, et al. Insufficient IL-10 Production as a Mechanism Underlying the Pathogenesis of Systemic Juvenile Idiopathic Arthritis. J Immunol 2018;201(9):2654–63.

110. Saper VE, Chen G, Deutsch GH, et al. Emergent high fatality lung disease in systemic juvenile arthritis. Ann Rheum Dis 2019;78(12):1722–31.
111. Schulert GS, Yasin S, Carey B, et al. Systemic Juvenile Idiopathic Arthritis-Associated Lung Disease: Characterization and Risk Factors. Arthritis Rheumatol 2019;71(11):1943–54.
112. Saper VE, Ombrello MJ, Tremoulet AH, et al. Severe delayed hypersensitivity reactions to IL-1 and IL-6 inhibitors link to common HLA-DRB1*15 alleles. Ann Rheum Dis 2022;81(3):406–15.
113. Nigrovic PA. Storm Warning: Lung Disease in Systemic Juvenile Idiopathic Arthritis. Arthritis Rheumatol 2019;71(11):1773–5.
114. Yasin S, Solomon K, Canna SW, et al. IL-18 as therapeutic target in a patient with resistant systemic juvenile idiopathic arthritis and recurrent macrophage activation syndrome. Rheumatology 2019;59(2):442–5.
115. Shimizu M, Nakagishi Y, Inoue N, et al. Interleukin-18 for predicting the development of macrophage activation syndrome in systemic juvenile idiopathic arthritis. Clin Immunol 2015;160(2):277–81.
116. Canna SW, Girard C, Malle L, et al. Life-threatening NLRC4-associated hyperinflammation successfully treated with IL-18 inhibition. J Allergy Clin Immunol 2017;139(5):1698–701.
117. Gabay C, Fautrel B, Rech J, et al. Open-label, multicentre, dose-escalating phase II clinical trial on the safety and efficacy of tadekinig alfa (IL-18BP) in adult-onset Still's disease. Ann Rheum Dis 2018;77(6):840–7.
118. Rood JE, Rezk A, Pogoriler J, et al. Improvement of Refractory Systemic Juvenile Idiopathic Arthritis-Associated Lung Disease with Single-Agent Blockade of IL-1beta and IL-18. J Clin Immunol 2023;43(1):101–8.
119. Verweyen E, Holzinger D, Weinhage T, et al. Synergistic TLR/IFNalpha/beta-Signaling Facilitates Escape of IL-18 Expression from Endotoxin Tolerance. Am J Respir Crit Care Med 2019;201(5):526–39.
120. Huang Z, Lee PY, Yao X, et al. Tofacitinib Treatment of Refractory Systemic Juvenile Idiopathic Arthritis. Pediatrics 2019;143(5).
121. Bader-Meunier B, Hadchouel A, Berteloot L, et al. Effectiveness and safety of ruxolitinib for the treatment of refractory systemic idiopathic juvenile arthritis like associated with interstitial lung disease : a case report. Ann Rheum Dis 2022;81(2):e20.
122. Record JL, Beukelman T, Cron RQ. Combination therapy of abatacept and anakinra in children with refractory systemic juvenile idiopathic arthritis: a retrospective case series. J Rheumatol 2011;38(1):180–1.
123. Ruperto N, Lovell DJ, Quartier P, et al. Abatacept in children with juvenile idiopathic arthritis: a randomised, double-blind, placebo-controlled withdrawal trial. Lancet 2008;372(9636):383–91.
124. Brunner HI, Foeldvari I, Alexeeva E, et al. Secukinumab in enthesitis-related arthritis and juvenile psoriatic arthritis: a randomised, double-blind, placebo-controlled, treatment withdrawal, phase 3 trial. Ann Rheum Dis 2023;82(1):154–60.

Targeted Treatment of Diseases of Immune Dysregulation

Smriti Mohan, MD

KEYWORDS

- Therapeutics • Treatments • Biologics • Management • Autoimmune
- Autoinflammatory

KEY POINTS

- Current treatments in innate immune dysregulation include inhibitors to proinflammatory cytokines interleukin (IL)-1ß and IL-18, as well as IL-6.
- Janus kinase inhibition treats some conditions of innate immune dysregulation such as interferonopathies as well as autoimmune diseases such as ankylosing spondylitis.
- Inhibitors of T and B cells are predominantly used to treat autoimmune diseases.
- Inhibitors to novel targets are in development to offer more precise therapeutic treatments.
- Increasing understanding of the overlap between autoinflammatory and autoimmune diseases may lead to new indications for currently available treatments.

INTRODUCTION: INNATE VERSUS ADAPTIVE IMMUNE SYSTEM

The immune system provides 2 layers, innate and adaptive, of defense against pathogenic organisms or endogenous dangers. Normally, the innate immune response is rapid (minutes to hours) but nonspecific to challenge, usually to predetermined stimuli (evolutionarily conserved sequences).[1] The adaptive immune response is slower (days to weeks) and highly specific to the antigens presented with each challenge. Cells of the innate immune system consist of phagocytes, dendritic cells (DCs), mast cells, and innate lymphoid cells, whereas the adaptive immune system consists of lymphocytes. Both arms of the immune system communicate, with the innate immune system providing the early signals to stimulate the adaptive immune system and the adaptive immune system enhancing innate immune responses.[1,2]

Innate immune system activation provides the fastest immunologic response to infectious triggers as well as endogenous damage and stressors. There are several layers to innate immunity, including physical and chemical barriers, cells, and blood

Division of Rheumatology, Department of Pediatrics, University of Michigan CS Mott Children's Hospital, 1500 East Medical Ctr Dr SPC 5718, Ann Arbor, MI 48109-5718, USA
E-mail address: smritim@med.umich.edu

Rheum Dis Clin N Am 49 (2023) 913–929
https://doi.org/10.1016/j.rdc.2023.07.002
0889-857X/23/Published by Elsevier Inc.
rheumatic.theclinics.com

proteins (such as complement proteins). Because of the rapidity of the response onset, mechanisms of innate immunity are evolutionarily conserved with various sensors known as pattern recognition receptors (PRRs) that detect internal and external abnormalities known respectively as damage-associated molecular patterns (DAMPs) and pathogen-associated molecular patterns (PAMPs). These patterns trigger the activation of a large protein complex consisting of PRR sensor proteins, adaptors, and pro-caspase-1, called the inflammasome.[3]

When PAMPs and DAMPs are identified by PRRs, they send signals causing assembly of the inflammasome complex, which causes cleavage of pro-caspase-1 to active caspase-1. Active caspase-1 cleaves pro-interleukin-1 (IL-1) and pro-IL-18 into active IL-1ß and IL-18, which are secreted through gasdermin-D pores formed in the cell membrane, leading to pathologic ion fluxes in a form of cell death called pyroptosis.[3] **Fig. 1** depicts inflammasome activation.

There are several PRR families, including nucleotide-binding domain- leucine-rich repeat receptors (NLRs), Toll-like receptors (TLRs), pyrin, and absent-in-melanoma 2-like receptors (ALRs). Most NLRs and ALRs can form inflammasome complexes.

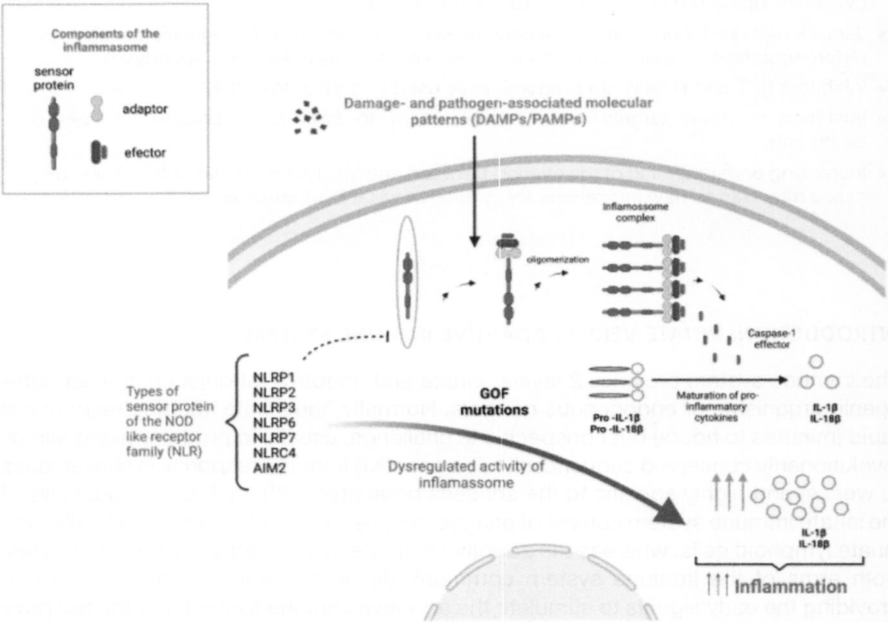

Fig. 1. Inflammasome activation and effect of gain-of-function mutations in the development of inflammasomopathies. Inflammasome activation starts after a trigger, such as damage-associated molecular patterns (DAMPs) or pathogen-associated molecular patterns (PAMPs), is sensed by a sensor protein of the Nucleotide-binding and oligomerization domain (NOD)-like receptor family (NLRP1, NLRP2, NLRP3, NLRP6, NLRP7, NLRC4, and AIM2), leading to the oligomerization and formation of multiprotein complex with the ability to cause the cleavage of caspase-1. This enzyme is responsible for the maturation of proinflammatory cytokines into their active form. Gain-of-function mutations (GOF) on the sensor proteins can lead to the dysregulation of the inflammasome, causing increased levels of proinflammatory cytokines (IL-1 β and IL-18), leading to uncontrolled and damaging autoinflammatory process. (*From* Pinto MV, Neves JF. Precision medicine: The use of tailored therapy in primary immunodeficiencies. Front Immunol. 2022;13:1029560. Published 2022 Dec 8.)

IL-1β and IL-18 induce and promote inflammation, locally or distantly, through activation of nuclear factor kappa B (NF-kB).[4,5] Increased NF-kB signaling results in production of proinflammatory cytokines such as tumor necrosis factor alpha (TNF-α) and IL-6.

The adaptive immune system, by contrast, generates a more diverse and specific response to pathogens. Antigen-presenting cells, such as DCs, interact with naïve T and B lymphocytes, leading to selection of antigen-specific clonal populations of T and B cells. Antibodies produced by B lymphocytes are the prime mediators of humoral immunity, the main defense mechanism for microbes and toxins located outside of the cell. Cell-mediated immunity is coordinated by T lymphocytes as a defense against intracellular organisms or phagocytosed microbes. T lymphocytes release inflammatory cytokines and partake in direct cell-cell interactions that help contain microbes but also lead to tissue inflammation. The process of tolerance to self-antigens is an important feature to prevent harm to self, and abnormalities in this process give rise to autoimmune diseases.[1]

Immune dysregulation leading to pathologic activity can occur in either the innate or the adaptive immune system, resulting in different disease phenotypes, which will be mentioned briefly here and are reviewed in detail elsewhere. This review focuses on currently available biological disease-modifying antirheumatic drug (DMARDs, referred to hereafter as "biologics") therapies in the treatment of immune dysregulatory syndromes, as well as potential novel candidates in development.

AUTOINFLAMMATORY DISEASES

Autoinflammatory conditions represent disorders of the innate immune system. As a result, autoinflammatory conditions are usually negative for autoantibodies or antigen-specific T cells; instead, these conditions are mediated by cells and molecules of the innate immune system and consist of episodes of "seemingly unprovoked inflammation." These episodes can be monogenic conditions, such as familial Mediterranean fever (FMF), cryopyrin-associated periodic syndrome (CAPS), TNF receptor–associated syndrome (TRAPS), and mevalonate kinase deficiency (MKD) with single disease–causing gene mutations or polygenic conditions with involvement of multiple genes. Many of the known monogenic autoinflammatory disorders present early in life, usually within the first decade, although functional differences in specific gene variants may result in decreased penetrance and later disease manifestations.

INFLAMMASOMOPATHIES

Mutations in inflammasome genes lead to conditions called inflammasomopathies, which result in abnormal activation of the innate immune system and release of IL-1 and IL-18 (see **Fig. 1**). These conditions include the prototypical systemic autoinflammatory diseases (SAIDs)—FMF, CAPS, MKD, and TRAPS. These conditions present with recurrent episodes of fever, rash, serositis, and arthritis, each with their characteristic presentations and symptom intervals. The autosomal dominant diseases in the CAPS category are caused by mutations in *NLRP3*, which presents with neutrophilic dermatoses, fever, arthralgia, and in more severe cases, sensorineural hearing loss and cognitive impairment. Abnormalities in *NLRP3* are the best characterized among the different inflammasomopathies.[2,6] There is increasing evidence of involvement of the NLRP3 inflammasome in diseases traditionally considered autoimmune, such as rheumatoid arthritis (RA), gout, and systemic lupus erythematosus (SLE).[2,3,7] This is in contrast to mutations in *NLRC4*, which result in life-threatening episodes of hyperinflammation (macrophage activation syndrome [MAS]). Those with *NLRP3* mutations typically produce excess IL-1ß, as opposed to IL-18, and are not prone to MAS. Gain-of-function (GOF) mutations of *NLRC4* lead to markedly elevated levels of IL-18 and recurrent episodes of MAS, although clinical presentation varies depending on the location of the *NLRC4* gene mutation.[8] Understanding the pathophysiology of the inflammasome led to the use of IL-1 antagonists in the treatment of these diseases.

INTERFERONOPATHIES

Gene mutations in type I interferon signaling pathways give rise to interferonopathies. Interferonopathies often present with systemic inflammation plus features of rash and lipodystrophy with musculoskeletal, neurologic, pulmonary, and metabolic involvement.[9] They bridge the divide between autoinflammatory and autoimmune conditions, as these disorders, although considered innate immune dysregulatory diseases, also display features more typically seen in autoimmune conditions such as autoantibodies.[10]

Interferons are produced on the detection of exogenous and endogenous nucleic acids and have a major role in fighting viral infections. There are 3 types of interferons (IFNs), with type I IFNs being the largest family, consisting of 5 subtypes, including interferon-alpha (IFN-α). Type I interferons bind the IFN-α/β receptor complex, which leads to activation of Janus kinase (JAK) pathways (specifically, JAK1 and tyrosine kinase 2 [TYK2]). These IFNs play a pathogenic role in SLE where production of autoantibodies and immune complexes lead to a vicious cycle of increased type I interferon production and more autoantibody-immune complex deposition.[5,10] New data suggest that disorders of the proteasomes also lead to elevated interferon levels and can be classified as interferonopathies. JAK inhibitors are now being used for treatment of type I interferonopathies.[9]

AUTOIMMUNE CONDITIONS

Autoimmune diseases are typically considered to be due to pathologic responses to self-antigens mediated through the adaptive immune system. Many autoimmune diseases have inherited susceptibility with clustering of autoimmune diseases in families, predisposing an individual to development of autoimmune disease, although there are often unknown environmental triggers that precipitate clinical autoimmunity.

Classic autoimmune conditions include RA, SLE, type I diabetes mellitus (T1DM), and celiac disease. Autoimmune diseases can be organ-specific, such as T1DM, or systemic processes, such as SLE. Increasing evidence demonstrates that aberrant innate immune system activation also plays a role in addition to an abnormal adaptive immune system in the development of autoimmune diseases.[2,11,12]

Tregopathies are disorders of regulatory T cells (Tregs), which are important to maintain immune tolerance; these disorders with abnormal Treg function give rise to diseases with autoimmune, atopic, and infectious presentations.[13]

OVERLAP CONDITIONS

Some conditions span the definition of autoinflammatory and autoimmune conditions. Interferonopathies, as noted earlier, are considered innate immune dysregulatory diseases but also have features of autoimmune conditions such as SLE. Coatomer protein subunit A (COPA) syndrome is a childhood-onset immune dysregulatory syndrome presenting with interstitial lung disease, high titer autoantibodies, and arthritis.[14] A hallmark of COPA syndrome is persistent type I interferon production, with clinical features resembling STING-associated vasculopathy of infancy, a known interferonopathy.[14,15]

Systemic juvenile idiopathic arthritis (sJIA) historically was categorized with other subtypes of autoimmune juvenile idiopathic arthritis (JIA), although it is now recognized to be more similar to autoinflammatory syndromes, as it responds to similar treatments as SAIDs. Although early features of sJIA indicate innate immune activation, untreated or treatment-refractory sJIA leads to a clinical presentation with chronic joint destruction that suggests an autoimmune process[16,17]; this is similarly true with adult-onset Still disease (AOSD).[16,18]

Suppressor of cytokine signaling 1 (SOCS1) haploinsufficiency is a new entity presenting with autoimmunity and immune dysregulation. Mutations leading to SOCS1 haploinsufficiency result in excess interferon production and a clinical phenotype with features resembling SLE including autoimmune cytopenias. However, SOCS1 haploinsufficiency can also present with atopic conditions, immunodeficiency, and lymphoproliferative disease.[19,20]

TREATMENTS: CYTOKINE BLOCKADE

Interleukin-1 Inhibitors

Understanding the inflammasome pathway and release of IL-1β has led to use of IL-1 inhibitors in the treatment of inflammasome-mediated autoinflammatory diseases. The Food and Drug Administration (FDA)-approved IL-1 inhibitors are anakinra, rilonacept, and canakinumab, and all are administered as subcutaneous injections. Anakinra is a recombinant human IL-1 receptor (IL-1R) antagonist with a short half-life (4–6 hours) that competitively binds to the IL-1R, resulting in inhibition of both IL-1α and IL-1β. It needs to be given at least daily.[18] Rilonacept is a dimeric fusion protein that functions as a soluble IL-1 decoy receptor by blocking IL-1β binding to cell surface receptors, thus blocking signaling. Rilonacept is administered once weekly due to its longer half-life than anakinra.[18] Canakinumab is a long-acting monoclonal antibody that binds specifically to IL-1β and prevents IL-1β binding to cell surface receptors.[21] Canakinumab is administered every 4 to 8 weeks. **Fig. 2** depicts the mechanism of action of the IL-1 inhibitors.

IL-1 inhibitors are approved in the treatment of SAIDs and RA and used to treat sJIA. Given that inflammasomopathies release excess IL-1β, IL-1 inhibitors have been used successfully in their treatment.[22,23] IL-1 inhibitors can also be used in the treatment of TRAPS, in which retention of misfolded mutated 55-kD TNF receptor protein in the endoplasmic reticulum serves as a DAMP signal activating the inflammasome with resultant release of IL-1β and IL-18.[24,25] Deficiency of IL-1R antagonist (DIRA) is an autoinflammatory condition resulting from lack of the endogenous IL-1R antagonist, leading to unopposed IL-1α and IL-1β release. Although anakinra and rilonacept can be used in the treatment of DIRA, canakinumab is less effective, as it cannot block unopposed IL-1α release due to its specificity for IL-1β. Side effects of IL-1 inhibitors include injection-site reactions, infection risks, and neutropenia, although the risks seem to be modest.[24] Anakinra can also cause hepatotoxicity.[26,27]

Although anakinra, rilonacept, and canakinumab are the predominant IL-1 inhibitors available on the market, several new IL-1 inhibitors as well as drugs targeting the IL-1 pathway downstream are in development.

Interleukin-18 Inhibitors

Activated inflammasomes release IL-18 in addition to IL-1β, so targeting IL-18 is one way to ameliorate the hyperinflammation observed with some inflammasomopathies. Specifically, elevated levels of IL-18 are seen with GOF mutations in *NLRC4*, where the most common clinical presentation is early-onset colitis and MAS.[8] IL-18 along with

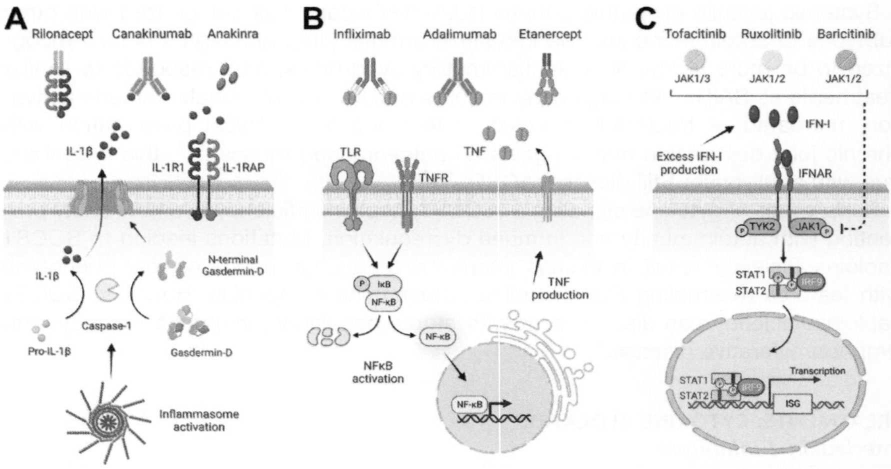

Fig. 2. Therapeutic targets and available agents for the treatment of systemic autoinflammatory diseases. (*A*) In inflammasomopathies, aberrant activation of the inflammasomes triggers the activation of caspase 1, which proteolytically generates active IL-1β and N-terminal gasdermin D. IL-1β is released through membrane pores formed by N-terminal gasdermin D and binds to IL-1 receptor to propagate the inflammatory response. IL-1 inhibitors include anakinra (recombinant IL-1RA), canakinumab (monoclonal anti–IL-1β), and rilonacept (dimeric fusion protein consisting of IL-1R1 and IL-1RAP conjugated to the Fc portion of human immunoglobulin G1 [IgG1]). (*B*) Disorders of NF-κB result in increased production of TNF among other proinflammatory mediators. Membrane-bound TNF is cleaved to form soluble TNF, which binds to TNF receptors to regulate cell death and promote NF-κB activation. TNF inhibitors include infliximab (chimeric human/mouse monoclonal antibody [mAb]), adalimumab (humanized mAb), and etanercept (dimer of soluble TNFR2 fused to the Fc portion of IgG1). Many innate immune sensors such as TLRs also induce inflammation via NF-κB activation. (*C*) Interferonopathies result from excess production of IFN-I, which binds to IFNAR to mediate JAK-STAT signaling. Inhibition of JAK by tofacitinib, ruxolitinib, and baricitinib is an approach increasingly used for the treatment of interferonopathies. IFNAR, IFN α/β receptor; IL-1R1, IL-1 receptor 1; IL-1RA, IL-1 receptor antagonist; IL-1RAP, IL-1 receptor accessory protein; IRF9, IFN regulatory factor 9; ISG, interferon-stimulated gene; TLR, Toll-like receptor; TNFR, TNF receptor; TYK2, tyrosine protein kinase 2. (*From* Du Y, Liu M, Nigrovic PA, Dedeoglu F, Lee PY. Biologics and JAK inhibitors for the treatment of monogenic systemic autoinflammatory diseases in children. J Allergy Clin Immunol. 2023;151(3):607-618.)

IL-12 enhances IFN-γ production, which is important in the development of hemophagocytic lymphohistiocytosis (HLH), and to a lesser extent MAS. IL-18 is tightly regulated by IL-18 binding protein, and shifts in this balance affect helper T type 1 (Th1), Th2, and Th17 cells.[28] Tadekinig alfa is a recombinant human IL-18 binding protein that downregulates secretion of IFN-γ.[29,30] It is currently being used in a clinical trial to treat patients with NLRC4-MAS (NCT03113760).[24,31] A recent phase II clinical trial of tadekinig alfa for the treatment of AOSD showed early clinical and laboratory improvements. Injection site reactions, arthralgia, and upper respiratory infections were the most commonly reported adverse effects in this clinical trial.[32]

Beyond tadekinig alfa, there are 2 more monoclonal antibodies currently in early trials. AVTX 007 is a fully human anti-IL-18 monoclonal antibody aimed to treat SAIDs including AOSD and sJIA as well as multiple myeloma. APB R3 is a long-acting recombinant fusion protein of the IL-18 binding protein attached via protein linker to antihuman albumin Fab fragment. Early testing of APB R3 is currently underway in treating AOSD.[31]

Novel Inflammasome Inhibitors

Other pathways in inflammasome activation are under active investigation for targeted therapies. These pathways include novel inflammasome inhibitors in varying stages of preclinical development (ie, NLRP3 inhibitors).[31] Dapansutrile (OLT1177) is an orally active beta-sulfonyl nitrile that acts as a direct inhibitor of NLRP3 and has also been developed into a topical gel. It is currently being tested in gout and completed phase II clinical trials for knee osteoarthritis.[11,31] MCC950 directly binds NLRP3 and inhibits inflammasome assembly. MCC950 is being trialed in several preclinical studies for non-CAPS NLRP3-mediated inflammatory diseases.[33] CY09 is another agent that specifically blocks assembly of NLRP3 inflammasome by binding to the NACHT domain and has shown in vivo and ex vivo efficacy in CAPS, pain, and gout.[6,34] There are current studies in CAPS for several novel inhibitors, which include inzomelid, an oral selective NLRP3 inhibitor; tranilast, an anthranilic acid that can bind NACHT domain; and diacerein, an anthraquinone compound that downregulates the inflammasome axis. The CAPS preclinical studies also include belnacasan and A1-AT, both of which directly target caspase I component and block IL-ß release.[33]

Interleukin-6 Inhibitors

IL-1 inhibitors are effective first-line treatments for inflammasomopathies, but they may be insufficient for the treatment of certain SAIDs or polygenic conditions such as sJIA/AOSD. A typical second-line agent is IL-6 inhibition. IL-6 is induced by IL-1R signaling, and IL-6 inhibition is used in SAIDs that are refractory to first-line treatments.[24,25]

IL-6 has pleiotropic effects on the immune system. Not only does IL-6 promote B cell activation and maturation[35] but it also directly stimulates hepatocytes to produce C-reactive protein and affects $CD4^+$ T-cell differentiation and activation. IL-6 also promotes Th17 cell differentiation and activates the JAK/STAT pathway.[36,37] Therefore, blocking IL-6 is an important part of reducing inflammation.

IL-6 inhibitors consist of tocilizumab, a recombinant humanized IL-6 receptor (IL-6R) monoclonal antibody, and sarilumab, a fully human IL-6Rα monoclonal antibody. Tocilizumab prevents binding of IL-6 to both the membrane-bound and the soluble IL-6R and prevents signal transduction and is administered by subcutaneous injection or intravenous infusion.[35] Sarilumab binds with greater affinity than tocilizumab to membrane-bound and soluble IL-6Rα[31] and as a result, binds at lower concentrations than tocilizumab.[35,38] Studies show that it can be effective in patients with AOSD who have previously failed tocilizumab therapy.[39]

IL-6 inhibitors are FDA approved for the treatment of sJIA, JIA, and RA. IL-6 inhibitors are also used to treat refractory MKD and other SAIDs.[24] Major side effects of IL-6 inhibitors include neutropenia, thrombocytopenia, increased serum lipids, and transaminitis. The infection risk is increased with both tocilizumab and sarilumab, although tocilizumab has a higher risk of diverticulitis, which can lead to gastrointestinal perforation in higher risk populations such as older adults with RA on concomitant corticosteroids or nonsteroidal antiinflammatory drugs.[40–42] Tocilizumab has also been associated with immediate and delayed hypersensitivity reactions.[43]

Th17 Cytokine Inhibitors

Th17 cells produce IL-17 and IL-22 that recruit neutrophils for defense against extracellular bacteria and fungi. IL-6 and IL-1 can stimulate cells toward a Th17 phenotype, and IL-23 is important in the proliferation and maintenance of Th17 cells.[44] Because of abundance of Th17 cells in mucosal tissues, abnormalities of Th17 cells result in autoimmune diseases of psoriasis, inflammatory bowel disease (IBD), and RA.[45] Inhibitors of IL-12/23 (ustekinumab), IL-17 (secukinumab, ixekizumab), and IL-23 (guselkumab) are now FDA approved for treatment of psoriasis and arthritis.

Ustekinumab is approved in the treatment of Crohn disease, ulcerative colitis, psoriasis, and psoriatic arthritis (PsA). In IBD, induction dosing is by intravenous infusion, with maintenance dosing as subcutaneous injection every 8 to 12 weeks. It is a fully human monoclonal antibody against IL-12 and IL-23. Adverse effects include hypersensitivity reaction, antibody development, infections (including activation of latent infections), and concern for posterior reversible encephalopathy syndrome.[46–48]

Secukinumab is a human monoclonal antibody selectively binding IL-17A, inhibiting its interaction with IL-17 receptor. Secukinumab is administered by subcutaneous injection monthly and is approved in ankylosing spondylitis (AS), psoriasis, and psoriatic arthritis. Interestingly, although Th17 cells are found especially in gut mucosa, secukinumab may trigger Crohn disease and therefore is contraindicated in treatment of IBD.[49,50] Adverse effects are similar to other biologics, with infection being the major adverse effect, as well as worsening or new development of inflammatory bowel disease. Ixekizumab is a humanized monoclonal antibody to IL-17A with a similar mechanism of action.

Guselkumab is a human monoclonal antibody against IL-23 approved in psoriasis and psoriatic arthritis. Its administration leads to reduction of IL-17A, IL-17F, and IL-22 levels. It is administered by subcutaneous injection. Adverse effects include upper respiratory tract infection, autoantibody development, transaminitis, and injection site reactions.[51,52]

Increased levels of IL-17 have been seen in AOSD and sJIA and may represent a possible therapeutic pathway in refractory disease. Mitrovic and colleagues reported complete remission in a patient with AOSD from secukinumab after loss of efficacy from anakinra and methotrexate.[16,31] There is Th17 dysregulation in COPA syndrome, but it is not yet known if this class of medications is effective in the treatment of COPA syndrome.[14]

INTERFERON BLOCKADE

Interferon-alpha

One possible therapeutic in the treatment of interferonopathies is anifrolumab, a fully humanized type I interferon monoclonal antibody that targets the IFN-α/ß receptor. It blocks all type I IFN/IFN-receptor signaling, thereby suppressing interferon gene response.[10] It is currently FDA approved in treatment of moderate/severe active SLE. However, it may present a possible treatment modality in interferonopathies.[24] Anifrolumab is administered as monthly intravenous infusion. Side effects of anifrolumab are upper respiratory infection, sore throat, and reactivation of herpes zoster.[53]

Interferon-gamma

Emapalumab is a fully human anti-IFN-γ monoclonal antibody that inhibits receptor dimerization and blocks signal transduction. It works on free and receptor-bound IFN-γ.[31] In addition to tadekinig alfa, emapalumab may be efficacious for treatment of NLRC4-MAS. Locatelli and colleagues tested safety and efficacy of emapalumab in children with primary HLH and found that 65% of previously treated patients had favorable response with improvement in clinical and laboratory markers of HLH, with 70% able to go on to hematopoietic stem cell transplantation (HSCT).[54]

Emapalumab administration is by intravenous infusion twice a week, with dosage increase to achieve clinical response until time of HSCT. Emapalumab has mild adverse effects, including infusion-related reactions, although more data are needed to confirm this adverse effect profile. In Locatelli's study, the adverse effects seen were mostly attributable to worsening HLH, coadministered medications, or coexisting conditions, as opposed to directly from the emapalumab itself.[54] Thirty five percent of patients entered the study with active infection. As a result, the recommendation is to test for latent tuberculosis infection and start appropriate prophylaxis for *Herpes zoster virus*, *Pneumocystis jirovecii,* and fungal infections.[54,55] There was a recent case report of use of emapalumab in treatment of refractory sJIA with MAS for disease control before HSCT.[56] Gabr and colleagues reported on the successful use of emapalumab in a young adult patient with newly diagnosed AOSD with MAS.[57]

Tumor Necrosis Factor Alpha Inhibitors

TNF-α is a major proinflammatory cytokine released during states of inflammation. TNF inhibitors were the first biological DMARDs developed as a targeted therapy toward the cytokines seen in active inflammation. The first 3 TNF inhibitors developed were etanercept, which binds soluble TNF-α (comprising 2 soluble human TNF receptors on immunoglobulin backbone), adalimumab, a fully humanized monoclonal antibody that binds to the TNF-receptor (TNF-R) on the cell surface, and infliximab, a chimeric monoclonal antibody that also binds to TNF-R on the cell surface (see **Fig. 2**). Second-generation TNF-inhibitors include golimumab (fully humanized monoclonal antibody) and certolizumab pegol (pegylated monoclonal antibody). TNF-α inhibitors are indicated for a variety of autoimmune conditions, including the treatment of JIA, RA, AS, PsA, IBD, uveitis and psoriasis.[36,46,58,59] Side effects include increased infection risk, especially reactivation of latent tuberculosis, malignancies, demyelinating conditions, hypersensitivity reactions, and autoimmune disease (drug-induced SLE).[59]

TNF-α inhibitors can also be used in treatment of some autoinflammatory conditions.[24,60] Specifically, etanercept can be used for TRAPS, although the monoclonal antibodies adalimumab and infliximab cause paradoxic worsening of disease flare,[61] potentially attributed to inhibition of caspase-induced apoptotic activity and resultant increase in proinflammatory cytokines such as IL-1ß, IL-6, IL-8, and IL-12. Deficiency of adenosine deaminase 2 (DADA2) is an autosomal recessive condition with loss-of-function mutation in *CECR1* gene that causes skewed endothelial cell development and resultant vascular fragility. Patients present with hematologic manifestations and vasculopathy. For those with the vascular phenotype of DADA2, TNF inhibitors are a cornerstone of therapy due to normalization of elevated type I interferon and NF-kB signatures, although the mechanism of action is not fully understood.[24,62]

Janus Kinase Inhibition

As noted earlier, JAK inhibitors block the JAK/STAT pathway, which has a broad range of effects, and are classified as targeted synthetic DMARDs. There are 4 JAKs (JAK1, JAK2, JAK3, and TYK2). Baricitinib and ruxolitinib block JAK1 and JAK2. Tofacitinib blocks JAK1 and JAK3. Upadacitinib and filgotinib selectively block JAK1 and therefore may have fewer side effects than the other broader JAK-inhibitors (see **Fig. 2**). Major side effects include increased infection risk, similar to biological DMARDs, with an additional risk of elevated lipids. Viral reactivation, especially of the BK virus, is a significant concern.[9] Myelosuppressive effects may be more pronounced with medications that inhibit JAK2.[63] In adults older than than 50 years with RA, long-term monitoring while on tofacitinib showed higher risk for cardiovascular events and malignancy as compared with TNF-α inhibitors, although it is not clear whether this risk extends to adults without underlying risk factors or the pediatric population.[24] There is a risk of acute cytokine storm syndrome from abrupt discontinuation of JAK inhibitors, which can be life-threatening, so gradual discontinuation or tapering is recommended.[24]

In the treatment of interferonopathies, JAK inhibitors have proved to be beneficial, although there are no randomized clinical trials.[9] Case reports and case series show partial response to standard dosing in most patients with interferonopathies,[64] and there seems to be better response in patients with AOSD or sJIA.[64] JAK inhibitors have been used successfully in the treatment of SOCS1 haploinsufficiency,[65,66] and there are reports of successful use in COPA syndrome.[14,15,67–69]

In autoimmune disease, JAK inhibitors have been FDA approved in the treatment of polyarticular JIA, RA, ankylosing spondylitis, and psoriatic arthritis. They are increasingly being used in dermatomyositis (DM), as DM has been found to have an elevated type I interferon signature, similar to SLE.[70–72] However, studies of baricitinib in SLE were unsuccessful.[73,74] JAK inhibitors also seem to be less efficacious in traditional inflammasomopathies, although there are reports of using it in refractory MKD.[1]

BIOLOGICS TARGETING T AND B LYMPHOCYTES

T-Cell Inhibitors

Beyond specific cytokine inhibitors, there are broader T- and B-cell inhibitors in clinical use. Abatacept is a recombinant CTLA-4 fusion protein. CTLA-4 is an inhibitory molecule that binds CD80 and CD86 on APCs, preventing association of CD80/86 with the costimulatory receptor CD28 on T cells, blocking T-cell activation and decreasing the inflammatory response in T-cell–mediated autoimmune diseases.[75] Abatacept's mode of action suggests indication for diseases of adaptive immunity. It is FDA approved in JIA, RA, and PsA and has been trialed in systemic sclerosis and localized scleroderma. Abatacept is also approved in treatment of acute graft versus host disease, and trials are underway in CTLA-4 haploinsufficiency.[21,76] Abatacept is administered as a weekly subcutaneous injection or monthly intravenous infusion. Side effects include nausea and infection (especially cytomegalovirus disease and reactivation) and has similar risks of infections and malignancy to other biological DMARDs.[77–79]

B-Cell Inhibitors

Rituximab is a chimeric monoclonal antibody against CD20 and depletes the peripheral B-cell population by promoting B-cell apoptosis,[36] as well as through membrane attack complex formation and complement-dependent cytotoxicity. Rituximab is FDA approved for RA treatment and is also extensively used in other conditions including SLE, Sjogren syndrome, antineutrophilic cytoplasmic antibody vasculitis, and autoimmune encephalitis.[80–83] Currently, it is administered as an intravenous infusion, with varying frequency depending on disease process. Side effects include infusion hypersensitivity reaction, hypogammaglobulinemia (with potential increased risk of infection), increased risk of cancer, and progressive multifocal leukoencephalopathy.[81,84–86]

Belimumab is a human monoclonal antibody that blocks B lymphocyte survival by inhibiting B lymphocyte stimulator protein binding to receptors on B lymphocytes. Belimumab is approved for treatment of SLE including lupus nephritis as well as autoimmune cytopenias.[87] It is administered as weekly subcutaneous injections or monthly infusions. Side effects include hypersensitivity reaction, infections, diarrhea, nausea, and psychiatric disturbances such as depression, anxiety, and insomnia.[88,89]

Bortezomib is a plasma cell inhibitor and blocks the 26S proteasome involved in degrading ubiquitinated proteins, resulting in cell-cycle arrest and apoptosis. Bortezomib is administered by intravenous infusion or subcutaneous injection. Adverse effects tend to be frequent, notably peripheral neuropathy (with higher intravenous dosing), gastrointestinal side effects, fatigue, thrombocytopenia, and fever.[90,91] It is currently approved in the use of multiple myeloma, although a recent case series suggested efficacy in treatment of childhood-onset neuropsychiatric lupus.[90,92] Another recent publication suggested efficacy of bortezomib in treating psoriatic inflammation by inhibiting NRLP3 inflammasome activity.[93]

SUMMARY

Autoimmune and autoinflammatory syndromes cause disease by different pathways, although increasingly, disturbances in both innate and adaptive immune pathways have been implicated in some diseases. These diseases should be treated mechanistically based on known pathophysiology. Treatment of inflammasomopathies is predominantly through inhibition of IL-1, although novel small molecule inhibitors are in development that block at the level of the inflammasome. IL-18 and IFN-γ inhibitors show potential especially for treating conditions at high risk of HLH/MAS. JAK inhibitors are currently the best available treatments for interferonopathies, often at higher than standard dosing, although more specific interferon inhibitors are under investigation. Autoimmune disease treatment is often aimed at T- and B-cell pathway inhibition, as well as inhibiting Th17 cytokines and TNF-α. Novel small molecule inhibitors and monoclonal antibodies are currently in development that block at different signaling levels in the immune system (ie, level of inflammasome) to provide more precise targeting. Increasing knowledge about the mechanisms of disease pathogenesis will allow for more targeted therapeutics and precision medicine treatments in the future.

CLINICS CARE POINTS

- Inflammasomopathies result in release of excess IL-1ß, IL-18, and IFN-γ, which can be targeted by those specific inhibitors or novel agents currently in development that block at the level of inflammasome.
- JAK inhibitors are increasingly being used in the treatment of interferonopathies, as well as immune dysregulatory syndromes with an overlap of autoinflammatory and autoimmune features, although they may need higher doses to reach therapeutic effect.
- Autoimmune diseases seem to respond to different cytokine inhibitors than autoinflammatory disease, with more evidence for use with Th17 inhibitors and TNF inhibitors as well as inhibitors of B and T lymphocytes.
- Side effects of biologics generally include increased infection risk, especially reactivation of viruses, hypersensitivity reactions, and increased malignancy risk. Anakinra, tocilizumab, and JAK inhibitors can also cause hepatotoxicity.

DISCLOSURE

No disclosures.

REFERENCES

1. Bindu S, Dandapat S, Manikandan R, et al. Prophylactic and therapeutic insights into trained immunity: A renewed concept of innate immune memory. Hum Vaccines Immunother 2022;18(1):2040238.

2. Zhang Y, Yang W, Li W, et al. NLRP3 Inflammasome: Checkpoint Connecting Innate and Adaptive Immunity in Autoimmune Diseases. Front Immunol 2021; 12:732933.
3. Chen C, Xu P. Activation and Pharmacological Regulation of Inflammasomes. Biomolecules 2022;12(7):1005.
4. Kaneko N, Kurata M, Yamamoto T, et al. The role of interleukin-1 in general pathology. Inflamm Regen 2019;39(1):12.
5. Kawakami A, Endo Y, Koga T, et al. Autoinflammatory disease: clinical perspectives and therapeutic strategies. Inflamm Regen 2022;42(1):37.
6. Blevins HM, Xu Y, Biby S, et al. The NLRP3 Inflammasome Pathway: A Review of Mechanisms and Inhibitors for the Treatment of Inflammatory Diseases. Front Aging Neurosci 2022;14:879021.
7. You R, He X, Zeng Z, et al. Pyroptosis and Its Role in Autoimmune Disease: A Potential Therapeutic Target. Front Immunol 2022;13:841732.
8. Alehashemi S, Goldbach-Mansky R. Human Autoinflammatory Diseases Mediated by NLRP3-, Pyrin-, NLRP1-, and NLRC4-Inflammasome Dysregulation Updates on Diagnosis, Treatment, and the Respective Roles of IL-1 and IL-18. Front Immunol 2020;11:1840.
9. Cetin Gedik K, Lamot L, Romano M, et al. The 2021 European Alliance of Associations for Rheumatology/American College of Rheumatology points to consider for diagnosis and management of autoinflammatory type I interferonopathies: CANDLE/PRAAS, SAVI and AGS. Ann Rheum Dis 2022;81(5):601–13.
10. Saulescu I, Ionescu R, Opris-Belinski D. Interferon in systemic lupus erythematosus—A halfway between monogenic autoinflammatory and autoimmune disease. Heliyon 2022;8(11):e11741.
11. Oliviero F, Bindoli S, Scanu A, et al. Autoinflammatory Mechanisms in Crystal-Induced Arthritis. Front Med 2020;7:166.
12. Pan L, Lu MP, Wang JH, et al. Immunological pathogenesis and treatment of systemic lupus erythematosus. World J Pediatr 2020;16(1):19–30.
13. Cheru N, Hafler DA, Sumida TS. Regulatory T cells in peripheral tissue tolerance and diseases. Front Immunol 2023;14:1154575.
14. Vece TJ, Watkin LB, Nicholas SK, et al. Copa Syndrome: a Novel Autosomal Dominant Immune Dysregulatory Disease. J Clin Immunol 2016;36(4):377–87.
15. Deng Z, Chong Z, Law CS, et al. A defect in COPI-mediated transport of STING causes immune dysregulation in COPA syndrome. J Exp Med 2020;217(11): e20201045.
16. Mitrovic S, Hassold N, Kamissoko A, et al. Adult-onset Still's disease or systemic-onset juvenile idiopathic arthritis and spondyloarthritis: overlapping syndrome or phenotype shift? Rheumatology 2022;61(6):2535–47.
17. Nigrovic PA. Review: Is There a Window of Opportunity for Treatment of Systemic Juvenile Idiopathic Arthritis?: Window of Opportunity in Systemic JIA. Arthritis Rheumatol 2014;66(6):1405–13.
18. Sfriso P, Bindoli S, Galozzi P. Adult-Onset Still's Disease: Molecular Pathophysiology and Therapeutic Advances. Drugs 2018;78(12):1187–95.
19. Lee PY, Platt CD, Weeks S, et al. Immune dysregulation and multisystem inflammatory syndrome in children (MIS-C) in individuals with haploinsufficiency of SOCS1. J Allergy Clin Immunol 2020;146(5):1194–200.e1.
20. Fujimoto M. Inadequate induction of suppressor of cytokine signaling-1 causes systemic autoimmune diseases. Int Immunol 2004;16(2):303–14.
21. Pinto MV, Neves JF. Precision medicine: The use of tailored therapy in primary immunodeficiencies. Front Immunol 2022;13:1029560.

22. Romano M, Arici ZS, Piskin D, et al. The 2021 EULAR/American College of Rheumatology points to consider for diagnosis, management and monitoring of the interleukin-1 mediated autoinflammatory diseases: cryopyrin-associated periodic syndromes, tumour necrosis factor receptor-associated periodic syndrome, mevalonate kinase deficiency, and deficiency of the interleukin-1 receptor antagonist. Ann Rheum Dis 2022;81(7):907–21.
23. Arnold DD, Yalamanoglu A, Boyman O. Systematic Review of Safety and Efficacy of IL-1-Targeted Biologics in Treating Immune-Mediated Disorders. Front Immunol 2022;13:888392.
24. Du Y, Liu M, Nigrovic PA, et al. Biologics and JAK inhibitors for the treatment of monogenic systemic autoinflammatory diseases in children. J Allergy Clin Immunol 2023;151(3):607–18.
25. Broderick L, Hoffman HM. IL-1 and autoinflammatory disease: biology, pathogenesis and therapeutic targeting. Nat Rev Rheumatol 2022;18(8):448–63.
26. Murray GM, Ng SK, Beasley D, et al. Severe hepatotoxicity as a rare side effect of anakinra in a patient with systemic JIA. Rheumatol Oxf Engl 2021;60(9):e307–8.
27. Ahmed O, Brahmania M, Alsahafi M, et al. Anakinra Hepatotoxicity in a Patient With Adult-Onset Still's Disease. ACG Case Rep J 2015;2(3):173–4.
28. Park SY, Hisham Y, Shin HM, et al. Interleukin-18 Binding Protein in Immune Regulation and Autoimmune Diseases. Biomedicines 2022;10(7):1750.
29. Kaplanski G. Interleukin-18: Biological properties and role in disease pathogenesis. Immunol Rev 2018;281(1):138–53.
30. Dinarello CA, Novick D, Kim S, et al. Interleukin-18 and IL-18 Binding Protein. Front Immunol 2013;4.
31. Galozzi P, Bindoli S, Doria A, et al. Progress in Biological Therapies for Adult-Onset Still's Disease. Biol Targets & Ther 2022;16:21–34.
32. Gabay C, Fautrel B, Rech J, et al. Open-label, multicentre, dose-escalating phase II clinical trial on the safety and efficacy of tadekinig alfa (IL-18BP) in adult-onset Still's disease. Ann Rheum Dis 2018. https://doi.org/10.1136/annrheumdis-2017-212608. annrheumdis-2017-212608.
33. Moltrasio C, Romagnuolo M, Marzano AV. NLRP3 inflammasome and NLRP3-related autoinflammatory diseases: From cryopyrin function to targeted therapies. Front Immunol 2022;13:1007705.
34. Jiang H, He H, Chen Y, et al. Identification of a selective and direct NLRP3 inhibitor to treat inflammatory disorders. J Exp Med 2017;214(11):3219–38.
35. Ogata A, Kato Y, Higa S, et al. IL-6 inhibitor for the treatment of rheumatoid arthritis: A comprehensive review. Mod Rheumatol 2019;29(2):258–67.
36. Shams S, Martinez JM, Dawson JRD, et al. The Therapeutic Landscape of Rheumatoid Arthritis: Current State and Future Directions. Front Pharmacol 2021;12:680043.
37. Rose-John S, Jenkins BJ, Garbers C, et al. Targeting IL-6 trans-signalling: past, present and future prospects. Nat Rev Immunol 2023. https://doi.org/10.1038/s41577-023-00856-y.
38. Lamb YN, Deeks ED. Sarilumab: A Review in Moderate to Severe Rheumatoid Arthritis. Drugs 2018;78(9):929–40.
39. Simeni Njonnou SR, Soyfoo MS, Vandergheynst FA. Efficacy of sarilumab in adult-onset Still's disease as a corticosteroid-sparing agent. Rheumatology 2019;58(10):1878–9.
40. Barbulescu A, Delcoigne B, Askling J, et al. Gastrointestinal perforations in patients with rheumatoid arthritis treated with biological disease-modifying antirheumatic drugs in Sweden: a nationwide cohort study. RMD Open 2020;6(2):e001201.

41. Curtis JR, Xie F, Chen L, et al. The incidence of gastrointestinal perforations among rheumatoid arthritis patients. Arthritis Rheum 2011;63(2):346–51.
42. Xie F, Yun H, Bernatsky S, et al. Brief Report: Risk of Gastrointestinal Perforation Among Rheumatoid Arthritis Patients Receiving Tofacitinib, Tocilizumab, or Other Biologic Treatments: GASTROINTESTINAL PERFORATION IN RA. Arthritis Rheumatol 2016;68(11):2612–7.
43. Soyer O, Demir S, Bilginer Y, et al. Severe hypersensitivity reactions to biological drugs in children with rheumatic diseases. In: Atanaskovic-Markovic M, editor. Pediatr Allergy Immunol 2019;30(8):833–40.
44. Tangye SG, Puel A. The Th17/IL-17 Axis and Host Defense Against Fungal Infections. J Allergy Clin Immunol Pract 2023;11(6):1624–34.
45. Abbas AK, Lichtman AH, Pillai S, et al. Cellular and molecular immunology. Tenth edition. Elsevier; 2022.
46. Feuerstein JD, Ho EY, Shmidt E, et al. AGA Clinical Practice Guidelines on the Medical Management of Moderate to Severe Luminal and Perianal Fistulizing Crohn's Disease. Gastroenterology 2021;160(7):2496–508.
47. Tan MG, Worley B, Kim WB, et al. Drug-Induced Intracranial Hypertension: A Systematic Review and Critical Assessment of Drug-Induced Causes. Am J Clin Dermatol 2020;21(2):163–72.
48. Papp KA, Langley RG, Lebwohl M, et al. Efficacy and safety of ustekinumab, a human interleukin-12/23 monoclonal antibody, in patients with psoriasis: 52-week results from a randomised, double-blind, placebo-controlled trial (PHOENIX 2). Lancet Lond Engl 2008;371(9625):1675–84.
49. Papp KA, Langley RG, Sigurgeirsson B, et al. Efficacy and safety of secukinumab in the treatment of moderate-to-severe plaque psoriasis: a randomized, double-blind, placebo-controlled phase II dose-ranging study. Br J Dermatol 2013; 168(2):412–21.
50. Fauny M, Moulin D, D'Amico F, et al. Paradoxical gastrointestinal effects of interleukin-17 blockers. Ann Rheum Dis 2020;79(9):1132–8.
51. Deodhar A, Helliwell PS, Boehncke WH, et al. Guselkumab in patients with active psoriatic arthritis who were biologic-naive or had previously received TNFα inhibitor treatment (DISCOVER-1): a double-blind, randomised, placebo-controlled phase 3 trial. Lancet 2020;395(10230):1115–25.
52. Blauvelt A, Papp KA, Griffiths CEM, et al. Efficacy and safety of guselkumab, an anti-interleukin-23 monoclonal antibody, compared with adalimumab for the continuous treatment of patients with moderate to severe psoriasis: Results from the phase III, double-blinded, placebo- and active comparator–controlled VOYAGE 1 trial. J Am Acad Dermatol 2017;76(3):405–17.
53. Sim TM, Ong SJ, Mak A, et al. Type I Interferons in Systemic Lupus Erythematosus: A Journey from Bench to Bedside. Int J Mol Sci 2022;23(5):2505.
54. Locatelli F, Jordan MB, Allen C, et al. Emapalumab in Children with Primary Hemophagocytic Lymphohistiocytosis. N Engl J Med 2020;382(19):1811–22.
55. Garonzi C, Chinello M, Cesaro S. Emapalumab for adult and pediatric patients with hemophagocytic lymphohistiocytosis. Expert Rev Clin Pharmacol 2021; 14(5):527–34.
56. Chellapandian D, Milojevic D. Case report: Emapalumab for active disease control prior to hematopoietic stem cell transplantation in refractory systemic juvenile idiopathic arthritis complicated by macrophage activation syndrome. Front Pediatr 2023;11:1123104.
57. Gabr JB, Liu E, Mian S, et al. Successful treatment of secondary macrophage activation syndrome with emapalumab in a patient with newly diagnosed adult-

onset Still's disease: case report and review of the literature. Ann Transl Med 2020;8(14):887.
58. Ramiro S, Nikiphorou E, Sepriano A, et al. ASAS-EULAR recommendations for the management of axial spondyloarthritis: 2022 update. Ann Rheum Dis 2023;82(1): 19–34.
59. Leone GM, Mangano K, Petralia MC, et al. Past, Present and (Foreseeable) Future of Biological Anti-TNF Alpha Therapy. J Clin Med 2023;12(4):1630.
60. Matsuda T, Kambe N, Takimoto-Ito R, et al. Potential Benefits of TNF Targeting Therapy in Blau Syndrome, a NOD2-Associated Systemic Autoinflammatory Granulomatosis. Front Immunol 2022;13:895765.
61. Cudrici C, Deuitch N, Aksentijevich I. Revisiting TNF Receptor-Associated Periodic Syndrome (TRAPS): Current Perspectives. Int J Mol Sci 2020;21(9):3263.
62. Deuitch NT, Yang D, Lee PY, et al. TNF inhibition in vasculitis management in adenosine deaminase 2 deficiency (DADA2). J Allergy Clin Immunol 2022; 149(5):1812–6.e6.
63. Bertsias G. Therapeutic targeting of JAKs: from hematology to rheumatology and from the first to the second generation of JAK inhibitors. Mediterr J Rheumatol 2020;31(Suppl 1):105.
64. Boyadzhieva Z, Ruffer N, Burmester G, et al. Effectiveness and Safety of JAK Inhibitors in Autoinflammatory Diseases: A Systematic Review. Front Med 2022;9: 930071.
65. Hadjadj J, Castro CN, Tusseau M, et al. Early-onset autoimmunity associated with SOCS1 haploinsufficiency. Nat Commun 2020;11(1):5341.
66. Michniacki TF, Walkovich K, DeMeyer L, et al. SOCS1 Haploinsufficiency Presenting as Severe Enthesitis, Bone Marrow Hypocellularity, and Refractory Thrombocytopenia in a Pediatric Patient with Subsequent Response to JAK Inhibition. J Clin Immunol 2022;42(8):1766–77.
67. Department of General Paediatrics, Centre for Paediatric Rheumatology, Clinic Sankt Augustin, Sankt Augustin, Germany, Krutzke S, Rietschel C, et al. Baricitinib in therapy of COPA syndrome in a 15-year-old girl. Eur J Rheumatol. 2020;7(1):78-81. doi:10.5152/eurjrheum.2019.18177.
68. Kumrah R, Mathew B, Pandiarajan V, et al. Genetics of COPA syndrome. Appl Clin Genet 2019;12:11–8.
69. Frémond ML, Nathan N. COPA syndrome, 5 years after: Where are we? Joint Bone Spine 2021;88(2):105070.
70. Rheumatology Unit, Meir Medical Center, Kfar Saba, Israel, Natour AEH, Department of Internal Medicine A, Meir Medical Center, Kfar Saba, Israel, Kivity S, Rheumatology Unit, Meir Medical Center, Kfar Saba, Israel. Biological Therapies in Inflammatory Myopathies. Rambam Maimonides Med J 2023;14(2):e0008.
71. Kim H, Gunter-Rahman F, McGrath JA, et al. Expression of interferon-regulated genes in juvenile dermatomyositis versus Mendelian autoinflammatory interferonopathies. Arthritis Res Ther 2020;22(1):69.
72. Le Voyer T, Gitiaux C, Authier FJ, et al. JAK inhibitors are effective in a subset of patients with juvenile dermatomyositis: a monocentric retrospective study. Rheumatology 2021;60(12):5801–8.
73. Guilpain P. JAK inhibitors in autoinflammatory syndromes? The long road from drug development to daily clinical use. Rheumatology 2023;62(4):1368–9.
74. Morand EF, Tanaka Y, Furie R, et al. POS0190 Efficacy and safety of baricitinib in patients with systemic lupus erythematosus: results from two randomised, double-blind, placebo-controlled, parallel-group, phase 3 studieS. Ann Rheum Dis 2022;81(Suppl 1):327–8.

75. Jayatilleke A. Immunosuppression in Rheumatologic and Auto-immune Disease. In: Eisen HJ, editor. *Pharmacology of immunosuppression*. Vol 272. Handbook of experimental pharmacology. Cham: Springer International Publishing; 2021. p. 181–208.
76. Krausz M, Uhlmann A, Rump IC, et al. The ABACHAI clinical trial protocol: Safety and efficacy of abatacept (s.c.) in patients with CTLA-4 insufficiency or LRBA deficiency: A non controlled phase 2 clinical trial. Contemp Clin Trials Commun 2022;30:101008.
77. Kremer JM, Dougados M, Emery P, et al. Treatment of rheumatoid arthritis with the selective costimulation modulator abatacept: twelve-month results of a phase iib, double-blind, randomized, placebo-controlled trial. Arthritis Rheum 2005;52(8): 2263–71.
78. Watkins B, Qayed M, McCracken C, et al. Phase II Trial of Costimulation Blockade With Abatacept for Prevention of Acute GVHD. J Clin Oncol 2021;39(17):1865–77.
79. Dominique A, Hetland ML, Finckh A, et al. Safety outcomes in patients with rheumatoid arthritis treated with abatacept: results from a multinational surveillance study across seven European registries. Arthritis Res Ther 2023;25(1):101.
80. Mariette X, Barone F, Baldini C, et al. A randomized, phase II study of sequential belimumab and rituximab in primary Sjögren's syndrome. JCI Insight 2022;7(23): e163030.
81. Chung SA, Langford CA, Maz M, et al. American College of Rheumatology/ Vasculitis Foundation Guideline for the Management of Antineutrophil Cytoplasmic Antibody-Associated Vasculitis. Arthritis Rheumatol Hoboken NJ 2021; 73(8):1366–83.
82. Fraenkel L, Bathon JM, England BR, et al. American College of Rheumatology Guideline for the Treatment of Rheumatoid Arthritis. Arthritis Care Res 2021; 73(7):924–39.
83. Dinoto A, Ferrari S, Mariotto S. Treatment Options in Refractory Autoimmune Encephalitis. CNS Drugs 2022;36(9):919–31.
84. Gottenberg JE, Guillevin L, Lambotte O, et al. Tolerance and short term efficacy of rituximab in 43 patients with systemic autoimmune diseases. Ann Rheum Dis 2005;64(6):913–20.
85. Higashida J, Wun T, Schmidt S, et al. Safety and efficacy of rituximab in patients with rheumatoid arthritis refractory to disease modifying antirheumatic drugs and anti-tumor necrosis factor-alpha treatment. J Rheumatol 2005;32(11):2109–15.
86. Marinho A, Delgado Alves J, Fortuna J, et al. Biological therapy in systemic lupus erythematosus, antiphospholipid syndrome, and Sjögren's syndrome: evidence- and practice-based guidance. Front Immunol 2023;14:1117699.
87. Krustev E, Clarke AE, Barber MRW. B cell depletion and inhibition in systemic lupus erythematosus. Expet Rev Clin Immunol 2023;19(1):55–70.
88. Furie R, Petri M, Zamani O, et al. A phase III, randomized, placebo-controlled study of belimumab, a monoclonal antibody that inhibits B lymphocyte stimulator, in patients with systemic lupus erythematosus. Arthritis Rheum 2011;63(12):3918–30.
89. Navarra SV, Guzmán RM, Gallacher AE, et al. Efficacy and safety of belimumab in patients with active systemic lupus erythematosus: a randomised, placebo-controlled, phase 3 trial. Lancet Lond Engl 2011;377(9767):721–31.
90. Sanz-Solas A, Labrador J, Alcaraz R, et al. Bortezomib Pharmacogenetic Biomarkers for the Treatment of Multiple Myeloma: Review and Future Perspectives. J Personalized Med 2023;13(4):695.
91. Cengiz Seval G, Beksac M. The safety of bortezomib for the treatment of multiple myeloma. Expet Opin Drug Saf 2018;17(9):953–62.

92. Modica RF, Thatayatikom A, Bell-Brunson DH, et al. Bortezomib is efficacious in the treatment of severe childhood-onset neuropsychiatric systemic lupus erythematosus with psychosis: a case series and mini-review of B-cell immunomodulation in antibody-mediated diseases. Clin Rheumatol 2023.
93. Chen X, Chen Y, Ou Y, et al. Bortezomib inhibits NLRP3 inflammasome activation and NF-κB pathway to reduce psoriatic inflammation. Biochem Pharmacol 2022; 206:115326.

UNITED STATES POSTAL SERVICE®

Statement of Ownership, Management, and Circulation (All Periodicals Publications Except Requester Publications)

1. Publication Title	2. Publication Number	3. Filing Date
RHEUMATIC DISEASE CLINICS OF NORTH AMERICA	006 – 272	9/18/2023
4. Issue Frequency	5. Number of Issues Published Annually	6. Annual Subscription Price
FEB, MAY, AUG, NOV	4	$377.00

7. Complete Mailing Address of Known Office of Publication *(Not printer) (Street, city, county, state, and ZIP+4®)*
ELSEVIER INC.
230 Park Avenue, Suite 800
New York, NY 10169

Contact Person
Malathi Samayan
Telephone *(Include area code)*
91-44-4299-4507

8. Complete Mailing Address of Headquarters or General Business Office of Publisher *(Not printer)*
ELSEVIER INC.
230 Park Avenue, Suite 800
New York, NY 10169

9. Full Names and Complete Mailing Addresses of Publisher, Editor, and Managing Editor *(Do not leave blank)*

Publisher *(Name and complete mailing address)*
Dolores Meloni, ELSEVIER INC.
1600 JOHN F KENNEDY BLVD. SUITE 1600
PHILADELPHIA, PA 19103-2899

Editor *(Name and complete mailing address)*
JOANNA COLLETT, ELSEVIER INC.
1600 JOHN F KENNEDY BLVD. SUITE 1600
PHILADELPHIA, PA 19103-2899

Managing Editor *(Name and complete mailing address)*
PATRICK MANLEY, ELSEVIER INC.
1600 JOHN F KENNEDY BLVD. SUITE 1600
PHILADELPHIA, PA 19103-2899

10. Owner *(Do not leave blank. If the publication is owned by a corporation, give the name and address of the corporation immediately followed by the names and addresses of all stockholders owning or holding 1 percent or more of the total amount of stock. If not owned by a corporation, give the names and addresses of the individual owners. If owned by a partnership or other unincorporated firm, give its name and address as well as those of each individual owner. If the publication is published by a nonprofit organization, give its name and address.)*

Full Name	Complete Mailing Address
WHOLLY OWNED SUBSIDIARY OF REED/ELSEVIER, US HOLDINGS	1600 JOHN F KENNEDY BLVD. SUITE 1600 PHILADELPHIA, PA 19103-2899

11. Known Bondholders, Mortgagees, and Other Security Holders Owning or Holding 1 Percent or More of Total Amount of Bonds, Mortgages, or Other Securities. If none, check box → ☐ None

Full Name	Complete Mailing Address
N/A	

12. Tax Status *(For completion by nonprofit organizations authorized to mail at nonprofit rates) (Check one)*
The purpose, function, and nonprofit status of this organization and the exempt status for federal income tax purposes:
☒ Has Not Changed During Preceding 12 Months
☐ Has Changed During Preceding 12 Months *(Publisher must submit explanation of change with this statement)*

13. Publication Title	14. Issue Date for Circulation Data Below
RHEUMATIC DISEASE CLINICS OF NORTH AMERICA	JUNE 2023

15. Extent and Nature of Circulation			Average No. Copies Each Issue During Preceding 12 Months	No. Copies of Single Issue Published Nearest to Filing Date
a. Total Number of Copies *(Net press run)*			131	128
b. Paid Circulation *(By Mail and Outside the Mail)*	(1)	Mailed Outside-County Paid Subscriptions Stated on PS Form 3541 (Include paid distribution above nominal rate, advertiser's proof copies, and exchange copies)	67	73
	(2)	Mailed In-County Paid Subscriptions Stated on PS Form 3541 *(Include paid distribution above nominal rate, advertiser's proof copies, and exchange copies)*	0	0
	(3)	Paid Distribution Outside the Mails Including Sales Through Dealers and Carriers, Street Vendors, Counter Sales, and Other Paid Distribution Outside USPS®	49	37
	(4)	Paid Distribution by Other Classes of Mail Through the USPS (e.g., First-Class Mail®)	11	14
c. Total Paid Distribution *[Sum of 15b (1), (2), (3), and (4)]* ▶			127	124
d. Free or Nominal Rate Distribution *(By Mail and Outside the Mail)*	(1)	Free or Nominal Rate Outside-County Copies included on PS Form 3541	4	4
	(2)	Free or Nominal Rate In-County Copies Included on PS Form 3541	0	0
	(3)	Free or Nominal Rate Copies Mailed at Other Classes Through the USPS (e.g., First-Class Mail)	0	0
	(4)	Free or Nominal Rate Distribution Outside the Mail *(Carriers or other means)*	0	0
e. Total Free or Nominal Rate Distribution *(Sum of 15d (1), (2), (3) and (4))*			4	4
f. Total Distribution *(Sum of 15c and 15e)* ▶			131	128
g. Copies not Distributed *(See Instructions to Publishers #4 (page #3))* ▶			0	0
h. Total *(Sum of 15f and g)*			131	128
i. Percent Paid *(15c divided by 15f times 100)* ▶			96.93%	96.88%

* If you are claiming electronic copies, go to line 16 on page 3. If you are not claiming electronic copies, skip to line 17 on page 3.

16. Electronic Copy Circulation	Average No. Copies Each Issue During Preceding 12 Months	No. Copies of Single Issue Published Nearest to Filing Date
a. Paid Electronic Copies ▶		
b. Total Paid Print Copies (Line 15c) + Paid Electronic Copies (Line 16a) ▶		
c. Total Print Distribution (Line 15f) + Paid Electronic Copies (Line 16a) ▶		
d. Percent Paid (Both Print & Electronic Copies) (16b divided by 16c × 100) ▶		

☒ **I certify that 50% of all my distributed copies (electronic and print) are paid above a nominal price.**

17. Publication of Statement of Ownership
☒ If the publication is a general publication, publication of this statement is required. Will be printed in the NOVEMBER 2023 issue of this publication. ☐ Publication not required.

18. Signature and Title of Editor, Publisher, Business Manager, or Owner
Malathi Samayan - Distribution Controller *Malathi Samayan* Date 9/18/2023

I certify that all information furnished on this form is true and complete. I understand that anyone who furnishes false or misleading information on this form or who omits material or information requested on the form may be subject to criminal sanctions (including fines and imprisonment) and/or civil sanctions (including civil penalties).

Printed and bound by CPI Group (UK) Ltd, Croydon, CR0 4YY
08/05/2025
01864748-0002